Advance Praise for *Food Shaman*

"Food Genius, Food Innovator, Food Scientist, Food Shaman. Dr. Mike brings a whole new element (excuse the quantum pun) to how we perceive food, both at a mind and body level. An extraordinary read."

—Thomas Jreige, B.Sc, SSCP, DipPM, AAICD; Physicist

"Dr. Mike has stirred the cauldron, he has done the research and presents factual evidence to back up what indigenous healers inherently know. He is on the cutting edge of connecting the bridge between science with ancestral healing pathways. He has ingested the three drops of inspiration, digested the medicine, and has served up a mighty fine brew in the form of *Food Shaman: The Art of Quantum Food.*"

—Andrew Steed, Celtic Shaman Practitioner, Educator, and Author

"Dr. Fenster knocks the ball out of the park once more with the book, *Food Shaman: The Art of Quantum Food*. He unleashes his incredible mind and writing abilities to entertain and educate at the same time. He has a voracious appetite for knowledge that is shared with the

reader in his unique, entertaining style! I really love this book!"

—Bernadette Fiaschetti,
Host of the nationally syndicated
One Life radio program, national
health and wellness expert

"*Food Shaman* is a terrific source of healthy cooking and amazing foods from the world's top cardiologist-chef. It's the Ultimate Almanac of Healthy Foods bringing a fresh perspective on eating healthy; a *tour-de-force* of healthy cooking and medical science."

—Marty Makary, MD, M.P.H.,
F.A.C.S., Johns Hopkins Surgeon
and *New York Times* Bestselling
Author of *Unaccountable*

"Michael Fenster's *Food Shaman* is an addictive read rich in detail and enlightenment. It is straight to the point and digs into the complexities of the human connection with food without being boring or preachy. Fenster provides a refreshing take on food and presents it as an overall experience for the mind, body, and soul. This book holds all the ingredients to help heal your relationship with food."

—Francesca Luca, Radio
Host of "Talk With Francesca"

FOOD
SHAMAN
THE ART OF QUANTUM FOOD

MICHAEL S. FENSTER, MD

Post Hill
PRESS

A POST HILL PRESS BOOK

ISBN: 978-1-68261-724-3
ISBN (eBook): 978-1-68261-725-0

Food Shaman:
The Art of Quantum Food
© 2018 by Michael S. Fenster, MD
All Rights Reserved

Cover art by Cody Corcoran

This book contains advice and information relating to health care. It should be used to supplement rather than replace the advice of your doctor or another trained health professional. If you know or suspect that you have a health problem, it is recommended that you seek your physician's advice before embarking on any medical program or treatment. All efforts have been made to assure the accuracy of the information in this book as of the date of publication. The publisher and the author disclaim liability for any medical outcomes that may occur as a result of applying the methods suggested in this book.

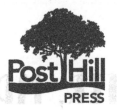

Post Hill Press, LLC
New York • Nashville
posthillpress.com

Published in the United States of America

DEDICATION

With greatest gratitude to Morrighan; for
new ideas to live, old ones must die;
Fulacht na Morrìgna; fulacht fìaðh.
As always, to The Queen of Stones; Mon raison d'être.

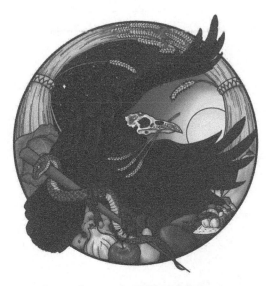

Figure by Jayde Hilliard-Simpson

CONTENTS

AUTHOR'S NOTE

An undertaking such as this book is always a bit of a balancing act. Controversial assertions that buck the conventional wisdom, guidelines, recommendations, and preconceived perceptions of the public best have some evidence to support them. Yet, the science can be technical, difficult, and oftentimes requires specific training or knowledge, a degree of expertise, to comprehend; it is a bit like speaking a foreign language. A superficial understanding schooled at Google University is most likely to lead to mistranslation and misappropriation of meaning.

Add to this the plain fact that every reader's background and demand for level of evidence will differ, and it quickly becomes a quagmire of navigating through the forest without getting lost in the individual trees. To help balance the burden of proof against the telling and the purpose of the story, there is located at the end of the narrative an appendix containing more scientific detail. The information is not necessary for telling of the tale, nor the implementation of the methods contained therein. However, for the curious, the skeptical, and the OCD among us (myself included), it is provided so that that no traveler of these pages need take my word and my interpretation of the data as the gospel. As the Buddha has advised, accept nothing lest it agree with your own experience and your own common sense. So, like any meal, partake of as much as you need to be satisfied.

Bon Appetit!

A SHAMAN'S PERSPECTIVE

By Andrew Steed,
Celtic Shaman Practitioner and Educator

Why scrap around and fight on the floor for leftovers when there is room at the banquet table for us all to feast?

It is one thing to acknowledge that each of us has a place setting at the table; it is another thing entirely to pick up the chair, unfurl the napkin, and join the celebration of life.

I first met Doctor Mike Fenster seated at the captain's table at a pirate feast deep in the catacombs of a Lancaster, Pennsylvania brewery.

I have since broken bread with him in three different countries as we have both sought to expand our own horizons.

What I love about Doctor Mike is his huge heart, with wisdom and wit to match. He blends traditional and indigenous medicine ways to serve a tasty repast for all who are willing to take responsibility for their lives.

Grabbing that chair and taking a seat requires courage. It also comes with a responsibility to wake up to the philosophy of "healer, heal thyself."

There is a great story in the Welsh tradition whereby a young boy is charged with stirring a cauldron of inspiration for a year and a day. The contents are meant for someone else, yet the boy does the work and ends up ingesting the three drops of inspiration himself. He infuses the medicine and becomes a wisdom keeper of the Isles.

Doctor Mike has stirred the cauldron, he has done the research, and presents factual evidence to back up what indigenous healers inherently know. He is on the cutting edge of connecting the bridge between science and ancestral healing pathways.

He has ingested the three drops of inspiration, digested the medicine, and has served up a mighty fine brew in the form of *Food Shaman: The Art of Quantum Food.*

When you take a heart surgeon and a gourmet chef and add the tasty roots of a shamanic pathway, magic happens.

To activate the magic requires us to be willing to suck the marrow from the bone and embrace the wisdom that has been marinated within the folds of these pages. A great recipe becomes a classic dish when we sharpen the tools, mix in the finest ingredients, and practice, practice, practice until we know the recipe by heart.

Many people succumb to the "quick fix" philosophy churned out in this fast-paced world. So busy desperately trying to get there that they miss the gift of life, the present!

Doctor Mike advocates that we fuel our bodies with real food to honour the relationships we have with the animal and plant nations that give up their lives so that we may live.

Around the time I met Doctor Mike, I was facilitating a diversity program with students at a local trade school. I shared with them that in 1998 I was traveling in Argentina and ended up staying on a farm in La Pampa. The farmer told me we were having lamb's eggs for dinner. At that time, I was a meat eater and lamb was my favorite meat. As we all sat around the dinner table, the farmer took a ladle and scooped it into the pot, exclaiming, "You did say you wanted lamb's testicles, Andrew?"

If you could have seen my face. The testicles had been boiled and the veins were sticking out. The faces of the audience members are always a delight to behold when they hear this part of the story. I often speak aloud what several of them are thinking, saying, "Did you eat them? Ugh testicle breath."

Around that table in Argentina, lamb's testicles were a delicacy and had I grown up on that farm, I would have partaken of them gladly. When they were placed in front of me, my own fears came bubbling to the surface. It was the look of them and the thought of eating them that got in my way.

I cut a sliver and started to nibble away until the farmer pointed to some ribs that were cooking on the barbeque. "If you don't fancy them we will polish them off," he chuckled. The farmer's family were delighted to have more testicles to feast on.

The next day the farmer castrated the bulls and those testicles were cooked on the barbeque. Without the veins I munched merrily upon them. They tasted like chicken!

Some of the faces in the audience were still horrified that people serve up testicles for a delicacy so I offered them this titbit: "You may think it odd that some people in the world eat testicles, yet they may find your eating habits just as strange. The testicles were fresh, the farmer raised his stock using organic methods, and he and his family knew exactly what they were eating. They look at some of your diets and scratch their heads at the fast food you cram into your bodies. And come on now, some of you eat hot dogs. You all know what goes into a mass-produced store bought hot dog don't you?"

Eating authentic food and being your authentic self is medicine to feed the soul.

I was delighted several years ago when Doctor Mike sought me out to wander into spaces between the spaces on an indigenous medicine pathway. I am excited to see how he has worked with the marriage of food and shamanism. Ancient medicine elders in all traditions have held a sacred union between themselves, the tribe, and the land.

Our species has been sleepwalking and in so doing has co-created a wounded wasteland. Our Earth, air, and water has been polluted. Doctor Mike calls us to wake up. It begins in honouring the temple of our own bodies so we can honour the temples of all beings around us.

Whether we are meat eaters, vegetarians, vegans, fruitarians, or anything in between, nurturing our relationship with the fuel that feeds us will allow us all to flourish.

Thank you, Doctor Mike, for sharing such a wholesome recipe of how to build this union within ourselves. For each of us has an opportunity to honour all life and co-create a thriving kingdom.

—Andrew Steed

A PHYSICIST'S PERSPECTIVE

By Thomas Jreige,
B.Sc, SSCP, DipPM, AAICD

In the last three decades, many diets, opinions, and ways to eat have been introduced into our lives, each one attempting to provide an easy solution to weight loss, or toward enhancing our existence. When I think of diet, I think of the different culinary attributes of cultures around the world and what makes them unique. From the ever-fresh Mediterranean diet to the raw and natural diet in Japan, food is a necessity for survival. The great thing about good food is that it brings people together. There is nothing more powerful than sharing a meal, with the effort of food preparation contributing to the enjoyment of the occasion. Ultimately, we consume food out of necessity; why not enjoy every meal putting a smile on our faces, enhancing the endorphins, and helping us all to live long and wholesome lives? The correlation of wholesome food and long life has been proven through generations of different cultures. However, there is more to this than just the food.

The title of this book *Food, Shaman: The Art of Quantum Food*, intrigued me. When I think of the shaman, I think of this person who has the skill to heal, summoning light and dark spirits. While we consume food as a necessity to live, other attributes of our human state can be nurtured through how much enjoyment we attain through the food and the enjoyment of the flavors which provide homage to our senses. This book delves into the world of the shaman, good food, and presents a quantum explanation around the ideas presented in this book.

Geoffrey Blainey, an Australian historian, philanthropist, and author of *The Tyranny of Distance* published in 1966, described how distance shaped Australia through its relations in trade in Asia and Africa. As technology is rapidly shaping our world, the tyranny is slowly diminishing, especially when it comes to meeting people and being part of people's lives through distance. I met Michael Fenster online through the wonderful food blogger Joumana Accad when Michael released his book *Fallacy of the Calorie*. I was one of the ever-passionate science nerds who contributed to discussions about the concept of why calorie counting is not an accurate way to look at how we digest food, but more the quality of the food. We have continued since then with banter and more discussion of food.

Food is the one thing that every human requires to function. What we eat does matter, and the way we consume food plays a big role in our mental health, physical health, and wellbeing. Michael draws on similarities between eating good food, and the feelings felt when experiencing this food. Behind this comparison is the message of enjoying your food to gaining higher psychological reviews and benefiting the body's nervous system. Our food should be an experience, one that we remember and savour. We all have an inner food shaman, one we should listen to when consuming food.

The key area of this wonderful manuscript is around the topic of quantum mechanics, food at a molecular level and drawing the comparison between the science and work of a shaman. When asked to review the manuscript, my curiosity was piqued, and I reminisced on my university education including Schrodinger's cat experiment and the interpretation of quantum mechanics on everyday objects. Schrodinger's experiment presents a topic called quantum superposition, being that the cat (in the context of this write-up) could experience simultaneously two states, dead or alive. Michael draws from science and shamanism through two simultaneous states: a state of physical satisfaction that the body has experienced when consuming a meal, along with the textures and the flavors. On the other hand, the mental state, psychological experiences, and feelings are nurtured and developed to provide the other end of the spectrum during the meal.

Looking at food consumption from the level of a shaman is no different than looking at food from a quantum mechanics (or quantum physics) perspective. This area of science looks at food from the natural perspective and the atom. It looks at the interactions of atoms that define our world. Looking at food at a quantum level can help us to understand not only what is physically occurring with food when we consume it, but provide us with an understanding of what makes us love food. Much like the quantum physicist, the shaman looks at the connection of nature with life (but sparing us from the quantum calculations, double and triple integrations, and complex mathematics that we all dread). A shaman looks to draw on spirits and attempt to heal us through looking at a balance of the light and dark forces that make up humanity. Understanding food from this perspective, quantum food allows us to understand how we heal when we eat; what is happening with the body's atoms when we consume our food. It is not only about dieting, but the other attributes that food provides. Happiness is one of those key areas.

Michael's work in the culinary sciences and education in food sciences and medical knowledge allows him to delve into these two areas and these two defined skills sets can be used to show both the light and dark sides of the food. Michael is a modern-day shaman, unlocking the mysteries of food, health, nutrition, and how we can achieve a higher-level state when consuming food, good health, the sciences and holistic approaches to consuming good food.

Michael and I share many common key things in life, having a passion and love for science and food. I look forward to the future, a day when we are sitting in a restaurant somewhere around the world discussing the finer elements of medicine, science and food. I hope that you enjoy reading this book as much as I have. It has been an honour to review this book and to be asked to validate the quantum science that appears in the manuscript and other scientific concepts. I could not put this book down, reviewing page by page, concept by concept as it confirmed the idea food is more than just nourishment for our bodies. What we choose to do with this information and how we choose to take future food experiences is up to us.

—Thomas Jreige
B.Sc, SSCP, DipPM, AAICD

WHY A FOOD SHAMAN?

"Where is your will to be weird?"
—*Jim Morrison,* The Lords and The New Creatures

This is not a book about teaching you how to become a shaman in the traditional sense. For those interested, there are many excellent references on the subject written by knowledgeable and reputable authors and expert practitioners. Likewise, there are many credible resources available on the web, social media, and through other modalities. It is important to understand I will not be teaching you how to become a shaman. If you are called, seek out a qualified instructor. As Sandra Ingerman observed, "The spirits choose a person who is to be initiated into the path of becoming a shaman for his or her community. It is not a profession you choose, rather it is part of one's destiny."[1]

That is not to say that we cannot use the *tools* of the shaman and the method to their madness for our own ends; to right our own ships and improve our own health, happiness, and wellness, and by extension that of our family, friends, community, and society at large. The shamanic process utilizes energy and intention to break a negative habit and replace it with a positive habit.[2] When we utilize such techniques the naturally efficacious result expands beyond our individual borders to productively affect cultural and societal concerns. When we make ourselves well we naturally improve the health of the system at large of which we are part and parcel.

Such action requires focus, passion, and effort. This triumvirate for success is found throughout the ages and across the globe by various names wherever humankind has sought to achieve its potential. Within certain circles of study in Japan, it can be referred to as a type of *sanshin,* a three spirit or three heart approach.

Because shamanism is a path of the heart, as well as the mind and spirit,[3] it lends itself naturally to working its transformative magic through the food experience. For the proverb as timeless as food and humanity itself acknowledges, the way to a man (or woman's) heart is through their stomach.[4, 5]

Roughly two decades ago, brilliant, brave, and talented young chefs inspired by revolutionaries like Alice Waters and Jeremiah Tower decades earlier turned their back on the status quo and industrial food conglomerate. Instead, they sought out authentic, organic, locally produced natural foods. Consumers had no problem paying more for real food that delivered taste and texture and invigorated the entire food experience with rediscovered fervor, flare, and flavor. The farm to table movement was here; again.[6]

In the wake of these epicurean explorers, the science of the food experience has likewise been transformed. Because of the popularity of this fresh approach to eating, the stark contrast between corporate commodities and native benefactions has been laid bare. It is only within the last decade that the scientific knowledge of the power and import of the entire food experience has begun to reveal itself.

Like the tip of an iceberg, we are only now beginning to peer below the surface and understand the enormity of the revelation below. With the power of logic and the scientific method, we have begun to unravel and examine the connecting threads that our forebears could only intuit. Yet in doing so, we have come upon the limits of our modern age's analytical methods.

We have reached the borderlands that theoretical physicists cast us toward when they launched us down the quantum rabbit hole. With strange realities like quantum entanglement and perplexing puzzles like Schrödinger's cat, the wall between the observer and the observed has begun to crumble. These are the days, as Einstein once opined, of "spooky action at a distance."[7]

However, this newfound barrier is the foundation stone of our modern logic, classical physics, and scientific method. What we recognize as scientific fact yields reliability, not certainty. Scientific fact must be reproducible and observer independent. Observer bias is one of the first and foremost potential errors that needs to be eliminated in the design of any experimentation to be utilized in hypothesis testing. Unfortunately, it is becoming increasingly apparent that reality does not operate within or recognize such arbitrary distinction. Waves of discovery simply wash away our self-scrawled half-truths in the sand. We must finally acknowledge the eight-hundred-pound gourmand in the room: it is simply impossible to have dinner without the diner.

This central tenet of human existence is what the ancients were able to perceive in observing our relationship with Nature. As in many ways the Earth is a microcosm of the universe, we are a microcosm of the world in which we exist. In our quest for sustenance, the daily act of consumption ties us to this reality as a microcosm within a macrocosm. We are all interconnected to one another like entangled particles. The shamans of antiquity knew this and it powered their work. We have forgotten.[8]

While they may not have understood the math behind the observable, our forebears nonetheless appreciated the ramifications of individual intention and action. They well understood as well the cultural and societal consequences of our interactions with the world around us as we assimilated it into a personal reality. This truth is a bond with Nature, and thus ourselves. It is a covenant we have sacrificed in our technological age on the Altar of Convenience. The story of food is the story of humankind. And of critical import, food binds us to nature for our sustenance and binds us to each other in a complex web of emotion, memory, and experience that ripples from the individual throughout society like waves from a pebble tossed into a clear, calm, mountain lake.

This is the food experience.

We do not need more RDAs, super foods, junk foods, food porn, or ultra-processed synthetic diets. While our modern age has yielded useful information by fractionating the food experience into its component parts and testing biochemical pathways in sterile test tubes, we have in the process fractured ourselves.

The food experience is not only the perfect place to examine and repair this splintered relationship, it is the most necessary one. We all must eat to survive, so there is not a human on the planet for whom engaging in this exercise is an option. What we choose to eat each day is the most intimate and powerful expression of the interaction between our environment and our genetics.

This simple daily activity is the fulcrum upon which we teeter between health and wellness or disability and disease. We have undone the machinery to glean an understanding of its inner workings. However, only through reassembly with complete integration can we move forward across the threshold. All the parts laying on the floor certainly help us understand form and function. But like a disassembled car, until the parts are reassembled and in working order, they can afford us no means of transport.

People are even more multifaceted. If you doubt that, take a large cauldron and fill it with seventy-three and a half liters of saltwater, add about a dollar's worth of hydrogen, oxygen, nitrogen, carbon, calcium, phosphorus, and a number of trace elements[9] and stir vigorously. Despite a complete recombination of the elements that comprise a human being in the saltwater that makes up roughly 70 percent of our bodies, neither a svelte and sultry Venus nor a handsome, tanned Adonis will emerge from such a sea.

Our humanity demands a complexity far in excess of such simple machinations. For living systems are always in a state of evolution or dissolution. They are infused with that essence of Spirit. We need to understand, if only for the simple act of self-preservation, to where and to what end have we headed our ships. There is Hell waiting for us there beyond these breakers. We are ordering disaster at the drive-through.

Our healthful approach to food has followed a predictably Western model. If someone has coronary disease, we give them a pill for their cholesterol and tell them to take an aspirin. If someone has depression, we give them a pill to increase the level of serotonin in their brain. Viewed across the population, depression accounts for roughly 15 percent of cardiovascular deaths. "That is comparable to the other risk factors, such as hypercholesterolemia, obesity, and smoking," according to researcher Doctor Ladwig. These factors cause, according to some estimates, over 20 percent of the deaths due to cardiovascular disease.[10] Studies have recently shown that depression is *as* potent a risk factor for the development of cardiovascular disease as any cholesterol level.[11] Yet there seems to be little emphasis on integrating a person and prescribing happiness.

And while we all suffer the slings and arrows of our hectic, crazy, way-too-busy modern lives, a recently completed seventy-five-year Harvard University study (The Harvard Happiness Study composed of The Grant Study and The Gluek Study) clearly demonstrated that the most important variable in terms of health and longevity was an intimate, deep, loving relationship.

In a face slap to Facebook, it is the *quality*, not the *quantity*, of relationships that count. To the probable surprise of many, variables like money, family history, intelligence, educational level, or socioeconomic status fell by the wayside. Lead investigator Doctor Valliant summarized; "The only things that really matter in life are your relationships to other people...Happiness is love. Full stop."[12]

To break the bread of the ancestors is to return to the nexus of our shared food experience. Humanity arose when the first creative chefs decided to grill a couple of mastodon burgers for the rest of us.[13] Those chefs became shamans and kept whole our humanity as among the world's very first healers. Examples of such relationships still survive in some indigenous cultures as various versions of the eating of the ancestors. In South America, members of certain tribes grind up the ashes and bones of dead parents and mix them in a soup. This meal is communally shared amongst all their relatives. It is a version of incorporating the ancestor or god into one's own body.

A pale shadow of this practice still haunts our modern ceremony and ritual. A modern corollary is the funeral feast, a variation of the sacred meal with the departed. Even today in Ireland a wake is an often lively celebration of the dead, where the deceased is seen to join in the merriment. At the other end of the spectrum, wedding feasts serve a practical purpose in feeding the guests. However, along with the practical there is sacramental purpose. The collective spread serves to unite all the attendants in the common act of eating, with all its rich, symbolic associations.[14]

Today, we return reinvigorated to take our place at the table. We engage with the totality of our senses and being, the plates laid before us. Through the lens of this food experience, the wisdom of the shaman can help us focus on the act of integration and affirmative transcendence, for it is what you feed that grows.[15]

Becoming a Food Shaman describes an approach to food and health that is beyond mere nutrition and more substantive than artless food porn. Currently, we approach food and health like we do everything else, with a convenient exclusionary dualism. What we consume can either be good for us *or* taste good, delicious or nutritious, but rarely, if ever, both.

Thus, as we stand at the horizon of a new postmodern age, we turn to the venerable techniques of humankind's first transpersonal and integrative healers; the shaman. We apply these methods without bias, judgment, or religion. It is not simply about breaking barricades, or wistful longing for long forgotten days that were never as idyllic as we recount.

To truly move forward, to evolve, requires fusion with our current state. We must transcend with inclusion, not rebuttal. We employ these practices to a most significant contributor to health and wellness; what, how, where, when, and why we choose to eat. We re-engage the culinary magic.

The journey forward is about recapturing humanity's birthright to the joy of the food experience. It is about healing and harmonizing our individual, societal, and cultural divisions with the natural world. For when we consume such real and wholesome Nature in authenticity, how can we transform into anything less than the Spirit which imbues her? Let us not suffer the shrunken palate modern convenience proffers, but strive to delight in the ample richness of this good Earth's august bounty.

SHAMANISM

"Shamanism is a healing pathway."
—*Andrew Steed; Celtic Shaman
Practitioner, Author, and Educator*

Many people view the shaman one dimensionally. Most often envisioned as a Native American medicine man, the shaman is much more. The stereotype of a half-naked, wizened old tribal elder clad in feathers, animal skins, and bones cavorting about with painted face, all the while incoherently claiming to communicate with spirits through a drug induced haze is about as accurate as most of the free health advice available on the Internet. That is to say, it is rather less than inaccurate.

Shamanism is an ancient, universal spiritual practice that reaches back to a time when our ancestors shared the planet with Neanderthals. Research suggests that the origins of shamanic practice can be dated to at least the Middle-Upper Paleolithic Period if not earlier, roughly seventy thousand years ago.[16] A skull which was excavated from the Middle Awash region of northern Ethiopia was found to be more than one hundred and sixty-five thousand years old. This skull had distinctive findings that clearly document a long history of ongoing human care and handling.[17] Reverence and cult of ancestor worship, closely associated with shamanic practices, has been a part of human history for an extremely long time.

The word "shaman" has its etymology deriving from the age-old Tungus tribe of Siberia. In their native language, this word translates as "spiritual healer" or "one who sees in the dark." Although the term shamanism may have originated in the remote hinterlands, the practice of shamanism is in the process. It is limited neither by time nor place. Archaeological and historical evidence for the practice of shamanism is found on Greenland and every continent except Antarctica.[18]

There is no doubt that at one time or another, *every* indigenous civilization had a shaman. Deep within every human being's original roots, is the ancient memory of such a connection. It is hard wired into our DNA because these people were our direct forebears. We are all the sons and daughters of some tribe.

Shamans were among the first human beings to explore the body-mind-spirit connection and transfigure the human species more than 35,000 years ago.[19] It was a time that saw the birth of art, consciousness, and transcendence.[20] One of the differentiating characteristics of shamanic practice is that it is not a mere exercise in erudition. Shamans are not mere mapmakers recounting the tales of others in the corner of some dusty library surrounded by stacks and tomes, information and exploits, written by others.

Shamanism is a practice of direct revelation.[21] The shaman does not draw on a tale told to him or her. They *are* the explorers and the authors. They *are* the story, and they tell the tale and inscribe the pages through direct experience. With relish and abandon, shamans taste the adventure. It is the difference between eating the meal or reading someone else's review.

These exploits are accomplished utilizing a form of meditation combined with focused intention to accomplish various goals. Shamanism is most definitely "not a religion, nor does it conflict with any religious tradition. It's a method.... (a) practice of direct revelation (that) is the ancestral precursor of all our religious and philosophical traditions, both ancient and modern."[22]

However unlike many religions, shamanism operates without religious denomination, dogma, or hierarchy. The pursuit is immediate, intuitive, direct. It is delivered without winnowing, defining, censoring, or judging. There is no bureaucracy of intermediaries. This effect can be like a spiritual body blow that focuses our attention on previously unrecognized or unseen issues. Quite often, these are the unseen roadblocks that inhibit our progress or prevent us from attaining our desired objectives. The shaman is a universal, pancultural messenger and healer that is often described as "the one who knows."[23] By applying these devices inwardly with every bite, we begin the process of knowing ourselves.

Such a technique is similar in many ways to the practice of Buddhism. And like Buddhism, it functions as a sacred tool. Michael Harner explains, "Shamanism ultimately is only a method, not a religion with a fixed set of dogmas. Therefore, people arrive at their own experience-derived conclusions about what is going on in the universe, and about what term, if any, is most useful to describe ultimate reality."[24] Ultimately, as we will discover, reality is about relationship—on all levels. The entire fundamental construal of the Universe is relational.

One of the most prevalent bits of misinformation regarding the shaman is their place within the historical pantheon of powerful personages and healers. It is a common, but inaccurate practice, to look back in time or at contemporary indigenous peoples and use a representative of the most advanced mode of consciousness at the time and conclude that this was the average *modus operandi*.

Not every Native American, nor tribal member, and certainly not the average *Homo sapiens* from one hundred thousand years ago, was a shaman. While every shaman is a medicine person, not every medicine person is a shaman. It is estimated that at most maybe 2 percent of the population is able to intuitively access these innate powers.[25] As Ken Wilber has observed, "A shaman was a very rare and gifted soul, and most people did not share this shamanic awareness. In fact, most people were terrified of the power of the shaman, and they hadn't a clue as to the higher mode of awareness that the shaman accessed."[26]

The Way of the Shaman is ancient, but time-tested. While the shaman may appear as a larger-than-life mystical wisdom warrior wielding change like a sword of truth within a fog enshrouded, visionary vortex, the truth is much more mundane. Shamanic practice, like many of the Buddhist pursuits, is about obtaining measurable outcomes in a timely fashion. Shamans are incredibly practical because they demand applicable outcomes that work in the here and now. Their conclusions are based on a percept; an absolute known based upon direct experience. They don't merely consume; they taste.

The form of the shaman tended to be of less significance than their function. This numinous role could be filled by either men or women. Accordingly, shamans filled many diverse functions within the numerous and varied cultures they served. However, according to Andrew Steed, a principal purpose of the shaman across all societies was to act as a vessel, or a "hollow bone between worlds."[27] It was in this capacity that they provided a pathway to commune with the natural world, a type of nature therapy.

Shamans were the originators of such remedies and they rightly take their place among the first spiritual heroes.[28] As the arbitrators betwixt and between the worlds of Human and Nature, this mediation invariably extended into the procurement, preparation, and consumption of food.

Prior to the Industrial Revolution, the history of humankind's social and cultural relationships defined themselves in terms of food production.[29] Yet from the onset of the Industrial Revolution in the eighteenth century, we have progressively and at an exponential rate unbound ourselves from this natural construction, even as we have increasingly tethered ourselves to our technology. Particularly in the last fifty to seventy-five years, we have altered our food and food pathways to such a degree that 60 percent of the modern diet consists of ultra-processed food.

Ultra-processed foods can be roughly defined as:

> *formulations of several ingredients which, besides salt, sugar, oils, and fats, include food substances not used in culinary preparations, in particular, flavors, colors, sweeteners, emulsifiers, and other additives used to imitate sensorial qualities of unprocessed or minimally processed foods and their culinary preparations or to disguise undesirable qualities of the final product. The most common ultra-processed foods (are) breads; soft drinks, fruit drinks and milk-*

*based drinks; cakes, cookies and pies; salty
snacks; frozen and shelf-stable plates; pizza,
and breakfast cereals.*[30]

This is the very definition of artificiality. It is synthetically derived food additives used to *disguise undesirable qualities* or *imitate the tastes and textures of real, natural foods.* This type of pseudo-food is responsible for over 90 percent of the sugar consumed in the modern Western diet. Such massive consumption of prepackaged, pre-prepared, and processed items is reflected in the fact that over 75 percent of all the sugar and high fructose corn syrup produced in 2014 was used by the food industry.[31] Chefs crafting foods and home cooks sourcing real ingredients simply do not construct meals this way. True chefs, like a true shaman, flourish only in authenticity.

The first shamans were likely the first chefs. What destined the first societies to move beyond the treetops was the communal meal, the first BBQ. Cooking was evolution, both in physiology and in humanity. The shared meal leads to transcendence and civilization.[32] Food is a bridge between the science and the spiritual—a bridge each of us must cross every day, several times a day.

Shamans and chefs can move us forward and break us through to the other side. They do this with a grace that simply cannot be accomplished within the confines of impotent, punitive guidelines that admonish, proscribe, and prohibit. The "healthful" edicts from governmental agencies, professional organizations, and self-proclaimed experts operate on the principle of limitation. As the Buddha himself might observe, there is no salvation in deprivation. We have allowed machines, technology, food alterations, and replacements to come between us and nature in the pursuit of convenience.

Though we are reaping in our current times the massive destructive potential of such consumptive patterns as a result of the global prevalence of such consumables, it is not a 21st century phenomenon. Jean Anthelme Brillat-Savarin, who can arguably be considered the father of the low-carbohydrate diet, labelled sugar and white flour as the cause of obesity. He reached this conclusion almost two hundred years ago in 1825. He is, though, perhaps better known for his equally applicable observation: "Tell me what you eat, and I will tell you what you are."[33] However, it cuts both ways. We not only are what we eat; we eat what we are. And what we are is seasoned by our culture and society, as much as it is by internal drivers.

If we continue to gorge ourselves on the false and inauthentic, it should come as no surprise that is what we become. In place of the authentic or actual self, we live a lie. We deceive ourselves with the mundane and trivial and we busy ourselves fashioning projects of deception. We are masters of the multitasking, all of which is to hide from ourselves the singular shocking truth of this existence: "The finite self is going to die—magic will not save it, mythic gods will not save it, rational science will not save it—and facing that cutting fact is part of becoming authentic."[34]

Like any true creative craftsman, the shaman operates from within his or her own veracity and sovereignty. The shaman learns to dance with authenticity. To execute their art, they draw from the gamut of physical, social, and psychological therapies, as well as from the spiritual domain. What is often overlooked in modern medicine is what the shaman incorporates; that true healing has both technical and symbolic components.

The technical element can be as straightforward as stitching a cut or performing a physical exam. But even simple techniques hold symbolic content. Roger Walsh further elaborates, "The symbolic component seeks to effect change—in the patient, the world, or the spiritual realm—via manipulation of symbols: objects that represent important forces or beings. Both technical and symbolic components can be therapeutic."[35]

The therapeutic aspect of the symbolic components is often referred to as a placebo effect. Recent research has demonstrated that placebo effects are genuine psychobiological phenomenon attributable to the overall therapeutic context, and that placebo effects can be robust in both laboratory and clinical settings. It is evident that placebo effects are real and that they have therapeutic potential. Furthermore, clinically relevant evidence demonstrates that placebo effects can have meaningful therapeutic effects, by virtue of magnitude and duration, in different patient populations.[36]

For the shaman, such therapeutic modalities are not limited to single patient applications. In the indigenous world, war dances, rain dances, or healing rites do not necessarily cause victory, bring rain, or cure a sick person. But the ceremony can and does bring about a remarkable (and measurable) physiological change in members of the group as tension and excitement rise, peak, and then subside.[37] For the Food Shaman, a meal—a wonderful food experience—may not cure cancer or stop world hunger, but it will measurably change all those who fully participate. And that is as good a place to start as any.

Participation is the key. For the Food Shaman, it is about much more than simply presenting a beautiful plate. It is about engagement. It is about moving the masses from mindlessly gobbling and grazing to actively participating in the food experience. Many people today misunderstand the healing work performed by shamans. There is a belief that shamanic healing is an active role for the shaman and totally passive for the patient. It is a misperception reinforced by the contemporary doctor-patient relationship where the physician is all knowing and all powerful. He or she hands out a pill or performs a procedure and the patient is healed.

Sandra Ingerman dispels that myth by drawing a clear distinction between curing and healing. "If a cure is provided by a shamanic practitioner," she observes, "it does not mean the work is done. Shamanic healing does not involve a practitioner passing a magic wand over you. You do have to take responsibility in your own process of healing."[38] While the shaman may provide a cure, it will be at best a temporary fix without participation from the patient. To truly heal, patients must become participants. They have a responsibility to take an active role in doing his or her personal work in the healing process. The meal may be prepared by others, but it is for us to dine.

Like an executive chef, the Food Shaman runs the spiritual pass between meal creation and consumption. Shamans stand at the gateways. Successful healing extends beyond the patient and reaches out to family, community, village, city, and eventually the world around us. This can be accomplished by utilizing the common core connection that all is ultimately one with Nature. The application of such shamanic practices ultimately leads to self-realization, personal development, and an evolution of consciousness, all of which is uniquely personal.

Shamanism is a tool, a practice in which each practitioner undergoes exceptional direction and guidance.[39] Two people may share the same meal, but their experiences, and thus their realities, will differ. Even if they both enjoyed the meal, there are measurable differences in the details. Like distinct fingerprints, each of our food experiences—even the shared ones—are unique and particular.

Nevertheless, although the effect resonates at the individual level, the process can be performed at the group level. A study performed at the University of Michigan explored the effects of shamanic practice on people who had suffered a heart attack. In this study one group learned shamanic principles and all participants received coaching on nutrition, physical exercise, and stress management.

The shamanic group had an immediate and sustained significant reduction on their depression score and a marked improvement on a test measuring hope. The conclusion was that shamanic practice could be used to increase hope while reducing depression in persons following a heart attack.[40, 41] Other recent research suggests that depression post myocardial infarction makes you twice as likely to have another heart attack.[42] These are real world, objectively measurable benefits.

Scientific research has shown that when we are in an ordinary state of consciousness, our waking state where we perceive the tangible world we live in, our brain waves are in a beta state. When we engage in thoughtfulness and mindfulness, we initiate an alpha state, which is a light meditative state of consciousness. Journeying deeper into a meditative state results in a further slowing of the brainwaves until we reach a deeper state called a theta state. Progressing even further results in the generation of delta waves. This state is associated with sleeping and dreaming. The shaman seeks to dwell in the betwixt and between of the theta state. Here it is believed that the shaman's soul journeys into the invisible realms, allowing access to helping spirits.[43]

Famously, Einstein sought to engage this dimension for his revolutionary thought experiments. As he explained in a letter to Jacques S. Hadamard, who was studying the thought processes of mathematicians at the time:

> *Words or the language, as they are written or spoken, do not seem to play any role in my mechanism of thought. The psychical entities which seem to serve as elements in thought are certain signs and more or less clear images which can be "voluntarily" reproduced and combined...but taken from a psychological viewpoint, this combinatory play seems to be the essential feature in productive thought—before there is any connection with logical construction in words or other kinds of signs which can be communicated to others.*[44]

His assessment of the shamanic state underscores its bridging importance:

> *I believe in intuition and inspiration. Imagination is more important than knowledge. For knowledge is limited, whereas imagination embraces the entire world, stimulating progress, giving birth to evolution. It is, strictly speaking, a real factor in scientific research....*[45] *In a certain sense, therefore, I hold it true that pure thought can grasp reality, as the ancients dreamed.*[46]

The methods of shamanism certainly cannot be neatly dismissed as the confused productions of primitive or pathological minds. The effects are real and serious and most certainly not an imaginary construct. Roger Walsh could be referencing the placebo effect when he correctly concludes that with respect to shamanistic outcomes: "Something much more remarkable, rewarding, and profound is going on."[47]

The Food Shaman employs similar reflection on the "what and how" surrounding our comestibles. At the simplest level, food provides nutrition and supplies us with energy. But along with the energy that our body stores from what we consume, we contain the stories of the corresponding experiences. Each of these contains thoughts, memories, emotions, and energy that is all their own. Shamans help people repurpose the unfavorable narratives their bodies contain, reclaiming it so the energy is useful again.

We have a complicated relationship with food because the food experience involves aspects of physics, nutrition, chemistry, biology, physiology, psychology, ecology, anthropology, history, theology, philosophy, sociology, and political science. Yet so often we are told to value our comestibles solely in terms of simple *in vitro* laboratory analysis. Nutrition is situational thinking; the food experience is conceptual thinking. Nutrition is an act of science; the food experience is an act of spirit. This distinction defines the objective relation versus the personal relations. Understanding nutrition is necessary for life, but what do we live life for?

Working with the food experience is a similar process to engaging the pan-disciplinary tools of shamanism. It incorporates nutrition, but that is only one mask from the crowded gallery. The many faces of the Food Shaman enable them to act as healers and doctors, priests or priestesses, harmonizers and psychotherapists, mystics and storytellers.[48] Of course, within this tale the most central personality to the ceremony is the chef.

However, in the contemporary telling of this story, the characters are dispersed, disparate, and dysfunctional. In our technologically wired world, we are more disconnected from our roots than ever before. We live in our heads and online without real emotion. Far too often, we strive vicariously to exist outside of ourselves like some digital voyeur. We become lost in logic, too rational, too obsessed with analytical measurements and analytical thinking, we become one-dimensional.

We become like fish in a lake. We are unaware of the entirety of existence beyond our watery world. Because we see neither sky nor land, oak nor owl, we deny their possibility. This is a dangerous form of bias. We lose awareness of the detail outside of our immediate attention and consciousness. Without integration and forward movement, we grow moribund and stagnant. In such a state wisdom fades to knowledge that fades to simply information. It is no wonder that we label our current moment The Information Age.

We need to breathe deeply both in *and* out. It is a complete rhythm that sustains life. If you try to put the sea in a box, it ceases to be the sea. There is no flow—it loses its heartbeat and its vitality. It is the water *of* the ocean, but *an* ocean no more.[49] In such a way we mark ourselves off either as having more than anyone else, or less, and either is made a virtue. We often use food to make such distinction because its emotional connection lends itself easily in the construction of such boxes: "By their food shall ye know them."[50] We need to look inward and feast with intention.

Observance, knowledge, and mindfulness are key practices. As an example, you start every day with water. Every morning there is an acknowledgment of the blessing of water, whether it be in the form of drinking it or passing it. Whether it's brushing your teeth, making some tea or coffee, or hopping in the shower, every day begins with water. Your body is mostly water.

Without water, there is no life. All living things are composed mainly of water. Therefore, the blessing of the waters become the blessing of the self, both to ourselves and nature. You can give thanks and bless the water you use. Starting with spirituality and gratefulness will start your day positively.

Being mindful and grateful for your food and nature will improve your food experience and life. Taste the food, embrace the flavor, savor the moment, and experience the mindful benefits. Appreciate the energy and intent of the chef who prepared it, for all is connected in the act of eating. Such simple action can raise your consciousness, allow you to appreciate the moments in your life, and help create a new, beautiful world. It's also why you never want to eat food from an angry chef.

As we experience the Universe, we must remember the Universe simultaneously experiences us. "There is a Tao, a Way, a Current of the Kosmos, from which we have not deviated and could never deviate," concludes Ken Wilber. "And part of our job is to find this deeper Current, this Tao, and express it, elucidate it, celebrate it. We are altogether fragmented in this modernity gone slightly mad."[51]

It is a simple path, but not an easy one. You must listen. To heal the land or others requires first a healing of the self. Like existence itself, this requires life-giving food. Compare the high and low of an artificial energy drink to natural endorphins of a romantic food experience. In one scenario, the cable snaps and the elevator falls violently from top to bottom: crash. In the other, the doors open silently, and a soft exit reveals pleasure brushed with the gentle sense of serenity.

Food is about a quality experience and shamanism is about a higher quality of life. You are in charge; learn to integrate. Shamanism is relevant precisely because these methods can be found in the profound works of transformation throughout the ages. Roots of these shamanic tools and methods are wrapped within the teachings of those whom Karl Jaspers refers to as The Axial Sages; Buddha, Lao Tsu, Parmenides, Socrates, Plato, Patanjali, and Confucius.

Shamanism is something everyone can do. A shamanic way of life is that which embraces a state of joy that bubbles up from a deep place within. It is a way of life that is utterly free of any religious overlay or dogma. The esoteric teaching "as above, so below; as within, so without" is a shamanic understanding. Harmony within always creates harmony without. The Food Shaman gets the body engaged through the physical act of consumption. The Food Shaman gets the mind engaged through the ceremony of the food experience.

Action requires no mystical supplies, no monastic retreat to perform ritual. Simply bring and engage your inner spirit. Such participation will carry and support you through the process. There is a focus created in performing and participating in such a ceremony as the food experience where body, mind, and spirit join together.[52] Yet it is paramount to always remain open and receptive to the unexpected, the unannounced, and the wyrd. Sometimes it needs to hit you from a totally unexpected angle, through a prism of strangeness. Through reflection, refraction, and rarefaction the cacophony becomes the song. It becomes a light that illuminates the work.

FOOD AND SEX: CAN YOU SMELL WHAT'S COOKING?

"Good food leads to good sex...as it should."
—*Anthony Bourdain*

You've had an annoying day.

No serious disasters on the home front, but enough nuisances to leave you quite piqued. The morning seems to trumpet in one fire after another, and after adding Smokey the Bear to your *curriculum vitae* accomplishments, you find yourself peckish as well as peeved as you trundle out for a long overdue lunch.

You figure you might as well try the new place. The way this day is going, if it is horrible it is but par for the course and certainly couldn't ruin your current mood. On the other hand, a good meal could turn your ship around. As you settle into your seat and pick up the menu, the waitress passes behind you with a grilled lamb steak exotically spiced with *ras el hanout*. The scent hits you like a blackjack to the head.

Without control, without direction, memories from years gone by cross the threshold into your conscious mind like an unwanted Jehovah's Witness. You had not thought about that intense, but short-lived romance in forever and a day. Now, all those pleasant recollections form an afternoon parade for one at your table. The mind's eye showpiece is multisensory; you see her face, hear her voice, feel skin warm with the glow of the Mediterranean sun, and smell her scent mixing with the salt of the sea.

It is that perfumed memory that burrows deep in your brain and unlocks emotions. The feelings wash over you, cleansing the grime and the angst of what had been up until now, a most terrible day. The recollection has mellowed with the years and like a wine that was once a bit harsh to swallow, it is now smooth, complex, and deeply satisfying. Close your eyes, and immerse yourself in the warm sensation of subtle pleasures. It is, as Barbara Streisand once sang, the laughter we remember.

Good times endure, if only in our mind.

Yet how could a simple scent unleash such a psychological tsunami?

Food and sex have been bestest roomies inside the human brain since the human brain has been concerned with food and sex. Which is to say pretty much forever. Of all the senses, only taste and smell are predominately hard-wired directly into our brain. When we hear something, see something, or feel something, it is generally filtered first. But taste and smell home in on command central like a well-guided drone strike.

It turns out smell and taste, and thus food and sex, are full of more rapid twists and turns than a python on crack. Not to mention they have us by the emotional and physiological goody-goodies the entire time.

We used to believe that certain areas of the tongue perceived certain tastes like bitter, sour, sweet, and salty. We used to believe that this was the extent of the sense of taste. We were wrong.

It is now recognized that there are taste buds located throughout the oral cavity, epiglottis, larynx, and nasopharynx. While the tongue may have the greatest concentration of taste buds, they are found in the soft palate and with a particular focus in that region between the hard and soft palate, which is known as the *geschmackstreifen*, or taste stripe.[53]

What is clear is that although there may be regional differences in terms of overall chemosensitivity, the idea of a "taste map" in which specific areas respond to specific taste is incorrect. It is likely that individual taste buds and even taste cells respond to multiple classes of what we call taste.

There is a difference between taste and flavor. If taste is defined as the visceral sensation of the classic four—sweet, salty, bitter, sour—then flavor is what we experience. It comprises the sensory data from smell, taste, and somatosensation that contribute to what we experience when we savor. Taste is a physical sense; flavor is a hedonistic sense.

Flavor acknowledges a fifth taste referred to as "umami." This newest palate pleaser is generally known as one that corresponds to the savory aspect of foods. It is derived from the Japanese who first described it in 1908, and coined the term as a neologism of *umai* which means "delicious" and *mi* which translates as "taste.[54]

Although we associate the tongue with taste, only about 10 percent of what we perceive as taste is derived from the tongue. Approximately 85 percent of taste is modulated through olfaction, or the sense of smell. In fact, we generally don't perceive taste as an isolated sensation. What we actually perceive is the flavor. Flavor incorporates taste, smell, texture, but is primarily driven by smell. The proof is in the non-tasting of the pudding. Just remember how bland everything you ate was the last time you had a cold and your nose was stuffed.[55]

Smell is so important that we acquire scent via multiple modalities. We smell with more than a sniff and a snuffle. Being carried in with inhaled air, the orthonasal route, is not the only way for odor molecules to reach the olfactory receptor cells. When we chew food, we generate a pressure gradient. Many of the odor and ultimately flavor molecules that are a result of this process are released and driven into the retronasal passage.

This is located at the back of the oral cavity extending through the nasopharynx into the back of the nasal cavity. Although the orthonasal route is the one usually used to test for smell perception, the retronasal route is the main source of the smells we perceive from foods and liquids within our mouths. For several reasons, it is likely that this is an important route for smell in humans. Among them is the reason stinky cheese like Époisses de Bourgogne smells like a high school gym locker but tastes delicious on the palate.

It is no small coincidence that the sensation of flavor is enhanced with the breath of life. Breathing in then out enhances the acquisition of molecules and their processing. Sommeliers perform this maneuver at a wine tasting so that they may experience the maximum depth and breadth the wine has to offer in terms of taste, texture, and flavor.

Smell is the process by which molecules known as odorants are detected by specific olfactory or odorant receptors (ORs). These are seven different types of receptors that function as chemo-sensors. The result is that we have the ability to differentiate individual smells, and thus tastes, among a staggeringly large universe of chemical compounds. (See appendix A1)

The cerebral processing of these smells is unique among all our senses. While all the other senses are acquired by specialized cells which transmit information that is filtered through the limbic system, the thalamus in particular, smell is mediated by primarily by olfactory neurons. These neurons are essentially the same neurons that comprise our brain tissue. Both operate via what is known as a GPCR, or G-Protein Coupled Receptor. To a large degree one can argue that olfaction, and taste by extension, is a direct expansion of our brain that reaches out into our environment.

Our olfactory neurons which perceive the smells from the environment then feed back into the olfactory bulb, which is located in the forebrain. This communicates directly with, among other brain structures, the pyriform cortex.

The pyriform cortex is where the majority of the sensory input from our sense of smell (and thus taste) is delivered via the olfactory bulb. It is the largest central olfactory processing area in the brain. The processing of smell in the pyriform cortex is unique. It is organized differently from any of our other four senses.

In other neocortical sensory areas, the cells that respond to a particular stimulus are clustered and their response properties vary smoothly across the cortex.[56] In the visual, auditory, and somatosensory systems, spatial information from the peripheral sense organs is maintained in the sensory cortex. You can feel where you are being touched when you are tapped on the shoulder, judge how far away your golf ball is from the green, localize to the sound when someone calls your name.

Yet with olfaction, the principal areas of the brain involved with smell and taste perception light up in a shotgun pattern of neuronal activity. This primary olfactory region (pyriform cortex, olfactory nucleus and tubercle, amygdala, and entorhinal cortex) along with the secondary olfactory areas (hippocampus, hypothalamus, thalamus, orbitofrontal cortex, and the cerebellum) helps explain the link between what we smell and the resulting mood and emotion, pleasure, sensation, and memory.[57] Among all our senses, we are built uniquely to experience smell and taste.

The area where this nearly uninterrupted relay occurs is located within the brainstem region of the central nervous system (CNS). This locale houses our animal brain; the pyriform cortex being present in amphibians, reptiles, and mammals. From perception in the environment to direct CNS stimulation, smell is only a two-synapse step in humans. This is in stark contradistinction to our other senses in which there are five to seven connections necessary before a similar endpoint is reached.

In addition to its direct CNS connection through the pyriform cortex, olfaction interacts with the limbic system. The limbic system is the collective name for the framework in the human brain involved in emotion, motivation, and emotional association with memory. The limbic system contains several distinct structures. Among these is the amygdala, which focuses on threats, emotional response, and directs attention. The amygdala receives the terminal ends of many olfactory bulb projections, specifically within the discrete amygdala sub-nuclei. Neurophysiologic recordings in animals and humans suggest that amygdala in particular is highly responsive to odor stimulation.[58]

The perception of olfaction involves other limbic system members such as the hippocampus, which deals with memories and learned behaviors, and the hypothalamus that functions in the release of hormones in response to emotion.

Finally, there is the orbitofrontal cortex which represents the main neocortical projection of the olfactory cortex. While not part of the limbic system, it receives the inputs that arrive from all primary olfactory areas. It supplies feedback projections that travel back to these areas. This is the area in which we become consciously aware of certain odors and interact accordingly. (See appendix A2)

It is in this nether cortex of carnal needs and neurons that food, sex, memory, and emotion collude, collide, coalesce, and conjoin. We understand this on a subliminal level. It was no coincidence that when *The Joy of Sex* was published, the title was a play off the previously released and hugely successful, *Joy of Cooking*.[59]

The exact pathways and mechanisms by which these interrelationships are formed is not known, but there is no question as to their existence. Food is more than nutrition, it is a defining human experience. It goes beyond the mere satisfaction of physiological needs. The sense of smell is so integral to our well-being that nearly 3 percent of the human genome of roughly twenty thousand and five hundred genes, or about one out of every fifty genes, is dedicated to making some type of smell, or odor receptor (OR). This only serves to highlight the critical role of taste and olfaction in our physiology and evolution.[60]

How we experience food and sex is physically linked within this hardwiring of the brain. Food and sex are integrated in the regions that control emotion, feeling, and memory; good food equals good sex. In this way, there is a sensuality to eating that is every bit as potent as any sexual urge. Like our attitudes toward sex, there is that aspect of food seduction that spurns the puritan and ascetic rejection of food pleasures.[61] It is why the rigors of diet restriction and food fads based on deprivation so often ultimately fail. It is the edible equivalent of prescribing abstinence from sex for the promise of beatitudes in the afterlife.

Such a Calvinist version of life equates "plain food" with a "good life."[62] These sixteenth century, puritanical remnants remain lodged in much of the rubbish that passes for healthful eating advice today. Such cultish behavior often targets sex as much as food. After all, as their reasoning goes, both can be counted among the seven deadly sins. (See appendix A3)

Such admonitions were popularized by Thomas Aquinas in the thirteenth century. His argument against the pursuit of these activities was essentially based on the fact that they are intimately associated with happiness.[63] This priggish viewpoint not only manifests in modern prudishness when it comes to sex, it pervades our approach to food. For it to be "healthful and good" for the body it must somehow deny us pleasure. Sex will damn the eternal soul and the road to Hell is apparently paved with delectable appetizers.

Yet if we travel even further back in time into the history of food and humankind before the Dark Ages, we recapture our direct and personal connection with the divine. We find the consumption of food as sacred. It originates with the idea of sharing a meal with God, or the gods. Some researchers view this act of heavenly communion as the etiology of sacrifice.

There has been a suggestion that this may have developed into the idea of consuming the god to gain their strength, virtue, or other characteristics. We still munch away looking for the baby Jesus in the king cakes of Mardi Gras. The Aztecs made huge loaves in the shape of the gods, and these were thrown down the temple steps to be devoured by the multitude.

The Aztecs participated in horrific human sacrifice and cannibalism, possibly linked again to the concept of the hallowed meal. In this case, their penultimate holy food was being used—human flesh.[64] Of the most basic things in our behavioral repertoire, eating is the most accessible and effective for conveying our messages to the gods and others. We can, of course, offer sex and violence, and sometimes like the Aztecs, we do. However, and fortunately, in our modern civilization, outstanding food served in superior ambience is almost universally preferred.

The play within the play of our modern dining dance relates to the sharing of food. It is through this act that we once again engage in ancient tribal ritual. We roast to boast; we cook to impress. As Robin Fox perceived:

> *To feed someone is one of the most direct*
> *and intimate ways to convey something of*
> *ourselves to the impressee. We are never just*
> *saying, "see how we can satisfy your hunger."*
> *We are saying more like "see how lavish and*
> *hospitable and knowledgeable we are."*[65]

But not all meals, foods, or company tempt us. Just as the idea of sexual congress with certain people engenders feelings of abhorrence, bad taste serves as an important warning system. Taste aversion is the opposite of flavor. It is the anti-hedonistic warning system. It is the flip side of taste's dual survival roles, for it becomes as important to know what to avoid when foraging as it is to find something edible.

If someone consumes a food and becomes ill, it is imperative that this association be learned and remembered. Think about food poisoning occurring hours after consumption. People who experience such foodborne illness may never again be able to eat that particular food. Being aware of things in the environment that may make you ill, or even kill you, is a vital survival tool. Even more primitive mammals exhibit this capacity.

John Garcia demonstrated this with coyotes. Coyotes were harassing sheep ranchers by preying upon the livestock. Instead of killing the coyotes, he laced a carcass with lithium chloride. While making the animals ill, it was not lethal. In essence, it replicated a bout of food poisoning. The coyotes ate the carcass, fell ill, and never bothered another sheep. In fact, the aversive memory was so strong that some coyotes ran away when they saw or smelled sheep.[66, 67] Humans may forever avoid a particular bar or tequila altogether after awakening to a coyote-ugly morning. It is nature versus nurture. Food is both reward and punishment. We describe pleasant things as tasteful, but an unpleasant thing causes disgust—literally an unpleasant taste.

As mammals, tastes and scent can strike us in unexpected ways. They motivate us through unconscious, subconscious, and primal pathways. Nonetheless, as humans, we possess a complex triune brain, which transcends and includes its predecessors. Our three-part brain not only has a reptilian stem and a paleo-mammalian limbic system, but it has something uniquely new and human; a complex neocortex capable of abstract logic, linguistics, and vision-logic.[68]

It is this complex construction combined with the processing power of our cerebral cortex that makes the food-sex-emotion-experience-memory so influential in affecting our intention and behavior. The taste-smell complexity of the involuntary memory is well described by Marcel Proust in his classic *In Search of a Lost Time* (previously known as *Remembrance of Things Past*). Such emotional, or Proustian, memory is long lasting, vivid, and stable. This in opposition to the voluntary memory of information, as anyone who has tried to recall information on an exam after spending the night cramming can attest. The memory of a lover long gone is as vivid and intensely emotional as the day it was formed as we catch the perfumed scent behind us; meanwhile, we can't remember our own cell phone number.

Recent scientific investigation across several different disciplines indicates that these potent central nervous system processes are even capable of altering our immune responses. Prior animal experimentation using rats or mice suggested a brain/immune system connection. The animals were given a conditioned stimulus, like a flavored water, that was paired with an immunomodulating agent.

This drug was known to have a physiological effect that resulted in alterations in humoral and cell-mediated immune responses to antigenic stimuli. After a time, the immune system of the mice would respond to the flavored water alone as if they had received a dose of the drug as well. The researchers concluded that, "Despite its capacity for self-regulation, it appears that the immune system is integrated with other psychophysiological processes and subject to modulation by the brain."[69, 70]

The interconnectedness and integration of these bodily systems is reflected in the development of cross disciplinary studies like psychoneuroimmunology, the study of behavioral-neural-endocrine-immune system interactions. There are at least two well-known pathways that link the brain and the immune system. There is the autonomic nervous system, which operates through direct neuron to neuron transmission. There is also the neuroendocrine outflow via the pituitary, which mediates its effects hormonally.

When we are in love, we are under the influence, hormonally speaking. Love can heal—and make us crazy. Everyone understands there is a relationship between sex, hormones, and desire. What is little appreciated is that great food spawns similar physiological responses.

What is well known is that certain regions of brain, especially within the hypothalamus and limbic system that are so integral to our processing of smell, taste, and flavor, have immunological consequences.[71] A research study examined whether utilizing a flavor stimulus, which would involve these pathways, could affect the immune response in healthy humans. Volunteers in this double-blind, placebo-controlled study were conditioned in four sessions over three consecutive days, receiving the immunosuppressive drug cyclosporine A as an unconditioned stimulus paired with a distinctively flavored drink, which served as the conditioned stimulus.

The following week, the participants received the drink, but it was now paired with placebo capsules instead of the immunosuppressive drug. Measurable suppression of immune functions was obtained by looking at markers associated with interleukin-2 (IL-2) and interferon-γ (IFN-gamma) as well as lymphocyte proliferation. The results clearly demonstrated that immunosuppression can be behaviorally conditioned in humans operating through the sensory inputs associated with smell, taste, and flavor.[72] Foods heal in ways that extend beyond traditional nutritional pathways.

Experimental data like this along with the experiential power of the Proustian memory would suggest a prominent role for smell and taste as a human sense. In contrast to this evidence, it continues to be conventional wisdom that human perception acquired through smell and taste is a poor substitute for visual input. In response to the constant barrage of movies, television, books, and computers, we've become a visual culture. This cultural and societal bias can easily and subtly color our perceptions and attitudes.

Not only is this general belief pervasive among the public, but it appears within the scientific community as well. And in the interest of full disclosure, there is some data to support this position. Recent genetic studies show a decline in the number of functional olfactory receptor genes as our more primitive primate ancestors made the evolutionary trek from *Homo erectus* to *Homo sapiens*.

Along the way there has been an apparent ascendance of vision with the reduction of smell. The evidence for this is based on the anthropological record. Over the course of our development there has been a progressive diminution of the snout as the eyes migrated toward the middle of the face, facilitating depth perception and a heavy pictorial dependence. Concurrently, our ancestors moved into the trees and began the adoption of an erect posture. All of this served to move our nose away from the ground, which is an environmental treasure chest of smells and odors.[73] Anyone who has ever had to take the dog for a walk can attest to that simple fact.

Humans currently have about three hundred and fifty different kinds of olfactory receptors, and that is on the low end for vertebrates. Mice and other animals that depend heavily on their sense of smell for finding food and evading predators have more than one thousand. From rodents through the primate series to humans there is a progressive reduction in the proportion of functional olfactory receptor genes. Mice have approximately thirteen hundred olfactory receptor genes, of which some eleven hundred are functional, and humans have about three hundred and fifty recognized functional OR genes.

However, the most recent investigations have suggested that it is not simply the number of genes that determine the keenness of sense of smell. In other words, it implies that three hundred and fifty genes in the human are more than enough to smell as well as a mouse. Other inquiry into comparing the data on smell detection thresholds shows that humans not only perform as well or better than other primates, they perform as well or better than other mammals. Additional research has demonstrated that in quantifying human olfactory abilities in tests of odor detection, humans can outperform the most sensitive measuring instruments such as the gas chromatograph.

The central olfactory brain regions that process the olfactory input; the areas that detect and process smell, taste, and flavor, are more extensive in humans than is usually realized. These dedicated olfactory regions include the aforementioned olfactory cortex, the olfactory tubercle, the entorhinal cortex, parts of the amygdala, parts of the hypothalamus, the mediodorsal thalamus, the medial and lateral orbitofrontal cortex, and parts of the insula. We make up for our limited receptors with the power of cognition. (See appendix A4)

We think, therefore, we smell. The experience of love is complicated—emotionally, physiologically, cognitively, and biologically. It is inclusive of, but more than, sex. The food experience is likewise complicated, and it appears may use similar, if not identical, neurophysiological and psychobiological pathways. Even our language reflects it; we hunger for affection and crave both sexual intimacy and a juicy burger, although not always in that order.

In the enlarged processing capacity for perceiving and discriminating odors, language plays a critical role. As Gordon Shepherd deftly recognizes:

> *This seems paradoxical, for we have great difficulty describing a smell in words.*

Insight into this difficulty comes from the finding that different smells are represented in the olfactory bulb by different patterns of olfactory glomerular activity. These patterns function as virtual 'odor images.' It has been hypothesized that these odor images provide the basis for discrimination between odors, analogous to the way that retinal images are the basis for discrimination of visual pattern stimuli. The complex patterns constituting odor images may be considered as analogous to the complex patterns constituting visual images of faces. And just as we are very good at recognizing a human face, yet have difficulty describing it in words, we have a hard time describing and verbally comparing odor images.[74]

Basically, we are really good at identifying, quantitating, and qualifying smells, tastes, and flavors precisely because we have the brain power to appreciate them. It is a type of cognitive work that only humans, among all the animals with olfactory organs, can perform. And much like facial recognition, it is a survival necessity for the tribe. It is argued that operating such a keen sniffer-taster is what humans are adapted to do.[75]

The advent of fire, perhaps as early as two million years ago, made the human diet more odorous and tasty.[76] From this time forward there is transfiguration of the human diet. From this moment hence, one can begin to speak of truly human cuisines, with all their diversity of smells. Professor Richard Wrangham voices support that: "[S]uch prepared cuisines based on cooked foods are one of the defining characteristics of humans."[77] It is also interesting to observe that from a shamanic perspective, fire is a living being whose nature is to transform and transmute.[78]

Next, added to the cooked cuisines, were fermented foods and liquids, with their own strong flavors. These developments occurred among the early hunter-gatherer human cultures and continued through the last ice age. With the transition to agricultural and urban cultures currently dated to about ten thousand to fifteen thousand years ago, human cuisines were again altered through the advent of animal domestication and plant cultivation. The use of spices and of complex preparatory procedures such as fermentation to produce cheeses, wines, slaws, and ales; smoking to flavor and preserve meats; and other various methods all produced foodstuffs that especially stimulate the smell receptors with their complex flavors.

Taken together, the evidence which includes the archeological and anthropomorphical records, indicate that humans are not poor smellers or microsmats, but rather are relatively good, perhaps even excellent, smellers or macrosmats.[79] Perhaps this helps explain why taste, smell, and flavor elicit such a profound sense of deep bodily experience. In light of the far-reaching effects of smell, it is not surprising that we are now identifying this primitive cellular reflex in various cells throughout the body. Odor receptors are among the most evolutionarily ancient chemical sensors in the body, capable of detecting a multitude of compounds, not solely those drifting through the air.[80]

Such a discovery is not surprising, because every cell of our being has its ancestral roots in the single celled organisms from which we originated. These wee beasties are still with us and manifest as our symbiotic organ; the gut microbiome (more on that later). To function and survive, these single cell organisms orient and feed by identifying variations in various chemical gradients within their environment. Our human cells can remember how to smell. There are smell receptors in our skin cells, lung cells, prostate cells, kidney cells, throughout the gastrointestinal tract, and even sperm are built to sniff.

Odorant receptors have been known to exist in cells not associated with classic mechanisms of taste or smell for a long time. For many years, their presence was viewed as a vestigial curiosity and their potential functions remained largely unknown. However, recent inquiry is demonstrating that these ORs are anything but curiosities. One of the first, and perhaps most intriguing, uses of olfactory receptors outside of traditional taste and smell pathways was discovered in sperm. Food and sex co-create the moment of our physical inception beyond just courtship through the romantic dinner.

The scent of lily of the valley may be the motivator that directs sperm to eggs. Conversely, the scent of citrus may act as a deterrent. Taken together, these results suggest an intriguing role for smell in procreation and adds an entirely new chapter to the food-sex-smell-taste-flavor story. It also explains the common use of this scent in perfumes. (See appendix A5)

Smell may not only be involved in creating life, but in protecting it as well. In 2009, Doctor Hanns Hatt and his team reported that exposing olfactory receptors in the human prostate to beta-ionone, a primary odor compound in violets and roses, appeared to inhibit the spread of prostate cancer cells by switching off errant genes.[81] It turns out what is good for the gander may be good for the goose as well, because β-ionone has also been shown to prevent the development of breast cancer.[82] (See appendix A6)

In other organs like the kidney, it appears that well-designed chemo-sensors such as ORs may function to regulate the excretion of certain substances. Therefore, it is no surprise that smell receptors have been discovered in the distal nephron and macula densa and that they may play a physiologically critical role in regulating fundamental aspects of renal function. Research has demonstrated no less than six different olfactory receptors that are expressed in the kidney. Animal studies have shown that mice whose kidneys lack the ability to "smell" can suffer from renal impairment, blood pressure abnormalities, and an unexplained propensity toward developing obesity.[83]

The lungs are another organ where olfactory receptors might be found, given that mammalian airways are sensitive to inhaled stimuli. Many airway diseases are characterized by hypersensitivity to volatile stimuli, such as industrial solvents among others. However, the identity and function of the cells in the airway that can sense volatile chemicals remain uncertain, particularly in humans.

Recent research has suggested that cells located in the lung known as pulmonary neuroendocrine cells (PNECs), are actually a type of OR cell. Such cells may not only be involved in the development of allergic reactions or acute asthma attacks, but may be responsible for acute exacerbations in people with chronic diseases like COPD.[84] (See appendix A7)

Given the central role of the gastrointestinal tract in everything food related, it should come as no surprise that smell receptors would extend naturally beyond the oral and nasopharyngeal region. Gastrointestinal enterochromaffin cells (EC) appear to respond to odorants present in the luminal environment of the gut. In an unsurprising twist, it has been discovered that we taste from kisser to keister. (See appendix A8)

These EC cells also secrete serotonin, the happy hormone. In the gut, serotonin controls both gut motility and secretion and is implicated in pathologic conditions such as vomiting, constipation, diarrhea, and irritable bowel syndrome. While much more research is needed, these olfactory receptors are potential novel targets for the treatment of gastrointestinal diseases and motility disorders.[85]

Odorant receptors (ORs) in the olfactory epithelium bind to volatile small molecules leading to the perception of smell. Smell receptors throughout the gut, controlling the speed of intestinal transport, makes sense. But what are multiple types of ORs doing in muscle?

A murine study found smell receptors involved in muscle recovery during myogenesis *in vitro* and muscle regeneration *in vivo*. Muscle cells need to smell where to go during muscle regeneration when muscle cells are extensively fusing. Once again, the scent of lily of the valley leads to an act of creation. In this case, the regeneration and repair of muscle tissue.[86] In fact, some experts speculate that genetic disease states like muscular dystrophy might be because our muscle cells don't smell correctly. (See appendix A9)

Given the wide and diverse dissemination of ORs throughout the body, our largest organ which is in constant communication with the environment would seem to be a logical repository of ORs. Indeed, research performed at Ruhr University Bochum in Germany found that human skin has more than fifteen different olfactory receptors. Exposing skin to specific fragrances like those found in sandalwood increased wound healing by 30 percent.[87] (See appendix A10)

Aromatherapy use as in the aforementioned example has long been snubbed by mainstream science as a baseless curiosity. However, in a circle of life sort of way, it appears on the verge of asserting its legitimacy in no uncertain measure. It makes us pause. Do we gather in the kitchen because it is a center of activity, or because the scents and smells begin the nourishing and healing before the first bite?

An essential oil with a long history of therapeutic benefits is lavender. It has been used in the treatment of anxiety disorders and related conditions. It is useful in making deliciously floral chocolate-dipped madeleines. In placebo controlled trials, lavender was superior to placebo in two hundred and twenty-one patients suffering from anxiety disorder. In addition, lavender improved associated symptoms such as restlessness, disturbed sleep, and somatic complaints, and had a beneficial influence on general well-being and quality of life.[88]

In another study comparing lavender to lorazepam in adults suffering from generalized anxiety disorder, lavender effectively ameliorated symptoms compared to 0.5mg/ daily of lorazepam. The use of aromas to modulate affect and mood is an ancient and well described practice. The olfactory impact of lavender on cognitive performance and mood was assessed in one hundred and forty-four healthy volunteers. A positive significant effect was found for lavender compared to controls for degree of contentedness, indicating that lavender is capable of elevating mood, or at least maintaining good mood, during the completion of challenging tests performed under laboratory conditions.[89]

Olfactory receptors are specialized chemical detectors that work like a lock-and-key system. When an agonist molecule comes along that fits the receptor's lock, the cells signaling machinery are engaged and switched on. When we realize how uniquely and intricately we are equipped to respond to smell, taste, and flavor sensations, the extent of OR distribution and the magnitude of their critical functions make perfect sense.

Olfactory receptors are only so named because that is where they were first discovered. It is perhaps more useful to view them in their likely evolutionary context as the original intermediary for interaction with our environment. They are a link, a direct connection, to our forebears and ancestors. When it comes to how we are wired and how our entire body operates, the nose knows and as we sniff is how we goes.

Despite the fact that odorant receptors are the largest subset of the family of G protein-coupled receptors found on the surface of cells, the precise role and function of the majority of ORs remains unknown. But we can certainly observe their macroscopic effects. Infants identify their mothers by sense of smell. Cheap perfume has authored many a tragedy. Pheromones can influence reproductive physiology and mating patterns. And smell, along with taste and flavor, is the most important determinant of food preference.[90] Food and sex are thus linked everywhere throughout the human body and the human experience.

Smell, taste, and flavor are integrative, flexible, and plastic, constantly molded and reshaped by new experience. Our intention and behavior are likewise shaped in concert. This implies that we are dealing with a fundamental problem in attempting to always relate genes to systems behavior: a given set of genes may not map directly onto a given behavior. In this respect, the mystery being addressed here is a caution for the new era of "systems biology" and against any belief that behavior can be related directly to genomes, proteomes, or any other type of "-ome." We are reminded instead that the functional ecology of the body is dependent on many factors.[91]

Sex is more than procreation. Food is more than nutrition. As humans, we are blessed with a consciousness that seeks to expand upward and outward into the universe. At the same time, we are hitched to a mortality driven by primal directives and unconscious underpinnings. We are...complicated.

Which returns us to the romantic dinner. The romantic dinner is still one of the most recommended forms of therapy for couples in counseling. The food-centric courtship ritual is a staple from the animal kingdom to our modern society. Some of the latest research demonstrates that that "eating may prime or sensitize young women to rewards beyond food."[92] In simpler terms, science has shown that the way to a woman's heart is through her stomach.

Gents, if you're looking for an insurance policy, make sure there's room for dessert. In related research from Purdue University, tasting something sweet made female study participants more interested in a potential partner. Sweet foods increase levels of dopamine, which according to the researchers is the gasoline for that amorous spark to ignite into "passionate love."[93, 94]

This combination of scrumptious victuals, pleasing music, proper ambience, and pleasant company is a formula for a successful food experience, good memories, and positive emotion. This, as the science has shown and Anthony Bourdain aptly observed, lends itself naturally to good sex. These all are atavistic motivators lodged deeply within our primitive brains.

Food and sex are inextricably linked as experiences we can all relate to, and often strive for. They so often keep company because they both are experiences that when we have that rare occurrence to engage them consummately and unfettered, we find that ultimately we cannot intellectualize them. They invariably reach beyond our conscious, cognitive brain and grab us by the basest, most primal parts. Food and sex become richest when we experience the gamut of possibilities—when we see, touch, taste, smell, hear—and perhaps most importantly, when it engages our higher self. It is then, put quite simply, that food, like sex, is an experience best shared.

HUNGER GAMES

No disease that can be treated by diet should
be treated with any other means.
—Maimonides

SAD But True: The Legacy of
The Standard American Diet

In order to maintain both our appetites and our health, we must have a diet that sustains both body and soul; nutritious and delicious must coexist and prosper together. A suboptimal diet is the leading risk factor for death and disability in the United States and worldwide.[95, 96] Such consumptive patterns that are seen in the modern Western diet are strongly associated with the development of many chronic illnesses. These disabilities and diseases are estimated to cause more than 17.3 trillion dollars of cumulative economic loss between 2011 and 2030 from healthcare expenditures, reduced productivity, and lost capital across the globe.[97] It is not just about individual titillation and toning; diet is a global concern of pandemic proportions.

Generally speaking, the working definition of a diet is that collection of consumptive patterns that represent the overall combination of foods habitually consumed, for good or ill. A healthful diet is one in which the combination of those food choices works together to produce synergistic health effects.[98] Evidence-informed beneficial diet patterns share several key characteristics. These include less processed and refined foods, as well as those with less added sugars.[99]

However, in constructing ways to assess and measure, advise and guide, as of late most of our mainstream modern resources for dietary advice have been at worst untruthful and focused on profit not performance, and have been at best rather simply less than unhelpful. What modern nutritional science has demonstrated are the limitations of drawing conclusions about health effects of any food product based on theories about its nutrient contents.[100]

Nutrition and policy science have advanced rapidly over the hundred plus years since the discovery of the first vitamins such as thiamine or vitamin B_1 around the year 1912. The term vitamin was originally *vitamine*, which was a shortened version of vital amine. All these life-giving compounds were believed to be based on the chemical amine moiety. Polish scientist Doctor Kazimierz Funk entered this term into the lexicon while describing the role of vitamin B_1 in the disease process known as beriberi Vitamin A was discovered about the same time.

Doctor Funk, along with English biochemist Sir Frederick Gowland Hopkins, formulated the vitamin hypothesis of deficiency disease. This theorem states that it is a lack of vitamins that cause disease.[101] While the deficiency theory of illness was helpful in the early days of nutritional exploration, continued adherence to this outdated approach has been a ball and chain holding back modern progress. It has often caused more confusion than cure.

Indeed, the first Recommended Dietary Allowances (RDAs) originated in 1941 by order of President Franklin Roosevelt. At that time, he convened the National Nutrition Conference on Defense *not* because there was a concern for the health of the US citizen, but to ensure there was a reasonable population of soldiers fit to fight the war. The goal of the conference was to identify ways to minimize nutrient deficiency diseases.[102, 103]

Dietary guidelines at this time were predicated on a historically successful approach. In 1747, Scottish naval surgeon James Lindin observed that citrus foods prevented scurvy. Limes were added to the diet of sailors in the British Royal Navy, which is how the British came to be known as "limeys." This method of attempting to isolate singular nutritional deficiency as the cause of specific disease states initially met with widespread success. Diseases like beriberi, kwashiorkor, pellagra, rickets, and many others were successfully identified and treated. Such a reductionist approach originating in the early twentieth century, however, still pervades our twenty-first century inquiry.

Since the onset of the Industrial Revolution, and particularly following World War II, the rapid modernization of agriculture, food processing, food formulations, and food pathways have relegated nutrient deficiencies to a much rarer occurrence in the United States and other Western nations. In place of diseases of deficiency, we have created a growing epidemic of chronic pathology. We traded acute, single nutrient deficiency diseases for the chronic disabilities and diseases of the modern Western diet. The problem in the United States and other Western nations is not that we do not get enough to eat, it is *what* and *how* we eat.

Continued blind adherence to such historical precedent has resulted in horribly oversimplified and inaccurate inferences on how diet influences such complex chronic afflictions that currently plague us: cardiovascular disease (CVD), diabetes mellitus, and obesity to name a few. Scientists and policy makers intuitively followed earlier methods that had been so successful in reducing deficiencies: identify the relevant nutrient, establish its target intake, and translate this to recommendations. Continued adherence to such a constricted approach contributed to some of the greatest nutritional misadventures of the last half-century; *e.g.*, saturated fat and cholesterol from the diet was the cause of CVD, and total fat was the cause of obesity.[104]

Therefore, when considering the many and varied diets both contemporary and historical that are available for evaluation, it is of paramount importance to examine the full diversity of diet-related risk pathways. It is not enough to simply measure blood lipids or check a body mass index (BMI). BMI is a measure that rather arbitrarily and inaccurately declares individual fitness or failure. The focus must be on foods and overall diet patterns, rather than single isolated nutrients. It is critical to recognize "the complex influences of different foods on long-term weight regulation, rather than simply counting calories, and characterizing and implementing evidence based strategies, including policy approaches, for lifestyle change."[105]

Firstly, it is now evident that dietary habits influence a plethora of diverse cardiometabolic risk factors, including but not limited to obesity, low-density lipoprotein (LDL) cholesterol, blood pressure (BP), glucose-insulin homeostasis, lipoprotein concentrations and function, oxidative stress, inflammation, endothelial health, hepatic function, adipocyte metabolism, cardiac function, metabolic expenditure, pathways of weight regulation, visceral adiposity, and the gut microbiome. Yet a predominant focus, reflected in the latest recommendations from the American College of Cardiology and the American Heart Association, continues to concentrate on dietary fat and blood cholesterol,[106] despite clear evidence to the contrary.[107, 108, 109, 110, 111] Their preoccupation with irrelevant measures like total calories and BMI ignores the gamut of impact that diet exerts across multiple pathways.

Another facet of investigation involves the importance of specific foods and overall diet patterns. So often modern investigation continues to focus on single isolated *nutrients*, as opposed to foods, in the context of cardiometabolic risk, often at the expense of the larger picture and common sense.[112] Repeatedly focusing on isolated nutrients leads to paradoxical dietary choices and unhelpful industry formulations.

A look at the mega-market grocery shelves stocked full of low-fat, fat-free, cholesterol free, gluten-free, low calorie, zero calorie, artificially flavored, artificially preserved, pre-prepared, and ready to serve microwavable offerings hint at the many monstrous offshoots that we have generated for the sake of convenience and profit. Such an army of deception congregates under the banner of "healthy choice."

For example, the US National School Lunch Programs in 2012 banned whole milk, but allowed sugar-sweetened chocolate skim milk.[113] This untested intervention in thirty-one million American children was based on hypothesized effects of total calories, total fat, and saturated fat in milk rather than empirical evidence on the health effects of whole versus skim milk. Results that when analyzed objectively show no untoward effect on health from whole milk.

Longitudinal studies suggest no harm from the consumption of whole-fat milk with respect to obesity, diabetes mellitus, or cardiovascular disease in adults.[114, 115, 116, 117, 118,] [119] Many additional studies suggest that dairy fat may actually have potential benefits for the prevention and treatment of diabetes mellitus. A simpler, authentically whole food-based approach better facilitates public guidance, minimizes opportunities for gimmickry and misdirection, and serves to limit industry manipulation.[120] (See appendix B1)

Specifically, poor diet quality is a driver of excess diet quantity. Furthermore, independently of energy balance, diet *quality* influences metabolic risk and propensity toward abdominal adiposity.[121] Mechanisms appear to include *calorie-independent* effects of different types of foods on satiety, glucose-insulin responses,[122] liver fat synthesis,[123] adipocyte function,[124] visceral adiposity, brain craving and reward,[125] and even metabolic expenditure.[126] In simple terms, it is not how much you eat or its caloric content; it's the *quality* of the food that matters. (See appendix B2)

Abdominal adiposity or "belly fat" which produces the largest metabolic harms, has increased to a greater extent than overall weight in many nations—yet another reason why BMI is misleading. Growing evidence suggests that energy imbalance is a consequence of multiple complex, upstream effects, in particular, poor diet *quality*. One again, what you eat is more important than how much. (See appendix B3)

While a simpler approach to dietary recommendations is most certainly warranted, it is an overly simplistic approach to understanding the problems of the paunch that has led us astray for decades. It is important to acknowledge our transformation from Mr. Rogers to Mr. Creosote; from sneakers and sweaters to churly and gluttonous obesity. It is not just Creosote's physicality that is so off-putting; his attitude is condescending and dismissive. In this setting, it is likewise imperative to also acknowledge the cultural and societal perspectives that shape our actions. It is a prevailing "thin is healthy" perception that drives our collective vulnerability to short-term solutions, fads, and gimmicks.[127]

It is fascinating to note that the significant rise in obesity and abdominal adiposity was only observed approximately thirty to forty years ago.[128] If we extrapolate backward using the current average annual weight gain of approximately one pound per year,[129] we add another twenty to thirty years to the calculation. We then arrive back where it all began, at the point of origin of our weighty increase. This of course places us in the post-World War II era, which is the point in time where many of the predominant characteristics of our modern Western diet first surfaced.

Current and accruing evidence suggest that the prevailing energy-imbalance concept of obesity is oversimplified.[130] The science of obesity is moving away from crude ideas of energy balance, willpower, and calories toward the more applicable elucidation of effects of foods and diet patterns on the complex physiological determinants of long-term weight regulation.

It is self-evident that total calories matter in the *short term*. The Robinson Crusoe regimen will shed pounds off anyone. It is why virtually anybody can initially lose weight on nearly any type of diet—and explains why so many fad diets seem to work at first. In the short term, the best predictor of success is adherence to one's chosen diet. Although short-term weight loss can be achieved by any type of calorie-reduced diet, the key point here is the *short-term* designation. Over 90 percent of these diets are complete and utter failures within five years of their inception.[131]

A meta-analysis of over eighty weight loss programs found weight loss of 5–9 percent after six months, yet half the weight was regained after four years.[132] Over one in four Americans report overeating or eating unhealthy foods to manage stress.[133] Animal, epidemiological, and mechanistic studies have linked stress to dysregulated eating, weight gain, impaired glucose metabolism, abdominal adiposity, and lipid abnormalities.[134, 135, 136] Individuals eat mindlessly in response to external cues and the rewarding value of food, overriding homeostatic hunger and satiety signals, all of which can be exacerbated by stress.[137, 138]

Dietary regimens which add stress and psychological strain to our already vulnerable systems do not stimulate long term success. By increasing the variables that drive us to such anguish, we simply set ourselves up for failure. We initiate a circle of negative feedback that only augments our suffering. The pursuit of a healthy life, a life-long endeavor, should bring us pleasure not pain.

The Buddha may well have observed our modern desire for the artificial endpoints of a "thin is healthy" outlook as a prime example of the Second Noble Truth; the cause of our suffering is the desire to have and control things.[139] He would no doubt applaud a pursuit grounded in The Middle Way. True scientific pursuit is such a path, a way of thinking or perception "placed between full adherence to a school and generic deprecation of ideas."[140] Music is composed of sound waves, vibrations, harmonics, arrangements, music theory, and a host of other technical components, but in the end what matters is the *music*. The Food Shaman correspondingly recognizes that with the food we consume, what is ultimately of consequence is the *experience*.

Over the long term, counting calories is neither biologically nor behaviorally relevant. Food is relevant. For long-term weight maintenance and for cardiometabolic health independent of adiposity, healthful food based patterns are most relevant.[141] Particularly, what is germane is the *quality* and types of foods consumed. This is what influences the diverse biological pathways related to weight homeostasis; satiety, hunger, brain reward, glucose-insulin responses, hepatic de novo lipogenesis, adipocyte function, metabolic expenditure, and the gut microbiome. (See appendix B4)

The simple take away is that in terms of healthful effect, including weight management, a calorie is not a calorie is not a calorie.[142] Not all calories are equal with respect to long-term adiposity. Certain foods impair pathways of weight homeostasis, others have relatively neutral effects, and yet others promote the integrity of weight regulation. Dietary influences are complex, including individual, sociocultural, community, agricultural, industry, governmental, and global contributors.[143]

Although scientific investigation of macro and micronutrients remains essential to elucidate biological mechanisms, the complex matrix of foods, gut microbiome interaction, food processing, and food preparation strongly modifies the final health effects.[144, 145, 146, 147] Critically, current investigation in nutrition science demonstrates that nutrient focused metrics are inadequate to explain most effects of diet on chronic diseases.

Instead, cardiometabolic diseases are largely influenced not by single nutrients like saturated fat or cholesterol, but by specific foods and overall diet patterns.[148, 149] That is why in 2015 the dietary guidelines advisory committee emphasized food-based, healthful diet patterns as a primary recommendation to address obesity and concluded that "low-fat diets have no effect on CVD and [we must] emphasize the importance of healthful, food-based diet patterns."[150] A cardioprotective diet pattern must be characterized by the healthful foods that are included, not simply specific items to be avoided.[151] (See appendix B5)

Is There a "Best" Diet?

Which brings us to the simple, but fundamental question: is there truly a *best* diet?

Like most subjective questions, it eventually comes down to individual preference. What do we actually mean by "best"?

For the adventurous foodie, professional chef, or those seeking a romantic night out on the town, the answer to that question may revolve completely around individual taste and preference. For the professional or competitive athlete, the answer may have to do specifically with the nutritional components, irrespective of tasteful considerations. For those with specific health conditions, it may have to do with the known health associations or implications of certain consumptive patterns. For the susceptible, it may focus on the avoidance of allergenic or offending specific or classes of comestibles. For yet others, there may be moral, ethical, or religious considerations that define that answer.

Despite the weight of these individual deliberations, currently across all forms of media and information distribution we are bombarded daily regarding the unbelievable effects of the latest superfood or miracle diet. And unbelievable is the key descriptor; the majority of such claims are unsubstantiated and baseless. Additionally, many of these products and programs are designed to facilitate weight loss which, as previously discussed, may function in the short term, but provide no direction for a long-term, sustainable, and sensible lifelong approach to food.

To answer the question of what is the "best" diet for us, we must first define the parameters by which we shall judge the contenders. A workable designation for this is a tripartite characterization:

- A collection of food and drink that gives us pleasure through consumption because it looks, smells, and tastes delicious. It makes life enjoyable and satisfies our soul.
- It should provide our bodies with the essential nutrients and minerals to maintain life. It sustains our bodies.
- It shouldn't kill us.

Given this definition, is there a "best" diet?

Can delicious and nutritious co-exist on the same plate? Is the relationship between delicious and nutritious akin to the never-ending battle between *tastes great* and *less filling*? Is this Holy Grail of Foodie-dom a reality, or simply a modern myth? If a "best" diet does exist, can we find it?

All of which is to say is that even if such a diet exists and we find it, should we even care?

Why *not* eat like a rock star, or at least a gourmand?

This brings us to an even more fundamental truism. Many people still try to apply the Rationale of Vices to the diet-health relationship as they cruise down the river de-Nile. It goes something along the lines of: "I've got to die of something. If I'm going to die anyway, why not maximize my pleasure in the present and if it means I live a year or two less so be it, but I've enjoyed myself?"

The problem with this excuse is that such a justification is based upon a faulty premise. Our mortal life, which defines our humanity, is framed by our birth and our death. We all will die. That is true and inarguable, and a key concept of acceptance for the authentic shaman.

The shamanic dietetic corollary is that a healthy diet is not an ambrosia or an elixir of immortality. Death is a threshold we will all eventually cross. However, the proper foundation upon which to ground our question is more along the lines of how do you want to traverse that finish line? Stride across under your own power and on your own terms or be pulled across like three-day old roadkill?

Making the logical and rational choice that we direct the manner of our crossing into Heaven's Gate, it follows that we next ask if such a diet needs be punitive in nature. What is the price of purchase, if there is one? What is the price of neglect?

In essence, what are the consequences of both adherence and inconsistency to such a regime?

What is at stake with such a decision is no less than our individual health, wellness, and happiness. The repercussions of our dietary choices that result within the physical realm lead us unto either health and wellness or disability and disease. For simplicity of discussion, the working definition of health is defined as the absence of disability and disease.

The development of any pathological state or disease can be reduced to an equation that depends upon two variables. These two variables are the genetics that we are born with and our interaction with our surrounding environment. Disease or wellness is the result of the interplay between these two forces.

While currently there is considerable limitation in addressing the genetic variable in the role of disease development, the environmental variable is highly mutable.

However, among the various contributors, there is no more powerful environmental influence than the cumulative effect of what we choose to consume each day.

While we think that we consciously control every aspect of our selections for sustenance; that is an illusion. To a degree, we are obviously knowingly involved in choosing what we wish to consume at the moment. However, these choices are guided by myriad unconscious influences. Such influences originate from within our survival instinct, our pleasure and reward center, our emotional state, and previous experience and memory. These in turn are impacted by cultural and societal forces. The result is a singular mindset.

These unique and personally deep-rooted interconnections are the reason why so many "one-size-fits-all" approaches are doomed to failure. It is why so many weight loss regimens are unsuccessful over the long term. While food may be examined and confined to a sterile laboratory and dissected into its component bits of protein, fat, and carbohydrate, and further reduced into percentage RDAs, vitamins, minerals, and other nutrients, a meal, and hence a diet, cannot be so dismembered. Much like us, our food experience is significantly greater than the sum of the individual parts.

Unlike most of the animal kingdom, people do not and have not for a long time eaten only for nutritional sustenance. We seek flavor and taste; we live for the *experience*. That is what food has become: an eating experience.

As an experience, it can only occur in the first person. The food experience parallels the shamanic approach in this regard. Our relationship with food is like that of the early explorers. The captain of a tall ship charting and exploring an undiscovered country lives an adventure that cannot be duplicated. The mapmaker in the corner of a dusty library may read the accounts and construct the atlas from the logs with great precision and accuracy, but he or she has never lived the event. Likewise, you cannot remove the diner from dinner. Simply reading a review will never fill your belly and lighten your heart.

In loop quantum gravity theory, it is understood that there is no isolationism. Quantum mechanics describes the reality of what things *are*, because nothing exists in and unto itself. Quantum mechanics describes reality because it describes how things occur and how they interact *with each other*.

Ours is not a universe of objects, but a universe of events. As physicist Carlo Rovelli explains, "It is only in interactions that nature draws the world. There is no reality except in the relations between physical systems. It is not things that enter into relations, but rather relations that ground to the notion of a thing."[152] It is both the diner and the dinner that define the food experience. The meaning is in the encounter, the life in the interaction. Which, as Nelson Goodman noticed, is a fortuitous occurrence, for just to exist as "a thing is a monotonous event."[153]

Which returns us to our initial query, but from a different perspective. If the best diet is subject to wide individual variation, is there a *worst* diet we all must avoid?

Cardiovascular disease remains the number one killer in the United States, birthplace of the standard American diet (SAD) or modern Western diet (MWD). One in three people in the United States will die of cardiovascular disease. However, research has suggested that a significant number of these heart attacks may be preventable.[154] In fact, a majority of the seven cardiovascular health metrics are those that are significantly impacted by our dietary choices. These include blood pressure, physical activity, healthy diet, body weight, and blood glucose (blood sugar) levels. If there is a strong association between SAD dietary practice and illness, what should we avoid?

All of which raises an even more fundamental question: What exactly is this thing we call the MWD?

To determine what it is about the modern Western diet that leaves us so vulnerable to the development of disability and disease, we must first determine the constituents of said diet. On the surface that would seem an easy affair, by simply asking people what they eat. Indeed, many of the current research studies that have been published rely on such dietary questionnaires. However, there is a caveat in that method of acquiring data. That other great observer of the human condition, and the human, Doctor Gregory House, correctly concluded that, "When you want to know the truth about someone, that someone is probably the last person you should ask."[155]

In a study that would not pass the test of political correctness today, one that was done over forty years ago, the results are still applicable. The researchers asked people to report in a dietary questionnaire format the foods they consumed. Unbeknownst to the subjects, the investigators sifted through their garbage to determine what they actually ate. The conclusion they reached is as relevant now as it was then; most people say they eat healthier than they actually do.[156]

Other studies which have examined the components of the average American diet have reached similar abysmal conclusions. There are several different methods that are used to assess what people eat and assign it a relative value. For example, the healthy eating index (HEI) scores ten equally weighted dietary components. There is a maximum score of one hundred and the higher the score the more ideal the consumptive pattern. Currently, less than one percent of US adults have an ideal diet score. The average score for US adults in 2010 was approximately fifty-one out of a possible one hundred. Even more frightening, essentially 0 percent of children currently have an ideal diet score.

This problem affects not just those involved in nutrition and health care. Over fifty cents of each food dollar in the United States is spent dining out. For the first time in history, chefs and restaurant owners are implicated in the disability and disease derived from the modern Western diet. Section 4205 as passed under the Affordable Care Act (ACA) defines regulations and responsibilities for certain restaurant owners and other establishments that are under the aegis of the community prevention of chronic disease portion of the ACA.

Interestingly, although it is often widely written and spoken about, there remains no standard definition of the modern Western diet. How do we avoid that which we cannot define or identify? It becomes a bit of a sticky wicket whose solution ends up looking a lot like what Justice Potter Stewart had to say about pornography: "I may not be able to define it, but I know it when I see it." Or in this case, when we taste it.

There are common threads found in all references of the MWD. These include a preponderance of foods that are highly processed, preserved, pre-prepared, and pre-packaged. These four "Ps" are the Four Horsemen of the Dietary Apocalypse. These foods are excessively high in added sugars and often rich in refined grains, carbohydrates, and oils.

Because such a diet contains a disproportionately high amount of carbohydrates and oils, other essential elements are often displaced. In the standard American diet, such a phenomenon results in a dearth of fresh fruits and vegetables. This lack of balance results in some of the defining characteristics of the modern Western diet. It is energy dense but nutrient poor.

The embrace of a convenience based utilization of foodstuffs in the post-World War II era has been associated with an increased incidence and prevalence of what have become to be known as the diseases of modern civilization. These include but are not limited to cardiovascular disease, obesity, diabetes, cancers (particularly cancers of the gastrointestinal tract), inflammatory bowel diseases, neurodegenerative diseases, and autoimmune diseases. Increasingly, science is demonstrating that these apparently unrelated conditions are bound together as differing manifestations that spring from the root cause of inflammation. Specifically, the inflammation tends to be of a subacute, chronic, and continuous nature. Tellingly, the point of origin seems to be the gut.

In countries and cultures that do not routinely consume a standard American diet, such a prevalence and incidence of those disabilities and diseases is not present. The Tsimane, an indigenous hunter-gatherer tribe from the Amazon in Bolivia, have the lowest reported levels of coronary artery disease of any population recorded to date.[157] Over the course of human civilization, and particularly the last several centuries, we have witnessed great societal and technological advancements. Despite our accomplishments, we have burdened ourselves with elder years of chronic disability and disease; and yet we have not increased the absolute potential for human longevity. This begins the tale of the current state and impact of the modern Western diet. This diet defines the predominant current approach to food in the United States and many industrialized Western countries.

A Tale of ALE

The health of the population can be determined by several metrics. One of most commonly utilized is the Average Life Expectancy, or ALE. The hypothesis is that the healthier a population is, the longer it lives. Therefore, the higher the ALE, the reasoning goes, the healthier the group.

Currently within the United States, the average life expectancy is 78.2 years. This is among the highest ALE ever recorded in this country. Hence, based on the aforementioned hypothesis, the current US population should be among the healthiest group of Americans ever.

Are we?

That depends on definition. If we look at a measurement known as the Healthy Average Life Expectancy (HALE), that value is only 68.1 years. The healthy average life expectancy represents the portion of your life that is free from suffering from a *major* complication of disability or disease such as a heart attack, stroke, cancer, or the like.

If we look at the average ALE of what we might term more "primitive" cultures, which in truth may be more accurately described as simply technologically bereft, we find a similar value. These numbers are particularly comparable when trauma, infectious disease, childbirth, and childhood illness, so effectively addressed within mainstream Western medicine, are accounted for.

In a non-invasive assessment of the prevalence of coronary artery disease (CAD), only 3 percent of Tsimane adults over forty had evidence of CAD.[158] In comparison, studies of similar groups in the industrialized West suggest a prevalence of greater than 50 percent.[159] With respect to elder years, the significant difference is that those "primitive" people tend not to spend the last decade of their life suffering from the major disabilities and diseases that we find so commonplace in our modern society.

If we drill down further to examine life expectancy without *significant* disease in our society, we find this value is only 42.7 years. This number represents the average number of years someone living in the United States is free from any significant disease or disability including things like arthritis, diabetes, hypertension, and other such maladies.

Currently in the United States, on average, one can expect that by age forty-three, they will be suffering from some significant disability or disease. The last three decades of their lives will be spent dealing with the complications and sequelae of such pathological conditions. In addition, the last decade of their lives will be spent battling a major complication like stroke, heart attack, or cancer until they finally die.

The results of these chronic disabilities and diseases of modern civilization have a great impact that extends beyond the personal level. These disabilities and diseases currently account for over half the healthcare burden in the United States. Such costs are estimated at over thirty-three billion dollars annually in direct medical costs. There's estimated to be over another nine billion dollars annually in lost productivity related to these conditions. Such figures derive from a direct dietary causality that leads to increased rates of disability and disease. All the while, none of our technology has improved our absolute maximum lifespan.

Absolute human longevity refers to the maximum amount of time a human being may exist. It is the human expiration date. While the Average Life Expectancy (ALE) reflects the average time we spend on the shelf before the Grim Reaper places us in his casket basket, the human Absolute Maximum

Lifespan (AML) reflects your ultimate shelf life. The AML is estimated at approximately 120 years due to a number of factors we are only beginning to understand. This is not far removed from the ancient Egyptian observation of approximately one hundred and ten years. Herodotus recounts reports from over two thousand and five hundred years ago of Ethiopians, subsisting on meat and milk, living to be around one hundred and twenty years old.[160] Such commentary suggests that the populations were able to observe enough people reaching this age, but no further, to draw a conclusion as to the limits. In a remarkably prescient quote, Genesis tells us that the time given our flesh on Earth "shall be one hundred and twenty years."[161]

So, while we may be spending more time on the shelf, we are also mouldering. Currently in the United States, just under half of our lifetime is spent dealing with complications and conditions that are a result of the disabilities and diseases of modern civilization.[162] These are disabilities and diseases that can be profoundly impacted by our dietary choices.

History, Tradition, and Science

Within the history of humankind there have been several seminal points which have profoundly affected the direction of civilization. Two of those in particular involve fundamental food transformations. The first of these was the agricultural revolution. This forever altered the human experience. Unlike any other animal species before or since, human beings took control of their own food sources. We moved from troops of hunter-gatherers dependent upon what we could find to producers in charge of our own sustenance. Some of the mechanisms and survival instincts which enhanced our survival as hunter-gatherers became superfluous.

The second great turning point was the Industrial Revolution, which set the stage for a number of the incredible technological and societal advances we've experienced over the last several centuries, in particular over the last fifty to seventy-five years. The Industrial Revolution has fundamentally transformed not only our food itself, but our food pathways.

With the onset of the Industrial Revolution for the first time ever it was possible, for example, for producers of grain to ship their product to a place like Chicago, and ranchers could do the same with their cattle. Such a singularity was previously an impossibility. The changes brought about by the Industrial Revolution gave birth to such modernizations as the industrial meat industry. It was the harbinger to our modern mega-food industry and agribusiness.

Yet during this time of tremendous technological and societal change that continues and accelerates into the modern era, our basic biology and physiology remains as it was hundreds of thousands, if not millions, of years ago. Those patterns of behavior that allowed us to survive as individuals and as a species and have become subsequently hardwired within us remain unchanged. Having become superfluous with the onset of the agricultural revolution, with the onset of the Industrial Revolution they became our liability, leaving us vulnerable to the modern food industry and agribusiness. Over the last fifty to seventy-five years they've became an exploitable weakness.

But as The Bard so adroitly observed, the hungers of humankind can lead to exploitation by more than mere physicality and physiology:

And my more-having would be as a sauce
To make me hunger more;
that I should forge
Quarrels unjust against the good and loyal,
Destroying them for wealth
(Macbeth 4.3.96-99).[163]

Profit and politics color the history of health and food throughout our society and across cultures. The history of food is truly the history of humankind. This is true even though we might wish it were not so. Ask most any cardiologist about saturated fat, cholesterol, and heart disease and they will tell you it is *science*, not tradition, which drives their decision making. But influences—political, financial, and even egotistical—can subtly bend the will and direction of the purest intellectual pursuit.

As irrefutable data accumulates and brings to light past transgressions and errors, we strive to appropriately adjust our course. However, we can only reach our destination by knowing where we are. And we can only know where we are by seeing where we have been. Our knowledge, like everything else in the here and now, must be held in a relational schema. A brief synopsis of the story involving fat, saturated fat, animal fat, polyunsaturated fat, vegetable oils, cholesterol, and cardiovascular disease over the last century is both intriguing and illuminating, if not a little disturbing in the telling.

The figure below gives a brief timeline of some of the major events and highlights that accompany this topic over the last century. A more detailed description provides a deeper understanding of why we flounder in our current dietary doldrums.

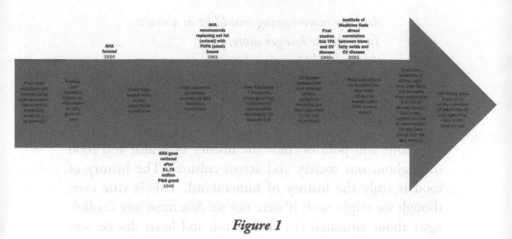

Figure 1

In the early 1900s, a German chemist by the name of Wilhelm Normann developed an inexpensive way to turn normally liquid vegetable oils into semi-solid and solid products through the addition of hydrogen, a process known as hydrogenation. Enterprising businessmen William Procter and James Gamble watched the lightbulb illuminate—literally. The soap and candle making duo realized that the invention of the lightbulb was going to seriously impact their bougie business, so they looked to alternatives.

Because the meat-packing industry in Cincinnati, Ohio (then known as Porkopolis) controlled the lard and tallow needed for candles and soap, P&G had secured their own supply of raw materials, and by 1905 owned eight cottonseed mills in Mississippi. With the help of another German chemist, E. C. Kayser, P&G was able to transform the liquid cottonseed oil into a solid that resembled lard.

Since hydrogenated cottonseed oil resembled lard, why not sell it as a food? Always a great scientific rationale for introducing new foodstuffs into the diet. We should all pause here and breathe a collective sigh that P&G was never in the roto-rooter/candy business. Thus it was that Crisco (CRYStalized Cottonseed Oil), was introduced to the American consumer in 1911. In 1924, The American Heart Association was formed. In 1948, thanks to the being the beneficiary of the P&G sponsored "Walking Man" radio contest, the AHA went national with a 1.75 million dollar windfall. A national fundraising campaign in 1949 netted another 2.7 million and the AHA never looked back.

Following World War II, Ancel Keys, who held PhDs in both biology and physiology, became interested in the rise of heart disease in the United States and the lack of a similar phenomenon in post-war Europe. He proposed the cholesterol hypothesis as the cause. This was the idea that saturated fat in the diet, mostly from animal sources, caused an increase in blood cholesterol levels. The increased cholesterol in the blood resulted in atherosclerosis. This was the suggested origin of cardiovascular disease (CVD) morbidity and mortality.

The die was cast and the Rubicon crossed. Keys vaulted to national and international acclaim. In 1961, he was on the cover of *Time Magazine* and appointed to the prestigious and influential AHA nutrition committee. Later that same year the AHA issued the first ever dietary recommendation to replace animal fats in the diet with plant based alternatives. The proposition was solidified when Keys published his Seven Countries Study in 1970, purportedly demonstrating beyond question the causal effect between animal (saturated) fat consumption, cholesterol, and heart disease.

Such was the confidence in this conventional wisdom that the US Senate adopted the low fat (30 percent of total dietary energy) and low saturated fat (less than 10 percent of total dietary energy) proposal. These were published in the United States Senate Select Committee on Nutrition and

Human Needs dietary guidelines and accepted as gospel by many. Even to this day it continues to be held sacrosanct by many healthcare practitioners and researchers. In truth, many experts at the time pleaded for more time and more research; their motion was denied. Unfortunately, much of the data and conclusions were taken at face value, because as Senator McGovern remarked at the time: "Senators don't have the luxury the research scientist does of waiting until every last shred of evidence is in."[164, 165]

The process of hydrogenation which transformed the liquid plant oils into solids and semi-solids created what are known as trans-fatty acids (TFAs). While TFAs occur naturally in miniscule amounts, mostly in the digestive system of ruminants, they do not normally comprise a significant portion of the diet. However, with the push over the last half century to move away from animal fats and toward fats constructed from plant based alternatives, the US diet contained increasingly more TFAs as a result of hydrogenated and partially hydrogenated vegetable oils.

They contained more liquid vegetable and seed oils as the push for polyunsaturated fats (PUFAs) derived from vegetable sources to replace saturated animal fats continued to mount. Many of these oils were derived from sources such as corn, safflower, sunflower, and so on, which are predominately omega-6 rich. Omega-6 PUFAs tend to feed the inflammatory pathway while the omega-3 PUFAs tend to counterbalance those effects via the body's anti-inflammatory pathway. These omega-6 rich oils remain a staple in the production of processed and fried foods.

Studies from as early as the 1970s suggested potential detrimental health effects from the consumption of TFAs. However, it was not until the 1990s that these studies began to yield evidence that could neither be ignored nor dismissed. In 2002, the Institute of Medicine (IOM) published an analysis irrevocably linking TFA consumption and CVD. That same year P&G divested of the Crisco brand. At the time, Crisco commanded 24 percent of an annual three-hundred-sixty-million-dollar market. It took the federal government almost a decade and a half to follow up on the IOM report and ban TFAs, although there are still substantial loopholes.

A recent analysis of a study performed in the late 1960s and early 1970s, the Sydney Diet Heart Study, evaluated the effectiveness of replacing dietary saturated fat with omega-6 rich safflower oil. This inquiry found that the vegetable oil group had statistically significant higher rates of heart attack and death than those eating animal fats.[166]

These are not isolated findings, either. Another study which was not published at the time, the Minnesota Coronary Experiment performed from 1968 to 1973, recently underwent a contemporary testing. The goal of this study was to determine whether replacing saturated fat with vegetable oil rich in omega-6 PUFAs reduced coronary heart disease and death by lowering serum cholesterol.

The vegetable oil group did achieve a significant reduction in their serum cholesterol. In other words, replacing the saturated animal fat with polyunsaturated vegetable oil alternatives *did* lower the blood cholesterol levels. However, there was no survival advantage for those who dropped their cholesterol level through this dietary maneuver. In fact, those who consumed the omega-6 rich vegetable oil and lowered their cholesterol had a *22 percent higher* risk of death for each 30 mg/dL (0.78 mmol/L) reduction in serum cholesterol. In other words, the more their cholesterol dropped, the *higher* their risk of death.

A further review of almost eleven thousand patients revealed that lowering cholesterol by replacing saturated animal fat with PUFAs rich in omega-6 fatty acids like linoleic acid yielded no benefit in reducing risk of death from CVD or any cause. The authors conclude that:

> *Available evidence from randomized controlled trials shows that replacement of saturated fat in the diet with linoleic acid effectively lowers serum cholesterol but does not support the hypothesis that this translates to a lower risk of death from coronary heart disease or all causes. Findings from the Minnesota Coronary Experiment add to growing evidence that incomplete publication has contributed to overestimation of the benefits of replacing saturated fat with vegetable oils rich in linoleic acid.*[167]

A contemporary of Keys, Professor John Yudkin, who served as Chair of Physiology at Queen Elizabeth College in London and later as a Chair in Nutrition, had argued that refined carbohydrates like sucrose were the primary cause of such modern maladies as obesity, diabetes, cardiovascular disease, and the like. Keys responded that:

> *It is clear that Yudkin has no theoretical basis or experimental evidence to support his claim for a major influence of dietary sucrose in the etiology of CHD [coronary heart disease]; his claim that men who have CHD are excessive sugar eaters is nowhere confirmed but is disproved by many studies superior in methodology and/or magnitude*

> *to his own; and his "evidence" from pop-*
> *ulation statistics and time trends will not*
> *bear up under the most elementary criti-*
> *cal examination....Unfortunately, Yudkin's*
> *views appeal to some commercial interests*
> *with the result that this discredited propa-*
> *ganda is periodically rebroadcast to the gen-*
> *eral public of many countries.* [168, 169]

Time, that final arbitrator of truth, has revealed it to be Keys' works that were constructed on feet of clay and wail the lament of Ozymandias.

We turn to science as the hand to guide us on a way forward from historical truth. We act on faith that it will lead us from undesired and unwise directions with a purity of purpose resilient to mortal temptations. Tradition is a gift to humanity; it provides bearing as it anchors us. It is rootstock gripping deep legacy. But when such resolution of purpose is corrupted, truth is twisted into false legacy. It can leave us adrift in the doldrums of dishonest narrative with neither bearing, nor compass, nor a way, for generations. That is why the path of the Food Shaman must always be one of authenticity and experience, no matter the so-called conventional wisdom of the time.

Once, it was conventional wisdom that the Earth was flat....

The Unhappy Triad: Salt, Sugar, and Fat

Salt

Such a situation that we find ourselves in today is known as evolutionary discordance. It is when previous strategies for individual survival and survival as a species that once conferred success find themselves at odds with the new environmental reality.

This evolutionary discordance has resulted in our modern-day Achilles' heel. These weaknesses have opened a Pandora's Box rife with the disabilities and diseases of modern civilization. The food industry and modern agribusiness profit from our vulnerabilities by constructing types of food that we crave; a perversion of a natural system that culminates in a destructive food addiction.

We have been hacked.

But what is the number of the beast?

It is three in number and they are salt, sugar, and fat.

Salt is necessary for life. Like herbivores, most omnivores, and our relatives the chimpanzees, we are built to seek out exogenous sources of sodium. The neural hardwiring that occurs naturally for the instincts and reflexes that promote survival involve the pleasure and reward centers of the brain. The need for salt is so strong, deep, and consequently fundamental that many scientists believe the desire for salt is the origin of all addictive human behavior.

In North America and Europe, most sodium comes from packaged, processed, and ultra-processed foods.[170, 171] The ill effects of salt consumption show a J-shaped relationship. What this means is that there seems to be a threshold, below which the mortality increases as you consume *less* salt. These more recent findings suggest that increased CVD risk can occur when sodium intake falls only slightly below our existing levels (<3000 mg/d). Likewise, concurrent studies have found that significant sequelae of excess sodium consumption may not manifest until intake exceeds 6-7000mg/day, even for those with hypertension. These revelations have generated controversy about the optimal lowest and highest levels of sodium consumption.[172, 173, 174,175, 176]

While the consequences of the current levels of dietary sodium intake, which is about 3,400 mg per day, is presently an area of contentious inquiry, the sources of sodium in the modern Western diet are not. The top five contributors to sodium in the United States are:

- Bread
- Pizza
- Sandwiches
- Cold cuts and cured meats
- Soup[177]

The usual suspects such as potato chips, pretzels, and other salty snacks were not far behind as they did make the top ten coming in at number seven. Just under half of all the sodium consumed comes from ten foods. Rounding out this top ten are burritos and tacos, salted snacks, chicken, cheese, eggs, and omelets. All in all, almost 75 percent of the daily dietary sodium intake comes from twenty-five highly processed, packaged, prepared, and restaurant foods.

Store-bought take away and restaurant foods alone contribute over 60 percent of the sodium consumed in the United States each day. McDonald's alone serves sixty-eight million people per day, roughly 1 percent of the entire world's population. This makes McDonald's itself the ninetieth-largest economy on Earth.[178] Various highly processed and ultra-processed foodstuffs have been correlated to an increased risk of malignancy as well as cardiovascular disease.[179]

Because what is consumed is highly processed, pre-packaged, pre-prepared, and preserved, there is a skewing of the naturally occurring sodium to potassium ratio. Studies have correlated an increased risk of cardiovascular and other complications when the dietary sodium to potassium *ratio* exceeds one. The danger is likely not in simply consuming too much sodium or salt, but in destroying the natural ratio and relationship that exists between sodium and potassium both in a natural, wholesome diet and in our bodies.

Fruits and vegetables are two of our most important sources of potassium. When they are eliminated from the diet, we negatively affect the expected balance. When we bend natural foods to our processing fancy, we further distort the normal equilibrium. A naturally raised piece of fresh pork prior to cooking contains a sodium to potassium ratio less than one. However, processing that piece of pork into a psychedelic pink deli ham reverses the ratio, yielding a sodium to potassium ratio greatly in excess of one. These types of machinations skew the balances and relationships that are found in diets that emphasize more wholesome and authentic food.

Unlike naturally occurring energy dense foods such as animal meats, many of these modern constructs are nutritional deserts. Increased energy intake, poor nutrition, and an increasingly sedentary lifestyle combine to set up the perfect storm for the development of disability and disease. Our connection to the world begins with what we eat.

Sugar

"Sweetness!"

The call goes out and we respond with Pavlovian ardor.

As we are genetically wired to desire and crave sweet substances, it is no wonder that such descriptive adjectives are the language we use to describe those closest to us. These are the monikers that please our ears and tickle our fancy most, when likewise turned upon us.

But when it comes to diet, those terms of affection can become terms of affliction.

In 1822, the average American consumed just over six pounds of sugar per year. Today, the average American consumes over one hundred pounds of added sugars per year, or roughly a quarter-pounder every single day that is composed completely of sugar. Within a month, we eat more sugar than our recent forebears did in a year. In less than two hundred years, the average person in the US and in most Western nations has increased their consumption of added sugars by roughly 1,700 percent![180]

However, this is not new news. Professor John Yudkin was warning us of the dangers of the overconsumption of highly refined carbohydrates like sugar over fifty years ago. Yet, we bit on the saturated fat switch and bait. As a consequence, we find ourselves fretting with the languor of a post sugar high, all the while promising ourselves improved dietary discretion *sine die*.

The current modern Western diet with its high sugar content has been documented to increase the risk of weight gain, excess body weight, obesity, type 2 diabetes mellitus, higher serum triglycerides, high blood cholesterol, higher blood pressure, hypertension, stroke, coronary heart disease, cancer, and dental caries.

The physiological conundrum is that our bodies were built to run on sugar. A mainstay fuel for our brain and other organs is the simple sugar molecule, glucose. Sugar, by which we commonly refer to table sugar or sucrose, is a compound consisting of one molecule of glucose and a molecule of another simple sugar, fructose.

When we consume sugar or other carbohydrates rich in natural sugars, we give our bodies access to an instant source of energy. The cerebral pathways involved in that response to the ingestion of sugar comprise the same reward and pleasure centers of the brain that respond to opioid narcotics, making this a powerful driver of behavior. Not only can this be a sweet survival advantage, but the excess can be stored as body fat for when times are lean. Thus, there is a natural attraction to consume such a versatile fuel source.

There is a method to the madness of adding a sweet sensation in the form of sugars to a wide range of foodstuffs. That addition extends to barely or imperceptible sweet perception; because regardless of awareness, it affects our behavior through our biochemical and neural networks. Baked goods like breads are often tinged with sugars (and salt and vegetable oils) to alter our response to them. These are contemporary products far removed from their original flour, salt, water, and yeast containing, naturally fermented ancestors. So conditioned are we, that we have become The Walking Un-bread, with baked goods a major supplier of the sugar as well as the salt and fat we consume as we take our daily loaf.

But it's not just that we eat more sweets. It is that highly refined and ultra-processed carbohydrates like breads and baked goods have replaced heartier, fiber-containing carbohydrates. While the level of carbohydrate consumption remains about what it was at the turn of the twentieth century, we have replaced over 40 percent of the fiber with refined carbohydrates. In 1909 Americans consumed approximately 500g per day of dietary carbohydrate. Almost 6 percent of that was in the form of dietary fiber. In 1997 Americans still consumed about 500g per day of dietary carbohydrate, but now less than 3 percent of that is in the form of fiber; the difference being replaced by refined carbohydrates.[181]

Furthermore, what is labeled and counted by governmental labeling agencies as fiber is not always naturally occurring fiber. Natural cellulose is insoluble in water. Manufacturing companies process the raw cellulose from industrial leftovers like wood and cotton pulp into sodium carboxymethylcellulose (CMC), which is soluble in hot or cold water. This is frequently added to foods and the CMC added is counted toward daily fiber on the nutritional labeling, and no doubt in the advertisements. CMC, as we will see in the following chapters, while not absorbed by our human gastrointestinal tract, can cause detrimental effects on our gut microbiome.

In simple terms, our current peptic pathway leaves us overfed but undernourished, addicted, and tasteless. This is because of the preponderance of the aforementioned processed and ultra-processed foods. It is not from categories of real foods like grass-fed pastured beef, fermented cheeses, freshly baked breads made with ancient grains, and the like. The vast majority of all the sugar and high fructose corn syrup produced is used by the food industry in the manufacture of processed and ultra-processed foods.

Ultra-processed foods can be further broadly classified (a detailed discussion follows shortly) as:

> *Formulations of several ingredients which, besides salt, sugar, oils, and fats, include food substances not used in culinary preparations, in particular, flavors, colors, sweeteners, emulsifiers and other additives used to imitate sensorial qualities of unprocessed or minimally processed foods and their culinary preparations or to disguise unde-*

sirable qualities of the final product. The most common ultra-processed foods (are) breads; soft drinks, fruit drinks and milk-based drinks; cakes, cookies, and pies; salty snacks; frozen and shelf-stable plates; pizza; and breakfast cereals.[182]

These ultra-processed constructions are many of the same foods that dump inordinate amounts of sodium into our daily diet while leaving us bereft of essential nutrients and minerals like potassium. We have been processing food since we threw the first ribs on the campfire. Cooking, smoking, drying, salting, fermenting, preserving, heating, milling, and refining has all contributed positively to our ascension as a species, and they are all forms of food processing.[183, 184, 185] But with the disingenuousness inherent in ultra-processing, we may have crossed a threshold in transmogrifying our food.

Sugar sweetened beverages (SSBs) are a particularly appropriate poster child for the consumptive tendencies of our modern age. Both long-term prospective cohorts and clinical trials demonstrate that SSBs increase adiposity. Per serving, SSBs associate with greater long-term weight gain than nearly any other dietary factor.[186, 187] SSBs are associated with increased incidence of diabetes mellitus and CHD.[188, 189] Worldwide, one hundred and eighty-four thousand cardiometabolic deaths per year are estimated to be attributable to SSB consumption.[190, 191]

As a result, there is increasing popularity of artificial sweeteners (*e.g.*, saccharin, sucralose, aspartame) and natural low-calorie (also termed high-intensity or non-nutritive) sweeteners (*e.g.*, stevia). However, based on animal experiments and limited human data, these artificial and non-nutritive sweeteners may not be benign, with potential for impact on cognitive processes (*e.g.*, reward, taste perception), oral-gastrointestinal taste receptors, glucose-insulin and energy homeostasis, metabolic hormones, and especially the gut microbiome.[192, 193, 194, 195]

The effects, potentially mediated through the gut microbiome, have recently been shown to significantly increase the risk of developing obesity and many of the other disabilities and diseases associated with the MWD. A recent meta-analysis examined the risk associated with consuming non-nutritive sweeteners like aspartame, sucralose, and stevioside. Almost forty studies and over four hundred thousand people were examined with a median follow-up of ten years. The researchers found consumption of non-nutritive sweeteners was associated with increases in weight and waist circumference, and higher incidence of obesity, hypertension, metabolic syndrome, type 2 diabetes, and cardiovascular events. They concluded that, "Evidence from RCTs does not clearly support the intended benefits of non-nutritive sweeteners for weight management, and observational data suggest that routine intake of non-nutritive sweeteners may be associated with increased BMI and cardiometabolic risk."[196]

Another recent finding echoed those results examining artificially sweetened beverages (ASBs). As part of the Women's Health Initiative observational study almost sixty-five thousand women were followed for over eight years. ASBs, at least two or more servings per day, were associated with a 21 percent increased risk of developing diabetes. However, substituting one serving of ASBs with water was associated with a significant risk reduction of 5 percent for developing diabetes.[197] To echo Andrew Steed, "Indigenous is indigenous, food is food," and natural is natural—and artificial is clearly not.

Fat

The demonization of fat as the dietary bogeyman for the last half century by the so-called experts has not translated into any tangible health benefits. Both prospective cohort studies and large randomized trials confirm that low-fat diets have no benefits for reducing major chronic diseases.[198, 199]

The large Women's Health Initiative (WHI) trial substantially lowered total dietary fat among nearly fifty thousand US women who were followed for nearly a decade. Despite a statistically significant reduction in fat intake the result was no benefit in any of the major end points including heart disease, stroke, cancers, diabetes mellitus, or insulin resistance.[200, 201, 202, 203]

In contrast, randomized trials have confirmed the many prior observational cohort findings that diets higher in healthful fats, including in excess of the recommended 30 percent limit, reduce the risk of cardiovascular disease and diabetes mellitus.[204, 205, 206, 207, 208]

The current focus on total fat shapes numerous government feeding programs and policies. It drives industry marketing of fat-reduced desserts, snacks, salad dressings, processed meats, and other products of poor nutritional value. Ultimately it leads most Americans to actively avoid dietary fat and instead consume far too many refined carbohydrates and artificial additives.

Fat is the packaging nature uses to deliver the densest form of available energy. At 9 kcal per gram, fat delivers more energy per equivalent weight than protein or carbohydrates (4 kcal per gram for protein or carbohydrates). Fat is required for the absorption of specific nutrients like the fat-soluble vitamins A, D, E, and K, as well as other important compounds. Any chef will tell you the flavor is in the fat. It is no wonder that we find fats, PHAT—pretty, hot, and tempting.

The modern food industry adds a majority of the fats in the foods they tender to us in the form of industrial vegetable oils, predominately consisting of the omega-6 PUFA kind. These oils are combined with salt and sugar in obscene amounts to triple whammy our weaknesses. Their offerings continually aim to satisfy our internal bliss points.

The bliss point is that combination of sugar, salt, and fat in a food that maximizes our pleasure response. The idea is to create these ultra-processed food-like substances based primarily upon layer after layer of sugar, salt, and fat. Such assembled constructs keep us coming back for more and more of what we need less and less of, increasing sales and profit margins all along the way.

This is the foundation of the modern Western diet: salty, sweet meats and greasy treats.

Ultra-Man: The SAD Effects of Ultra-Processing

The result of the MWD is the consumption of massive amounts of refined and ultra-processed foods rife with additives and built upon never-ending slabs of sugar, salt, and fat at the expense of other dietary components. Consuming the modern Western diet affects us both directly and indirectly. By its nature, the nutrient poor, energy dense modern Western diet is disproportionately constructed of fats, oils, and refined carbohydrates. This means other essential dietary components like fresh fruits and vegetables are excluded.

The growth of agribusiness and the food industry has resulted in the industrialization of food production. This transformation of the food and food pathways affects the complete spectrum of edibles. The stockyard method and grain finishing of beef cattle for example, alters not only the amount of fat but changes the qualitative composition of fats when compared to their pastured and grass-fed brethren. We are altering both the quality *and* the character of our food. It is not just that you supersized the burger and fries; it is that that the burger and fries only bear a superficial resemblance to a similar repast consisting of grilled pasture-raised grass-finished heritage beef and organic heirloom vegetables.

It is only within the last decade that we have begun to appreciate the indirect effects of what we choose to eat. It is estimated that each person consists of approximately ten trillion human cells. It is estimated that we coexist in a symbiotic fashion with almost one hundred trillion bacterial cells, a vast majority of which exist internally in our gastrointestinal tract. This collection of bacteria is referred to as the gut microbiome or gut microbiota. It can be rapidly and deeply affected by what we eat. This in turn can have serious health implications for us.

For example, for many years a relationship has been observed between the consumption of artificially sweetened beverages and an increased risk of obesity, diabetes, and cardiovascular disease that the aforementioned studies have recently confirmed. Additionally, those women consuming artificially sweetened beverages often suffered more serious cardiovascular complications. Yet until of late, artificial sweeteners were believed to be inert in terms of their interaction with the human body once ingested.

Not long ago, it still remained a complete mystery as to how choosing a "healthier" low or no calorie alternative could correlate to a risk level comparable to those consuming sugar sweetened beverages. What has been revealed is that while it is true that these compounds do not interact with human cells, they can have a profound effect on the gut microbiome. The ingestion of these compounds causes changes in the gut microbiome that result in ongoing, continuous low-level inflammation.[209] This state can lead to the development of obesity, diabetes, and complications such as cardiovascular disease.

Numerous compounds that have been added to foods for decades often do not require detailed testing or oversight. They are released under the auspices of generally recognized as safe (GRAS). Since 1958, the government has allowed companies that place additives into food to be the ones determining whether they are safe or not. Many of these compounds are ubiquitous and found in a variety of commonly purchased modern foods. It is estimated that there are more than 10,000 additives allowed in food, 43 percent of which are GRAS additives.[210] Such components are omnipresent in the manufacture of the ultra-processed constituents of the MWD. Two such compounds were recently studied to examine their specific effects on the gut microbiome.

Polysorbate 80 (P80) and carboxymethylcellulose (CMC) were found to alter the gut microbiome. The changes they induced ranged from a chronic low-level inflammation to overt colitis. This transformation correlated to an increased risk of developing obesity and metabolic syndrome, a precursor of diabetes.[211] The gut microbiome will be discussed in greater detail in the following chapter.

The dialogue clearly requires more than a simplistic "eat this, don't eat that" approach based on broad food categories. How the food is assembled and prepared is more critical a variable in our modern times than at any other point in history. Building on the post-World War II stimulation of modern food processing, in the 1980s technology accelerated and created a class of products identified as 'ultra-processed.' They are ready-to-consume, are entirely or mostly made not from foods, but from industrial ingredients and additives, and are extremely profitable.

They are more fully defined and characterized as follows:

> *Ultra-processed products are made from processed substances extracted or refined from whole foods—e.g. oils, hydrogenated oils and fats, flours and starches, variants of sugar, and cheap parts or remnants of animal foods—with little or no whole foods. Products include burgers, frozen pasta, pizza and pasta dishes, nuggets and sticks, crisps, biscuits, confectionery, cereal bars, carbonated and other sugared drinks, and various snack products.*
>
> *Most are made, advertised, and sold by large or transnational corporations and are durable, palatable, and ready to consume, which is an enormous commercial advantage over fresh and perishable whole or minimally processed foods...[They] are typically energy dense, have a high glycaemic load, are low in dietary fiber, micronutrients, and phytochemicals, and are high in unhealthy types of dietary fat, free sugars, and sodium.*
>
> *When consumed in small amounts and with other healthy sources of calories, ultra-processed products are harmless; however, intense palatability (achieved by high content of fat, sugar, salt, and cosmetic and*

other additives), omnipresence, and sophis-
ticated and aggressive marketing strategies
(such as reduced price for supersize servings),
all make modest consumption of ultra-pro-
cessed products unlikely and displacement
of fresh or minimally processed foods very
likely. These factors make ultra-processed
products liable to harm endogenous satiety
mechanisms and so promote energy over-
consumption and thus obesity.[212]

These pseudo-foods go viral, in the old-fashioned small-pox way, wherever they are introduced. In the early 2000s, ultra-processed products accounted for over half of all calories consumed in Canada; in the US, they currently account for over 60 percent. In industrially emerging countries like Brazil, they have just started to establish a beachhead. In the early part of the twenty-first century, they already accounted for over one-quarter of the total calories consumed in Brazil. This was a stark increase from much lower levels in the not too distant past.

With aggressive marketing and a Western allure, the common descriptor of such industrial comestibles, "packaged foods"—such a label is a reasonable proxy for ultra-processed products—reap tremendous profits, and deliver huge sales. Ultra-processed products continue to increasingly displace previous healthful, natural, staple foods such as legumes, milk, vegetables, and fruits in any environment into which they are introduced.[213]

Displacement of foods and authentic culinary ingredients by ultra-processed packaged foods transforms food supplies and ultimately the food culture and subsequent dietary patterns. The consumption of ultra-processed products correlates to a reaping of ill-health, the disabilities and disease of modern civilization.[214] These manufactured constructs are often packaged and sold as meals. They are energy-dense, containing undesirable fats, excessive sugars, and salt. They are nutritionally barren with less fiber and nutrients than unprocessed or minimally processed naturally occurring foods. Their flavor profile ranges from banal to unpalatable. It's gastro-meth with a direct link to obesity and metabolic syndrome.[215]

As the nature of food has changed, so have food pathways. Instead of ingredients, purchases are increasingly made and consumed as the meals just described. Many ultra-processed products are consumed as snacks, available anytime and anywhere. Snacking is a relatively new cultural phenomenon, arising in the post-World War II era.

It is a trend that is growing as fast as our waistlines. In countries ranging from the United States to China, products in snack form amount to up to a quarter of all calories consumed. In China, since 2000, snacking has tripled every two years.[216, 217] While corporate food and beverage giants used to strive to "teach the world to sing," now the global strategy of transnational food manufacturing corporations is to "teach the world to snack" from infancy to old age.[218]

Along with convenience, there are potent economic drivers as well. Since the 1980s, national food systems have been shaped by dominant international economic policies designed to promote the flow of capital and the rapid expansion of trade. International and global trade agreements, intensified since the 1990s, have enabled transnational food manufacturing, retailing, fast food chains, and associated corporations, to become colossal.[219, 220]

The annual turnover of some transnational manufacturing corporations, collectively sometimes known as Big Food, Big Soda, and Big Snack, is on a level with the gross national products of middle-size countries.[221] The Director General of the World Health Organization (WHO) warned, "Market power readily translates into political power. Few governments prioritize health over big business. As we learned from experience with the tobacco industry, a powerful corporation can sell the public just about anything."[222]

The Sampler: Diets From Around the World

The presence or absence of disease is a function of genetics and environment. The single most important modifier of the environmental component is our diet. Diet is determined not only by the sources of food available, but by individual palatability, values, and habits. These in turn are subject to socioeconomic, cultural, and environmental influences.[223, 224, 225] It is clear that the modern Western diet (MWD) or the standard American diet (SAD) is the epitome of a "worst" diet. It is clearly associated with the development of ongoing, low-level, continuous chronic inflammation and the disability and diseases associated with it. Its financial successes are orchestrated through backdoor, addictive formulations and shadowy politico-corporate operations. It appeals not to our taste buds nor a true food experience, but to convenience, sloth, and an acceptance of mediocrity.

In the larger context of evidence-based personalized nutrition, it appears that greater opportunity for positive change depends more on non-genetic characteristics like diet than genetic factors. Diet, like personality, counts for a lot. This gives our dietary choices weightier influence and heavier impact over the course of our lives.

This in turn puts us at increased risk of developing significant illness if we choose poorly. Dietary choices affect us both directly through the effects of dietary constituents on our physiology and indirectly through the component impact on our individual gut microbiome. The MWD is engineered to specifically tickle our pleasure centers and addict us in an ever-increasing consumptive cycle. All of which deposits us back at our initial question in a search for alternatives: Is there a singular "best" diet?

In searching for the best approach, it is imperative to define exactly what we are seeking.

The term diet has come within the vernacular to be associated with the verb. When the average person hears "diet," the immediate thought is the active pursuit of consumptive patterns designed to reduce weight. However, here the term refers to a sustainable, authentic, lifetime approach to food. Through examining the ingredients that comprise the modern Western diet and revealing their untoward effects, it becomes clear that a dietary approach questing for the best outcomes must focus on the *quality*, not just the quantity, of the food.

A hundred years ago, a chicken was pretty much a chicken. Pastured, naturally raised, and organic by today's standards, a piece of chicken was exactly that—a concept easily understood by all. In today's environment, that piece of chicken may take the form of a pastured, naturally raised chicken of old, a highly industrialized and processed bird raised on GMO feed under conditions outlawed by the Geneva Convention, or worse still, an adulterated and assembled fast food facsimile consisting of a reformulated nugget manufactured from artificial and undisclosed bits. Clearly, in our modern times the *quality* of the comestibles has taken on a penultimate significance.

As an example of a potential "best" diet, one of the most rigorously tested and highly recommended dietary approaches is the Mediterranean diet. Features of the Mediterranean diet include a high intake of fresh fruits and vegetables. It is extremely rich in the consumption of legumes, nuts, and pulses. It is quite diverse in its palate, incorporating whole grains, olive oil, fish, poultry, and dairy products. The beverages consumed consist predominantly of wine and water. While the Mediterranean diet is often believed to be high in fish and shellfish, this is true only in certain regions. For example, in the landlocked, mountainous northern areas of Italy you are much more likely to find red meat on the menu than seafood. However, it is specifically scanty in its offerings of *processed* meats and sweet desserts.[226]

The Mediterranean diet and its many variations have been shown to improve a range of health-related risk factors, reduce long-term weight gain, and are consistently associated with lower risk of adverse clinical events.[227, 228, 229, 230, 231] Much work regarding healthful outcomes in the Mediterranean diet has been performed by the *Prevención con Dieta Mediterránea* (PREDIMED) group. In one of their studies, a Mediterranean approach including supplementation with extra virgin olive oil or mixed nuts, combined with lifestyle advice, led to significant reductions in cardiovascular events and the risk of developing diabetes compared to a traditional low-fat diet approach. Of critical import, there was no calorie counting. People on the Mediterranean diet could eat as much as they liked without restriction.[232, 233]

Other research has shown the Mediterranean diet results not only in a lower incidence and prevalence of diseases like

diabetes, but less significant complications like strokes associated with such diseases, and in some circumstances, reversal
of diabetes and related conditions.[234, 235] The Mediterranean
diet is associated with a significantly lower risk of developing
many of the disabilities and diseases associated with modern
civilization like Alzheimer's dementia.[236] (See appendix B6)

This is particularly impressive in light of two common
targets of dietary restriction or elimination in the United
States: fat and salt. The Mediterranean diet is historically high
in both fat *and* salt. About 35 to 40 percent of the energy is
derived from fat, a major portion of which is tied to olive oil
consumption. This is actually more fat than is found in the
modern Western diet, which clocks in at about 30 percent.

The Mediterranean diet is more about a general approach
than the consumption of specific food items. This is because
the Mediterranean Sea is bordered by twenty-one different
countries and three continents: Africa, Asia, and Europe.
This makes for an extremely diverse collection of cultures
and cuisines. Even though the bulk of the Mediterranean
diet influence comes from eleven countries, this still leaves a
wide range of ingredients, preparatory methods, spices, and
seasonings that span the entire spectrum of possibilities.

What is universal to any of these Mediterranean
approaches is a consistent emphasis on fresh, wholesome,
and authentic food that is minimally processed. Because it
focuses on these ingredients, the meals are both nutritious
and delicious. The appetizing food is paired with positive
social interaction and communal fellowship; it is a proper
food experience. This is what makes it sustainable as "it constitutes a set of skills, knowledge, practices and traditions ranging from the landscape to the table, including the crops, har-

vesting, fishing, conservation, processing, preparation and, particularly, consumption of food." [237]

It is a sustainable food experience for the individual, community, and planet. A true Mediterranean approach reaches well beyond a narrow sea of choices into an ocean of possibilities. While steeped in history, it embodies many of the characteristics we will subsequently designate as Quantum Food.

It is a fascinating correlation that a foundation of a new age modern approach to the food experience, quantum food, may owe its origins to the Ancient Mediterranean in much the same way that modern loop quantum gravity theory finds its birth in the venerable teachings of Democritus from Miletus, twenty-six centuries ago.[238] In recognition of its importance, the Mediterranean diet was awarded a place on the Intangible Cultural Heritage List of the United Nations Educational, Scientific and Cultural Organization (UNESCO) in 2013 by the Intergovernmental Committee of the Convention, as an intangible heritage of humanity.[239]

In contradistinction, both observational cohorts and randomized trials confirm little clinical benefit of diets focused exclusively on isolated nutrient targets, such as low-fat, or low-saturated fat diets, which produce no significant benefits on cardiovascular disease, diabetes mellitus, or insulin resistance.[240, 241, 242, 243] Based on the evidence, the 2015 Dietary Guidelines Advisory Committee concluded that low-fat diets have no effect on CVD and emphasized instead the importance of healthful, food-based diet patterns.[244] It is a well-accepted fact that we will eat food until we die, so we must come to terms with our relationship within those confines.

The wheels of time move inexorably forward. They drag us onward, grinding our lives with the surety of a new sunrise. Yet it is a march of attrition, not the rapid explosion of new birthing. Upon certain circumstances, they may seem to move so slowly as to suspend belief in the passage of time at all. Thus giving rise, if even for a brief moment, that is the entirety of our existence, in our own immortality. If someone has mentioned looking back a decade ago and you've immediately conjured up the 1990s, you've experienced this phenomenon.

It is within such periods of fancy that other fables take hold. An unproven statement becomes a recommendation. A recommendation becomes a guideline. A guideline becomes a meme. A meme becomes a fact. A fact becomes a commandment, and to question the commandment is to commit the sin of heresy.

Eventually, as Shakespeare perceived, we must all confront our own mortality. As a society, there comes a time when we must critique the origins that motivate our behaviors, particularly when those behaviors appear to run counter to their original objectives. Kusunoki Masashige, a fourteenth-century samurai, observed that:

> There will be a time when critics appear.
> The man without ability will complain
> about criticism. The man of ability will
> laugh. The inferior man will seek to silence
> all criticism. The superior man will be
> inspired to improve and overcome valid
> criticism.[245]

In January 2016, the United States Department of Health and Human Services, along with the Department of Agriculture, released the latest dietary guidelines. These guidelines continue to promulgate the mythos created over a half century ago, that the wholesale limiting of dietary fat begets good health.

Forging an unproven hypothesis that quantity mattered more than quality, the culpability for the incidence and prevalence of the disability and diseases that were manifesting as a result of the modern Western diet was laid at the feet of the consumers. It was proclaimed that people consumed far too many calories and got fat. When they got fat, they got obese and sick. Packing over twice the punch of either protein or carbohydrates, fat is nature's most energy dense provision. For the regulators, the cause was Krystal Burger clear; what we ate too much of was fat. Their belief was, in perfect iambic pentameter, that "it is the fat, in fact, that makes us fat."

Thusly have we crusaded for over half a century. And thusly we continue, despite critical evidence to the contrary from such trials done by the PREDIMED group that have clearly demonstrated that a Mediterranean approach to diet results in a lower risk of cardiovascular disease, diabetes, strokes, and the other ills that plague consumers of the modern Western diet. This is despite the fact that the Mediterranean diet generally derives about 40 percent of its total energy from fat—more than that seen in the modern Western diet. This, despite the fact that the Mediterranean diet historically delivers more salt than the average American consumes. This, despite the fact that the benefits were received without any type of caloric overseer or consumptive limits.

Several studies including a meta-analysis that examined forty-four different studies of a Mediterranean approach scrutinized its effect on health outcomes. What is specifically unique in the meta-analysis is that it only included those Mediterranean approaches that had no restriction on fat intake. Expressly, these studies prescribed the traditional

Mediterranean approach of procuring high-quality goods based on their innate characteristics. It is an approach that eschews the traditional Western tactic toward dietary health of eliminating fat (and many would argue taste) and counting calories. What they found in a saturated fat laden nutshell is that such an approach significantly reduces the risk of cardiovascular events, certain cancers, and type II diabetes mellitus.[246, 247, 248, 249]

Despite an ever-increasing pharmacologic armamentarium, advances in diagnostics and treatments, such chronic inflammatory conditions continue to be the major source of morbidity and mortality in industrialized Western countries like the United States. Globally, from 1990 to 2013 deaths due to cardiovascular disease and the prevalence of diabetes increased by more than 40 percent. In 2012, deaths resulting from diabetes, cardiovascular disease, and cancer amounted to more than twenty-seven million worldwide. Consumption of the modern Western diet is correlated with an increased incidence and prevalence of certain types of cancer, including breast and colorectal cancer.[250]

The true Mediterranean diet defies stringent classification. The modern term was coined by Ancel Keys in the 1960s after observing dietary patterns in the Mediterranean basin for several decades following World War II. His observations were primarily confined to Greece, and, in particular, the island of Crete. Modern studies have expanded not only the observations but the inclusion of the cuisines of the twenty-plus different countries that currently border the Mediterranean. Add to this the many diverse cultures, geographies, and ethnicities within these countries and it soon becomes readily apparent that there is no singular Mediterranean diet.

What is apparent is that there is a consistent Mediterranean approach. There are factors and practices common to the more ancient, traditional Mediterranean diets, as well as some of the modern practices which often utilize non-traditional ingredients. One of the key observations is that no matter the original provenance of the comestible, what is highly valued is its freshness and quality. There is an appreciation of the terroir that defines all real food, not just the wine, a Mediterranean dietary staple.

A partial checklist highlighting the Mediterranean approach would likely include the following five points:

- Impeccable Sourcing: All the great chefs follow this pillar of the Mediterranean approach to cuisine. It means evaluating the value of your food in terms of quality first and quantity second. Ask yourself the following five simple questions for anything you are thinking about eating:
  - Is it fresh?
  - Where did it come from?
  - How was it grown/raised?
  - Was it processed? If so how?
  - What was added, or removed?

We will discuss sourcing in greater detail in later chapters.

- Taste the rainbow: We're not talking beast mode sugar supplements here. We're talking fruit and veg. Vary not only the amounts, but the types. Use the local seasonality to determine what goes in your basket and on your plate.

- Olive oil: A common misconception is that you cannot enjoy anything crispy, golden brown, and delicious because there is minimal deep frying in any healthful approach to food. However, cooking with olive oil can certainly yield these textural treasures that we have become accustomed to. Using a cold first press extra-virgin olive oil as a condiment eliminates a major source of the omega six pro-inflammatory fats that pervade the modern Western diet. Many areas of the Mediterranean historically used tallow and lard, saturated fats less prone to instability and the formation of TFAs seen with modern vegetables oils used in deep frying.

- Plates and Portions: With respect to the Mediterranean approach, eating should be like dating. Partake of what attracts you, sample lightly, frequently, and don't miss out on variety.

- Wine-ing: Another often overlooked dining staple across the many Mediterranean cultures, and indeed many cultures worldwide, is the moderate consumption of wine or its equivalent.

A study applied these types of Mediterranean principles to the local and regional cuisines found in Switzerland, a most non-Mediterranean location. The results of applying the Mediterranean approach were as suspected. As a result of the positive food experience, there was high adherence, satisfaction, and improvement in a number of health markers.[251]

The answer is not simply to be found within one food or even one food group. While the Mediterranean diet emphasizes increased consumption and enjoyment of fruits and vegetables compared to what is consumed as part of the MWD, it is not *only* about fruits and vegetables. Vegetarianism *per se* is neither necessary nor sufficient for a good diet. Indeed, French fries and soda are vegetarian, as are other harmful factors such as refined grains, starches, added sugars, sweets, trans-fats, and excess sodium. With a typical Western exclusionary approach, such unwanted guests often find themselves at the table.[252] Plant-based diets with a high intake of sweets and refined grains may in fact increase heart disease risk.[253]

Thus, a vegetarian diet is not a guarantee of health, whereas a non-vegetarian diet can be rich in healthful foods. The Tsimane, with the lowest incidence and prevalence of CAD ever recorded in a population, consume a traditional hunter-gatherer diet rich in meat and fish. With that being said, all healthful approaches begin with generous portions of vegetables, fruits, grains, and legumes. A balanced diet does not mean equality of portions amongst different food groups. A plant-based—not necessarily plant *exclusive*—diet is a solid starting point for any meal or cuisine. Contemporary or historical, indigenous or industrialized, New World or Old World, a plant-based approach is a commonality among sustainable, delicious, and nutritious cuisines.[254, 255, 256]

The Paleo diet is a popular approach based on assumptions regarding the diet of hominins prior to the agricultural revolution. It focuses on wild sourced meats and plants. The approach includes lean (often wild game) meat, fish, eggs, fruits, vegetables, nuts, and seeds. It excludes cereal grains, legumes, dairy products, potatoes, vegetable oils, sugar, and processed foods. It is quite possible that the avoidance of the latter three on the list are responsible for significant proportion of the purported health claims.

The low-carbohydrate diet eschews refined grains, starches, and added sugars. In doing so it addresses a majority of the total carbohydrates and ultra-processed foods in modern diets. While the gluten-free approach encourages avoidance of refined carbohydrates in the form of certain breads, it has some potential drawbacks. Gluten is a protein found in foods made with wheat, barley, rye, and triticale. However, due to cross-contamination concerns, oats and certain other foods are often added to the *verboten* list.

In many of the foods that are consumed on this diet, the processing to remove gluten modifies macro and micro nutrient composition. Gluten-free products tend to be lower in iron, folate, complex B vitamins, and fiber. Comparatively, they tend to have a higher glycemic index. As a final insult to injury, the tastes and textures can be quite off-putting, and the products usually cost significantly more than their gluten-containing counterparts. Outside of those who must adhere to it for true diagnosed celiac disease, potential benefits remain unclear. Utilizing organic ancient grains may be a simpler and more cost-effective strategy. To wit, simply concentrate on the principles of wholesome, authentic, organic, real food.

This tenet holds true when we examine other dietary regimens that are associated with positive health outcomes. When compared to the Western emphasis on a low-fat and caloric restriction formula for healthful eating, these approaches often seem paradoxical in nature. But when examined in light of remaining true to principles of virtuous victuals, it follows logical suit, even when we eliminate variables like fresh fruits and vegetables.

The Inuit diet is what the indigenous peoples of the harsh northern clime have existed on for centuries, if not millennia. It is extremely low in carbohydrates, because the cold and unforgiving nature of the terrain forbids any significant plant cultivation and limited plant growth. It may be the original "low carb," or "Atkins" diet.

While an oversimplified conclusion of the Mediterranean diet approach may be that we simply need to eat more fruits and vegetables (which we actually do), the Inuit diet has minimal fruit and vegetables. It consists of over 50 percent meat and fat. Despite that, the cardiovascular disease rates are over 50 percent less than that found in the United States. There is a similarly impressive reduction in other disabilities and diseases like hypertension and diabetes.[257]

The new Nordic diet is an offshoot of the Inuit diet based on native Scandinavian foods and dietary patterns. Unlike the Inuit diet, the new Nordic diet emphasizes a plant-based foundation. It encourages generous portions of fish and seafood, and includes other marine derived foods like seaweed. Finally, there is an emphasis on more natural foods such as game or other wild crafted comestibles.[258] If there is any doubt how delicious such an approach can be, simply visit NOMA—*if* you can get a table. This is the two-Michelin-star Scandinavian restaurant run by Chef René Redzepi in Copenhagen, Denmark. Their new Nordic approach and menu has garnered them the best restaurant in the world award a remarkable four times between 2010 and 2014. It has been one of the top five best restaurants in the world consecutively since 2009.

Another delicious dietary paradox which has received significant attention is what is known as the French paradox. In the 1990s, a comparison of the rates of cardiovascular disease between middle-aged men in the United States and France was performed. It was found that the French consumed not only more fat, but more saturated fat compared to their American counterparts, along with significantly higher consumption of butter and cream. There was a significant dairy component, and in keeping with the Mediterranean approach, copious enjoyment of a variety of cheeses.

But the food, like the cheese, tended to be wholesome, natural, and authentic. The category of cheese in France does not include the Day-Glo orange processed cheese like food substance in individually packaged slices otherwise known as American cheese. Undeterred by alarmists across the pond, the French at the time were eating everything American cardiologists were telling their patients to avoid. The result of such Gallic audacity was that the French cardiovascular event rate was 50 percent of that seen in the United States.

Even more impressive was the fact that the lowest area of cardiovascular disease in France, with an event rate 25 percent of that seen in the United States, was the Gascony area. This is the home to France's foie gras production and more of the fatty duck liver is consumed here than anywhere else in France. No matter what the ingredient, the traditional French approach demands quality, fresh comestibles, many of which are produced and sourced locally.[259]

Halfway across the globe, the traditional Japanese diet is a world away from traditional French ingredients and techniques, and there is a galaxy of separation from the modern Western diet. Despite the differences between their techniques and ingredients, the Japanese, like the French, exhibit a significantly lower rate of cardiovascular events. Their average life expectancy is among the highest in the world and thus, if you subscribe to this measure of population health, they are among the healthiest people in the entire world. Not only do they live longer, but compared to the average American they have a significantly longer HALE. They also consume significantly more salt than their US counterparts. Among ethnic subgroups, Japanese women are only surpassed by the Tsimane with respect to the delayed appearance of CVD.[260]

The Japanese diet, like many island cuisines, is rich in fish and seafood, potent sources of omega-3 fatty acids. The omega-6 polyunsaturated fatty acid (PUFA) to omega-3 PUFA in the Japanese diet is estimated at 4-8:1. Like many of the healthful cuisines around the world, such a fresh approach unsurprisingly leads to an omega-6: omega-3 PUFA ratio more in line with that seen naturally. That ideal ratio is anywhere from 1:1 to 3:1. In stark contrast, the MWD is anywhere from 16:1 or even higher.[261]

Japanese cookery, like many other Asian cuisines, tends to emphasize vegetables, soups, and broths served with large amounts of rice or beans. There are entire food cultures within Japan and Asia dedicated to fermented or pickled foods, which supplement the diet with high concentrations of short chain fatty acids. The portion size is generally smaller than that seen in the modern Western diet, but the emphasis, reminiscent of the Mediterranean approach, is on freshness and flavor as opposed to huge quantities.

Within the Japanese nation, the Okinawan people exhibit the highest average life expectancy and healthy average life expectancy. Not only are they among the longest-lived peoples on Earth, but they are among the groups that maintain extended good health. Okinawa, as chronicled by the National Geographic Society, is considered a blue zone. Such areas are pockets where there are abnormally high concentrations of centenarians in good health and are felt to represent possible models for favorable lifestyle emulation.[262]

Unlike mainland Japan, the Okinawan diet is based on the sweet potato, *Ipomeoea batatas,* introduced roughly four hundred years ago from China, not rice. This sweet potato is one of most nutritious vegetables available, rich in fiber, carbohydrates, proteins, vitamin A, vitamin C, vitamin E, thiamine, riboflavin, vitamin B_6, potassium, iron, and calcium. It is delicious, especially with pork.

The Okinawans exhibit the highest pork consumption of anywhere in Japan. Pork is their most important meat source. However, the pork tends to be heritage breed, pastured, and raised locally on sweet potatoes grown on the islands. They tend to use up all the pork they produce, but will rarely import commercially produced pork as the local and regional supplies run out.

The Okinawans use everything but the oink, consuming all parts of the pig including the offal in a variety of stews and other dishes. Specifically, the Okinawans eat more than bacon. A rich source of vitamin B_1, thiamine, pork is utilized in dishes like *soki* (a spare rib dish), *tebichi* (boiled pigs' feet), *mimiga* (crunchy pig ears), and *rafute* (pork with soy sauce and brown sugar).

Once an island kingdom known as Ryukyu, mention of it first appears in Chinese texts dating to 605AD, during the Chinese Sui dynasty. Chinese envoys began arriving in the fourteenth century. During the fifteenth century, the Sappo envoys from China numbered over five hundred and might have stayed as long as six months. For this reason, chefs from Ryukyu were sent to China to learn how to prepare acceptable foods. In seventeenth century Ryukyu was annexed by the Satsuma clan of Japan. Chefs were then sent to Japan to learn Yamato cuisine. Modern Okinawan cuisine is the result of an ancient royal court cuisine. However, as modern Western dietary habits are increasingly adopted by younger generations, the average life expectancy and healthy life expectancy are falling. The younger generation seems to have a penchant for Western high GI foods, particularly breads.

The traditional diet is a great example of functional foods approach. Food is understood as *nuchi gusui*: medicine for life. This traditional view is echoed in ancient texts that reveal the highest ranking doctor was the diet doctor, then the internal medicine doctor, then the surgeon, and then the veterinarian. Roughly 39 percent of the Okinawan diet is derived in one form or another from the sweet potato. However, there is substantial consumption of fish and fish paste. Given its history, particularly as a participant in the spice trade as an independent kingdom until 1879, it draws from varied ingredients and cooking styles.

In addition to pork and the Satsuma sweet potato, other staple ingredients include different tubers like *konnyaku*, *goyu* (bitter melon), shiitake mushrooms, *gobo* (burdock root), *hechima* (sponge cucumber), and seaweeds like *kombu*. There is wide use of various spices and herbs, including mugwort, sweet potato leaves, fennel, green seaweed, bitter leaf, *hihatsu* (a member of the pepper family; *Piper hancei Maxim*), and turmeric. The result is a flavorful, texturally pleasing diet that is high in vegetables, legumes (via soy), and accompanied by moderate alcohol consumption. Similar to the Mediterranean diet, but a galaxy away in terms of ingredients, it is rich in omega-3 PUFAs, EPA, DPA, DHA, phytonutrients, fiber, calcium, magnesium, potassium, vitamin A, vitamin C, vitamin E and most critically—piquancy. (See appendix B7)

Even pig's blood is used by combining it with starch and salt to produce a jelly, which is then stored in pig's fat. Since, as the Okinawan saying goes, "You eat every part of the pig apart from the oink," there is consumption of not just meat, but lots of collagen, elastin, and other components missing from a bacon-centric Western plate. A study examined mice genetically predisposed to develop high blood cholesterol levels that were fed a pelletized form of the Okinawan diet, complete with Okinawan pig bits; feet, ears, stomach, intestines, and such. This freeze-dried powder significantly reduced their blood lipid levels, like that seen with pharmacologic agents in the West.[263]

Perhaps the observation from Sasamori Gisuke, visiting Okinawa in 26th year of Meiji era (1894), said it best; "They say one sort of pig is enough to produce dozens of different marvelous dishes. The delicacy of the pork cuisine here would be enough to shame into silence those Westerners who eat meat as their main dish." Yet once again, like the Mediterranean food experience, it is not just what they eat, but how. Many older Okinawans practice *hara hachi bu*. This is the Confucian concept of eating until one is 80 percent full, and then stopping.

The Okinawan love affair with pork flies in the face of the Western conventional wisdom that paints red meat as yet another dietary devil. Although this topic will be covered in great detail in the following chapters, it is important to briefly mention a few pertinent facts here. One of the seminal studies to date was a meta-analysis performed by Harvard University. They defined red meat as that coming from beef, pork, or lamb. This was one of the first large analyses to look at the difference between fresh red meat and processed red meat.

The sample size was over 1.2 million people from around the world. The findings were startling. Fresh or unprocessed red meat was *not* associated with any increased risk of coronary heart disease or diabetes. This finding was in agreement with a large body of data suggesting that saturated fats *per se* did not contribute to an increased risk of heart disease or diabetes. The researchers did find that processed meat like the industrially produced bacon, hotdogs, or deli salami was associated with a 42 percent increased risk for coronary heart disease and a 19 percent increased risk for the development of diabetes.

The authors concluded: "Findings suggest that unprocessed red and processed meats have differing relationships with cardiometabolic outcomes, and that differences in preservative contents, rather than fats, could at least partly account for these findings."[264] It is neither the calories nor the quantity of food that matters, but its quality.

Another trial performed in Europe examined almost four hundred and fifty thousand people from twenty-three different countries. Like the previous Harvard study, the EPIC trial found a correlation between ill health and processed meats, but not fresh meat. There was *no* correlation between unfavorable health outcomes including cardiovascular disease and cancer and the consumption of fresh meat at any level. In contrast, the consumption of processed meat increased the risk of early mortality from any cause. Researchers estimate that about 3.3 percent of deaths could be prevented if all participants had a processed meat consumption of less than 20g/day.

The study found an association between processed meat consumption and rates of cardiovascular disease and cancer. There was an association that was linear in nature such that the higher the consumption of processed meat the more likely the development of cardiovascular disease, cancer, and the risk of earlier mortality. The authors concluded that, "The results of our analysis support a moderate positive association between processed meat consumption and mortality, in particular due to cardiovascular diseases, but also to cancer." [265]

There are any number of other dietary approaches that are proffered about as best diets, the healthiest diets, or some miracle diet variant. Some are geared toward health, some toward weight loss, and some seem to merely offer vagaries of hope. Regardless, the commonality that binds many of them is that they are restrictive and exclusionary in nature. They focus on trying to identify a single "bad guy" like red meat, eggs, dairy, fat, gluten, and once the offending agent is eliminated all will be well with your belly, your health, and the world.

Many such programs focus on offering a miracle pill or a superfood. They offer a path to Epicurean enlightenment by chanting the chorus of "you must eat this, you must avoid that." But as Harold Draper, a noted biochemist and nutrition expert, noted, there are no essential foods—only essential nutrients. [266] This is true. Accordingly, by simply keeping it real you can entertain a wide variety of palate pleasing guests at your table. But bar your door from the dark Faustian stranger offering white castles in the sky under the guise of convenience.

How The Convenience Culture is Killing Us

For the vast majority of the timeline that is human civilization, food was hard to come by. But what you got, less the spoilage, was what today might be considered high end: local, organic heritage breed proteins, heirloom fruits and vegetables. In terms of food value at that time, the primary driver in this equation was quantity. But the times they are a'changin'. Over the last century, *quality* has become the defining variable.

Real, authentic, and wholesome food that supports the human body and the human gut microbiome that has co-evolved to co-metabolize such a diet with us is clearly revealing itself to be the cornerstone of health and wellness, along with the authentic flavor. It is the bulwark against the disabilities and diseases associated with the modern Western diet. Such comestible choices are a decision that remains entirely within our purview.

The oft artificially preserved, highly processed, pre-prepared, and pre-packaged food-like stuffs that make up the majority of the modern Western diet are highly correlated with a number of maladies. Such illnesses are not prominent in cultures in which such a gustatory approach is not prevalent. Dietary approaches like the Mediterranean diet have demonstrated the ability to profoundly make an impact on such disabling end points. (See appendix B8)

The results of a 2016 study reinforce the benefits of such a method, not only in preventing a first heart attack or stroke, but in preventing recurrent events in those diagnosed with disease. Such secondary prevention highlights the magnitude of benefits conferred from undertaking a true *food value*, as opposed to *food as fuel* (or caloric/quantitative) approach. It is never too late to start.

The study examined over fifteen thousand patients with known, stable coronary heart disease (CHD) from thirty-nine countries enrolled in the STABILTY trial. Those indulging their appetite with a Mediterranean attitude saw an approximately 30 percent relative reduction (absolute 10.8 percent in controls versus 7.3 percent in the most intensively immersive Mediterranean group) in heart attack, stroke, or risk from death due to major adverse cardiovascular events (MACE). Specific foods associated with a lower risk of MACE included fruits, vegetables, fish, alcohol, dairy food, and tofu/soybean.[267] (See appendix B9)

However, as Booker T. Washington noted, "Nothing ever comes to one that is worth having, except as a result of hard work." Tasty food and the healthful benefits as the result of working with nourishing and genuine ingredients are no exception. It takes a bit of interest to read a label, a smidge of effort to source your sustenance, and perhaps a dram of desire to rally your inner Emeril into the kitchen. All in all, it is not much effort when measured against the return on such an investment. But we have become a culture of convenience. When we drive around a parking lot for forty minutes to park six spaces closer to the entrance to the gym, something is askew.

The restaurant industry has seen the writing we paid someone else to write on the wall. We want it *now*, quality be damned! According to Yum Brands CEO Greg Creed, who oversees Pizza Hut, Taco Bell, and KFC brands, the motto is "easy beats better." In the bloody arena in which eateries compete for your discretionary dining dollar, many choose a strategy based on convenience. They believe this is more important than quality or better tasting food. They believe that is what the public prefers.

To back their claims that this is a winning strategy, Taco Bell points to sales over the last several years that have been buoyed by such an approach. Instead of competing by offering higher-quality, and thus often more expensive ingredients, the focus is on convenience. This is predominantly reflected in the areas of delivery and digital innovation. While trained chefs work long hours sourcing and preparing prime ingredients to prepare a meal both sumptuous and salubrious, industrial chains assemble intestinal incendiaries with ever more facile delivery systems.

In addition to building more brick and mortar stores in pursuit of omnipresence, there is a focus on delivery. In fact, delivery was the number one demand from their customers. We don't just want it now—we don't want to be bothered to pick it up either. In addition to home delivery, ordering was made simpler and more efficient by taking the process online and mobile. That way when you order your flat-line fries with an emoji sent at digital speed, you can group text EMS on the request. No separate additional 911 call needed—convenient *and* efficient!

Taco Bell's sister company, Pizza Hut, adheres to the "easy beats better" philosophy. Recently, Pizza Hut executives switched their focus from making a pizza that customers might actually enjoy to simply cutting down delivery time. The result was an impressive 5 percent same-store sales growth. With 46 percent of the carryout orders originating from digital channels, the consumer demand is on convenience not quality. Despite impressive numbers, competitors Papa John's and Domino's exhibit even greater digital dominance with over 50 percent of their carryout orders originating digitally.

Creed observed that in the past Pizza Hut had not paid much attention to making life easier for customers as it focused on being "better." Sales slumped even though Pizza Hut was often listed as a consumer favorite. Apparently the public is fickle, and thirty seconds are not only for sound bites, but for real ones too. Even those who prefer Pizza Hut pizzas are only willing to wait about two minutes longer to receive their share of the pie. Since Pizza Hut takes more than two minutes longer to deliver than its competitors, focus shifted to faster. It is *not* about better ingredients, a better pizza, or product. It is about the illusion of instant gratification and emotive entitlement.

Nothing satisfies cravings of convenience more than supersizing that instant delivery.

Perhaps the most important feature on the convenience train and the one thing that drove the recent sales boom at KFC, Taco Bell, and Pizza Hut was an emphasis on inexpensive *quantity*. KFC released the five dollar boxes, Taco Bell boosted sales by 8 percent with a new one dollar breakfast menu, and Pizza Hut bolstered growth with a five dollar flavor menu. Such marketing continues to blur the distinction between value and quantity, between worthwhile and worthless.

Creed remarked that there was a time when the way to beat the competition was to have a better product. He now believes that convenience trumps quality.[268, 269] A lazy argument for lazy minds, but one that is all too easily proven true in the face of public ignorance and wilted effort. It is pervasive not only in the fast food industry, but extends into ingredient procurement and meal preparation.

The irony lies in such a stratagem where we strive to save seconds from a meal we should be spending *more* time to savor. We remove days, if not years from our lives by eating such easy fixins'. Like some modern Circe, these peddlers of misapprehension prey upon our weakness and sloth. Our indolence and apathy are rewarded with disability and disease, metamorphosing us from Pizza Hut through our own acedia into Jabba the Hutt.

Such comestibles of convenience may be consumed, but not enjoyed. Heed well the siren song of expediency. Strive like Odysseus against the easy temptation and make the effort of authenticity:

Though much is taken, much
abides; and though

We are not now that strength
which in old days
Moved Earth and Heaven, that
which we are, we are;
One equal temper of heroic hearts,
Made weak by time and
fate, but strong in will
To strive, to seek, to find,
and not to yield.[270]

Siren Songs of Supplemental Seduction

The clouding of fact and fiction perfumed with convenience is perhaps nowhere on display like it is in the world of supplements. While some supplementation is necessary and beneficial—pre-natal vitamins with folic acid come to mind—not all that glitters is gold; or in the case of supplements, a product that works. The caveat is in the title. These are supplements, not replacements. Far too often supplements are taken as a replacement for a proper diet or peddled as an antidote for rampant indiscretion. In typical Western fashion, we tend to think that if one or two is good, eight or ten must be better. One of the fundamental principles in the practice of medicine applies here. The poison is in the dose. You simply cannot supplement your way to good health.

While there are many illustrative examples of the folly of pursuing such a route, the calcium story is particularly applicable. Osteopenia and osteoporosis are devastating diseases that afflict our elderly population. These conditions are associated with an increased risk of significant bone fracture, which in turn significantly increases morbidity and mortality. Like so many of the disabilities and diseases of our modern civilization, there is a connection between diet and inflammation in the etiology of these pathologies. Like so many of the disabilities and diseases of our modern civilization, we tend not to see anywhere near the incidence and prevalence that we experience in societies and cultures that don't partake of the modern Western diet.

We are constantly breaking down and rebuilding our bone structure. About 92 percent of our bone matrix consists of forms of calcium like calcium phosphate and calcium carbonate. Diets rich in natural sources of calcium and lifestyles that include regular exercise helps strengthen our bones and their functionality well into our later years. Conversely, lifestyle stressors including excessive alcohol intake, smoking, obesity, and a sedentary lifestyle increase our vulnerability to potentially fatal fractures.

If the problem is that as we age our bones lose calcium, then simple logic would suggest that by consuming more calcium the problem could be easily remedied. But as Albert Einstein intimated, everything should be made as simple as possible, but no simpler. For every one problem we overcomplicate, there are nine problems we oversimplify.[271] This is one of those nine.

The consequences of excessive oral calcium intake first came to light in the 1920s. During this time, milk and antacids made from bicarbonate were recommended for treatment of underlying peptic ulcer disease—the so-called Sippy regimen.[272] The overconsumption of calcium with antacids led to milk-alkali syndrome—hypercalcemia leading to metastatic calcification and renal failure.

Overconsumption of calcium supplements can result in hypercalcemia by consuming too much calcium in a single dose, even with normal kidney function. According to some studies, over one third of women currently taking calcium supplements exhibit overconsumption with evidence of excessive calcium in their blood and urine.[273]

The recommended daily allowance (RDA) for adults ranges from 1,000 mg to 1,200 mg per day.[274] Calcium supplements are used by 43 percent of US adults and a substantial number are consuming total amounts of calcium in excess of 1200 mg/day. Among supplement users, daily intake of calcium just slightly in excess of this has been reported to be associated with higher death rates from all causes, including from CVD. While the exact mechanisms by which this might occur are unknown, one potential pathway may be through progression of atherosclerosis. Excess calcium may exert a detrimental effect through multiple pathways, including metabolism, insulin secretion and sensitivity, inflammation, thrombosis, regulation of body weight, and vascular calcification.

What has been found after years of dietary recommendations and supplementation is that:

> *"Little of the additional calcium provided by calcium supplements…is incorporated in bone by adults, but it may lead to a positive calcium balance and contribute to ectopic calcification. Because of the widespread awareness and treatment of osteoporosis with calcium supplements among older adults, this population would appear to be at greater risk of developing the adverse consequences of positive calcium balance, including vascular calcification."* [275]

A landmark study evaluated both men and women of various ages and ethnicities without a history of clinical CVD for their risk of developing significant coronary artery disease. They followed the group for ten years and classified calcium intake not only by amount, but by method—supplementation or diet. In their sample, the overall mean calcium intake was slightly *less* than currently recommended in US guidelines, with mean intakes of 1081 mg and 908 mg for women and men, respectively.

Their results were nothing less than Earth shattering and common sense at the same time. They clearly demonstrated that the risk of developing cardiovascular disease was dependent on the *source* of calcium intake, through artificial supplementation or a natural diet.

Their results are consistent with other smaller studies which have shown that consuming natural foods rich in calcium was *not* associated with any increased CVD risk. However, this study went even further and clearly demonstrated there was a significant protective effect or *decreased risk* of developing CVD, with a natural diet rich in calcium.

Conversely, an increased risk of CVD among calcium *supplement* users was plainly documented. In what seems almost ironic, increasing *dietary* calcium may actually *decrease* risk the risk of kidney stones. As already mentioned, calcium *supplementation* appears to *increase* the likelihood of developing kidney stones. One explanation for this apparent paradox may be that large boluses of calcium intake through supplements may transiently elevate serum calcium concentrations, which in turn may lead to vascular calcification and other adverse health effects.

This study, which followed patients for the development of CVD over a decade, documented a 27 percent *lower* risk of heart disease with a natural diet rich in calcium containing foods. Yet just trying to supplement your way to health by ingesting calcium in pill form was associated with a 22 percent *higher* risk of heart disease. This was not only about the total amount of calcium consumed. The highest risk for CVD was in the group of patients who consumed the lowest amount of calcium in the diet and took supplements. In perfect concordance with the rest of the data, the lowest risk group had the highest calcium rich diet and took no supplementation.

A healthful, natural, and delicious diet rich in calcium is good for body and soul. In the particular case of calcium supplementation, it is not a benign or neutral effect, but a significant health risk for major disability and disease. Without clarifying the method of calcium intake, increasing total daily calcium intake through supplementation might seem the logical extension and thus be misconstrued to be protective of heart disease.

What seems a natural and simple extension of logic, to replace missing calcium in the bone by consuming excess calcium in the form of supplements, achieves the exact opposite of its intended aims. This research highlights that:

> *The relationship between calcium intake and CVD risk is complex and appears to depend on the source of calcium intake, with dietary calcium generally showing a protective effect, but calcium supplement use being associated with increased risk.*
>
> *Rather than promoting bone health, excess calcium from the diet and supplements is postulated to accrue in vascular tissues. Pathological changes, presumably resulting from atheromas…increase the risk for adynamic or low bone turnover… When low BMD [Bone Mineral Density] is identified in older osteoporotic patients, they are typically treated with additional calcium and vitamin D as supplements.*

Rather than increase skeletal mass, excessive calcium consumption may contribute to cardiovascular calcification. [276]

Strict calcium supplementation is not only ineffective in treating the condition for which it was recommended, but it may kill you. In complete contradistinction, simply eating a natural diet that contains wholesome and authentic foods rich in calcium can help preserve your bones, your heart, your overall health and well-being. [277, 278, 279] Partnering with Nature in the kitchen and at the table is never a bad idea.

The woeful tale of calcium supplementation should serve as a grim warning for any and all unsubstantiated nutritional claims. Nutrient claims are a commonly used marketing tactic, but the association between claims, actual outcomes, and the nutritional quality of the products is often unknown. With respect to unsubstantiated nutritional, superfood, or miracle diet claims, there is nothing new under the sun. Scilicet *Caveat Emptor*! (See appendix B10)

Is there a "Best" Diaita?

Although when it comes to food and health we are often bludgeoned over the head like a baby harp seal with all the nutritional information meant to make us buy a particular product, the critical fact to remember is that we do not order nutrients at our table. We eat food. This is the basis of our food experience. Our food experience is our life experience, and it should not have to be austere and depressing. As the Buddha came to understand, the path of asceticism will not lead to enlightenment. As the shaman knows, the strings of joy must be plucked along with the strings of sorrow.

Our path to Epicurean enlightenment lies in finding the common threads that exist within the many delicious and diverse cuisines and cookery approaches that deliver us from the ills of our modern Western diet. These threads reveal a focus on fresh, local, sustainable, wholesome, authentic, and minimally processed ingredients. While we often think we know everything there is to know about food, nutrition, and health, as the recent revelations regarding the gut microbiome have taught us, the fact is that "everything we know today is an approximation of something else we don't yet know."[280]

The sensible journey is moderation and the Middle Way. It is not the middle way because it lies in between two extremes as a compromise between excess and frugality, but because it rises above them. As such, it is free from their errors, their imperfections, and the blind alleys of disability, disease, and despair into which they lead.

To follow the Middle Path means to provide the body with what it needs to be in a strong and healthy condition. To allow it to exist in a state of balance and maintain that homeostasis, avoiding that shift from harmony that is disease. Yet at the same time to rise above mere bodily concerns and appreciate how these threads intertwine into the larger experience of life. When we seek real and authentic food, we engage our mind and our spirit in the right conduct, concentration, thought, and wisdom.

In fact, by pursuing such a course we are embarking upon a way of training the mind to commune with Spirit. It is about neither compromise nor renunciation; there is no salvation in deprivation. It is about exploration, creation, and true enjoyment free from the demands of craving and clinging.

Our modern word diet, which has become synonymous with weight loss methods, needs to return to its original Greek roots. The original Greek word, *Diaita*, meant a "way of living." Our diet reflects not just a consumptive pattern, but a lifestyle.

Unfortunately, our modern lifestyle, like our modern Western Diet, has fallen ironically out of balance. George Carlin wryly observed that:

> *The paradox of our time in history is that we have taller buildings but shorter tempers, wider freeways, but narrower viewpoints. We spend more, but have less, we buy more, but enjoy less. We have bigger houses and smaller families, more conveniences, but less time. We have more degrees but less sense, more knowledge, but less judgment, more experts, yet more problems, more medicine, but less wellness.*
>
> *We drink too much, smoke too much, spend too recklessly, laugh too little, drive too fast, get too angry, stay up too late, get up too tired, read too little, watch TV too much, and pray too seldom.*
>
> *We have multiplied our possessions, but reduced our values. We talk too much, love too seldom, and hate too often.*
>
> *We've learned how to make a living, but not a life. We've added years to life not life to years.*[281]

George might perhaps turn to us, the audience, and in conclusion ask us to consider: Is there a "best *Diaita*?"

The answer is both yes and no. No, in the sense that there is not a strict list of "eat this, not that." There is not a single book of recipe wisdom to follow. There are no ten kitchen commandments to get us through the pearly gates.

The best diet is neither ascetic nor indulgent in practice. It is not exclusive or exclusionary in ingredients or methods. It does not merely navigate between extremes but transcends them as a comprehensive lifestyle approach.

It's a lifestyle based on local fresh agriculture, quality ingredients, recipes, cooking methods, and secrets passed from generation to generation, seasoned with a deep appreciation of the pleasure of authentic food, shared meals, and fellowship. The best diet is a kind of "diet of everything." Ken Wilber explains,

A "diet of everything" is just that: if we assume that all the world's cultures and cuisines have important but partial truths, then how would all of those truths fit together into a richly woven tapestry, a unity-in-diversity, a multicolored yet single rainbow? If we seek to have a truly integral view, we want to take the very best of the ancient wisdom and combine that with the very best of modernity.[282]

The alternative is a partial, fragmented, and often contradictory approach which can only yield partial, fragmented, and incomplete results.

The best diet is not a diet at all; it is an attitude. It is seasoned with a deep appreciation of the pleasure of real food rooted in Nature. It is an authentic experience and a sacred, sovereign life reclaimed from an addiction that only leads unto disability and disease; an addiction that is all too real, all too sad, and all too true. An addiction to despair, disease, and disability, that is the legacy of the Modern Western Diet.

It is never too late to change. That starts with a look deep inside ourselves for answers....

FIRE IN THE BELLY:
THE GUT MICROBIOME

"All disease begins in the gut."
—*Hippocrates*

There is an old proverb that states "The way to a man's heart is through his stomach." As was pointed out earlier, modern science has confirmed that applies to the fairer sex as well. In fact, within the last decade there is a rapidly growing body of evidence that disorders of the bowel are at the center of the explosion of the disabilities and diseases associated with the modern Western diet, including cardiovascular disease, which is the number one killer of both men and women in the United States and many other industrialized countries.[283]

As formerly mentioned, such disabilities and diseases can be defined in a broad sense as originating from an interaction between our genetics and our environment. For example, there are people who are born with a genetic variant of a certain enzyme known as a lipo-oxygenase. This enzyme is involved in the way we metabolize certain types of fats.

Omega-six fatty acids are a type of polyunsaturated fatty acid often found in liquid vegetable oils, like the commonly used safflower oil.

If these people with a genetic variant consume high amounts of omega-six fatty acids, they are susceptible to an inflammatory reaction that results in atherosclerosis of the carotid artery. These blockages in the carotid artery can cause a stroke. In contrast to the people with a genetic variant, those without the genetic variant do not significantly exhibit such pathology.[284, 285]

Foods like safflower oil are quite abundant in the modern Western diet and often come in hidden forms like mayonnaise, salad dressings, breads, and deep-fried foods. One can easily imagine two people living in the same house, eating the same regimen rich in commercial breads, salad dressings, deep-fried foods, and condiments like mayonnaise.

If one person has a genetic variant, it is perfectly plausible that based on their genetics one may suffer a stroke while the other does not. Conversely, both could consume a more balanced diet with significantly fewer omega-six polyunsaturated fatty acids, a diet that would likely be higher in the anti-inflammatory omega-3 polyunsaturated fatty acids. In this scenario, *neither* may develop any atherosclerotic disease that results in a stroke. It is the unfavorable environment, the diet, which unmasks the genetic susceptibility.

The short time period over which our diet has been altered from the Industrial Revolution to the present does not allow for genomic adaption. Many of the polymorphisms that are now associated with certain disease states have likely been part of the original human genome. For the most part the genes associated with the diseases of Western civilization do not manifest as such unless they are exposed to an unhealthy environment. It is perhaps more useful to view this genetic-environmental interplay as genes that will manifest in a negative environment. This seems to be a more accurate labeling than the current conventional approach which is to simply label these as *disease-causing* genes.

Such a label as *disease-causing* genes places all the responsibility in the hands of fate; that is the genetics with which we were born. Such labelling removes our power for change. While it is true that we may be born with certain vulnerabilities, it is our actions, our decisions to engage or not engage, that determine whether we manifest that destiny or forge a new one.

Short of ecological catastrophe, our diet is the most important environmental interaction we experience. We are quite literally bringing the outside environment into our own bodies several times a day, every day of our lives. As we ingest this food, the only thing running interference for us is the razor thin layer of wee beasties known as the gut microbiome or gut microbiota.

This gut flora that has coevolved to co-metabolize our food with us is a partnership that dates back millions of years. With our nuclear DNA changing at the rate of only about 0.5 percent per million years, our DNA is essentially unchanged from that of the first *Homo sapiens* that appeared over two hundred thousand years ago on the East African plains. A likely pivotal evolutionary moment in our gut microbiome partnership occurred even earlier with the development of fire and cookery, which occurred at least five hundred thousand years ago, though more likely originated at least one to two million years ago, if not further in the past.

Once the first chefs started slinging mastodon burgers around the campfire, the internal rules for breaking down food changed. Cooking now acted as the first part of digestion. Plant starches were much more easily broken down and the ability to chew and extract nutrients from meat was greatly enhanced. As Harvard Professor Richard Wrangham hypothesizes, at this point we may likely have adapted as a species to specifically metabolize *cooked* food.[286]

This strategy requires developing a commensal community of bacteria specifically geared to deal with the biochemical challenges of Maillard and caramelization reaction products. Compared to raw food, we can currently extract approximately sixteen times more energy from the same items when they are cooked. For some comestibles, the differences can be profound. We digest about 94 percent of the protein if an egg is cooked, but only 55 to 64 percent if it is consumed raw.[287]

Our wee minions help operate the machinery of the entire digestive process, not just feeding on our leftovers like a dog begging at the table as we thought for so long. The bacterial gut microbiome is a collection of characters that have gotten comfortable and efficient squatting in their long-term surroundings—our bodies. Over millions of years, these residents have gotten accustomed to a delivery service distributing a varied but naturally derived diet, including barbecue.

Although the existence of our indispensable internal minions may have eluded them, our ancestors were well aware that all things were connected, and a properly functioning digestive system was the key to health. In the ancient city of Ostia, the port city of Rome, there are the remains of what was once a communal lavatory. Still legibly inscribed upon one of the remaining walls is the Latin phrase: "*Amice fugit te proverbium Bene caca et irrima Medicos.*"[288] This loosely translates as "Buddy, don't you know the saying? Shit well and bugger the doctor!"

The microorganisms that inhabit our gastrointestinal tract exist from our oropharyngeal cavity to our anus; from pie hole to poop shoot. For the purposes of discussion will focus primarily on the bacteria that inhabit our intestine, and particularly the large intestine. Likewise, the types of microbes that comprise the microbiota include not only bacteria, but protozoa, yeast, fungi, and viruses. Again, for the purposes of discussion we will focus primarily on the bacteria. This is not to say that the other areas and other types of critters are not important, but in many cases we know significantly less about them than we do about the bacterial gut microbiome of the large intestine. One could define the sum total of that knowledge by saying we barely know the difference between our gut microbiome exit portal and a hole in the ground.

This remarkable collection of commensal organisms has evolved with us over the millennia as humankind has evolved. While the human body is composed of approximately ten trillion cells, the gut microbiome consists of approximately one hundred trillion cells. That means ninety percent of the cells that make up your body are not you. To give you an idea of the enormity of their foreign presence, consider the fact that there are approximately one thousand times more bacteria in your gut than there are stars in our galaxy. This does not even begin to account for the additional fungi, protozoa, and viruses that inhabit our inner nooks and crannies.

According to the Human Genome Project, you are composed of approximately twenty thousand five and hundred genes that make up our exclusively human genome. These are located within our human cells. This is what makes you a unique creature. Your accompanying gut microbiome contains well over a thousand different species that comprise the one hundred trillion bacteria present.

The human gut yields a bacterial metagenome of around 3.3 million bacterial genes, more than one hundred and fifty times larger than the human gene complement. It is now hypothesized that human beings could not even survive if it were not for the existence of our gut microbiome. There is more bacterial DNA in our metagenome (the DNA that includes everything inside us; our entire being) than human DNA. Although they only contribute about 1 to 3 percent of our body mass, about 1–2 kg of bacteria, they exert a powerful biological and physiological impact, along with generating approximately 30 percent of our daily energy.

Between populations, societies, and even between individuals there is variation in the gut microbiome. Diet, environment, host genetics, and early microbial exposure have all been implicated in the development of such diversity, yet much remains to be elucidated. What is apparent is that the human gastrointestinal tract, including the gut microbiome, is one of the most concentrated and complex ecosystems on the planet.

Since we cannot develop, function, or survive without our symbiotic organ, we have to re-examine the definition of ourselves; what it really means to be a human *being*. We are not an isolated organism, we are a supraorganism composed of our human cells and our minions, the human genome and the microbiome metagenome.[289] The human population is now being broadly classified into three entero-types by scientists according to the gut microbiome. We can be defined and grouped by our bacterial cohorts. Although each one of us remains singular, we are all, each one of us, bound together as a microcosm of Nature. Each one of us is a micro-ecosystem, not isolated and independent, but connected and interdependent.

Our petite partners produce vitamins we do not even possess the genes to make. They co-metabolize what we ingest and extract nutrients we need to survive. A healthy gut microbiome not only directs our immune system on how to recognize potential pathogens, but they even directly act to maintain our intestinal integrity. There is evidence they may produce anti-inflammatory compounds that have wide-reaching systemic effects.[290]

The entirety of these tiny beings is in constant communication with our gut, which functions like a second brain. But what we call second actually came first. It is argued that from an evolutionary perspective, our entire cerebral capacity developed with the sole purpose being to deliver more food to the lower brain.[291] There are direct neural connections between the brain and the gut via the vagus nerve. Our innards are wired with over two hundred million neurons belonging to the enteric nervous system. Ask any cat or dog owner if they consider their pet to be a sentient, intelligent creature. They will tell you more than you care to know about how their pet is just like a little person. Your gut contains the equivalent brainpower.

We now know that this communication between the brain and the gut is bidirectional. Previously it was thought that emotions originating in the brain would travel via the vagus and enteric nerves to influence the gut. It was viewed as a hierarchical, boss-drone, one-way type of relationship. It is now been shown that communication can originate in the gut and move via the bloodstream to affect the brain, predominately acting through the hypothalamus.

If the gut shares anatomic, neural similarities, to the brain it raises the question of whether some diseases can be "shared" disease states. In Parkinson's disease, digestive symptoms can predate neurological appearance by twenty years. New evidence suggests that Parkinson's disease may originate in the gut. In 2006 at the University of Nantes in France, biopsy of lesions in gut neurons revealed classic Parkinson's disease pathology identical to that found in brain neurons.[292]

Not only are the GI tract neurons similar to brain neurons—so are the neurotransmitters. There is tremendous communication that occurs through the release of hormones, neuropeptides, and neurotransmitters. Many of the neurotransmitters are the same but can have different effects depending on their location. Serotonin in the brain is associated with well-being and a happy mood. Serotonin in the gut relates to the transit time of food through the intestine, and is tasked with helping to set immune function.[293]

Such neurotransmitters can get there from here, from GI tract to brain. The gut microbiome communicates constantly with our gastrointestinal tract like a cell phone communicating via Wi-Fi. For example, the gut microbiome produces serotonin. In the gut, about 95 percent of the serotonin is associated with gastric transit. When bacteria in the gut secrete serotonin, they affect that transit time and nutritional parameters, as well as the immune status.

However, not all the serotonin stays within the gut. This bacterially produced serotonin can reach our brain. In the brain, that same serotonin is associated with the production of a positive mood and a sense of well-being. Thus, a truly happy belly does quite literally make us feel pleased.

By increasing serotonin and the delivery of other such compounds to the brain, bacteria influence a wide range of emotive states. Strictly speaking, due to the bidirectional capacity built into the system, the gut microbiome affects emotion and mood. Attention, concentration, happiness, anxiety, and depression are all affected by the gut. The gut is a contributor to the subconscious. The idea of a "gut feeling" takes on a whole new, an eerie inkling of subtle, outside, non-human influence when understood in this context.

Because the gut microbiome is not only populous, but active, it is powerfully wired into not only our central nervous system and the brain itself, but also into our immune system. As previously mentioned, bacterially produced serotonin is associated with determining the state of immune function. Within the immune system, the gut microbiota plays an important role in regulating the immune function of the entire body. Roughly 70 percent of the body's total immunity is located within the gastrointestinal tract, predominately within an area known as GALT, or gut associated lymphoid tissue. The GALT is among the largest reservoirs of infection fighting cells in the body.[294]

Quite simply, the gut microbiome functions in our body as an endocrine organ, every bit as essential as a thyroid, a pancreas, or a brain. The gut microbiota generates biologically active metabolites which are produced in response to specific dietary inputs. They elicit effects not only locally, but can act at a distant site within the host. It is just an endocrine organ that we rent; we don't own it nor is it completely within our charge.

However, there are distinct elements within our purview and over which we exhibit considerable influence. The current composition of the modern Western diet can alter our inner garden like a troupe of wandering orcs. Instead of healthy populations of bacteria that help protect us from disability and disease our inner Eden can come to resemble the plains of Mordor, "a barren wasteland, riddled with fire and ash and dust."[295]

Consuming a more natural diet, one that resembles the consumptive patterns of the pre-Industrial Revolution, can help prevent disease. It has been shown to aid in the prevention and treatment of osteoporosis, muscle wasting, kidney stones, hypertension, and asthma. It has been shown to retard the progression of age-related chronic renal insufficiency.[296, 297, 298, 299, 300, 301, 302, 303, 304, 305]

Injury to the gut microbiome and gastrointestinal lining can lead to detrimental changes that result in increased intestinal permeability and initiate an ongoing cycle of chronic, continuous low-grade chronic inflammation.[306, 307] Increased intestinal permeability is a condition where the normally tight seals between the cells that line the gut wall no longer perform that function. The entire gut becomes leaky and all manner of bacteria and toxins can enter the bloodstream and circulation. It's like leaving the Walmart doors unlocked on Black Friday.

An ever-growing number of studies have demonstrated that changes in the composition of our microbiome correlates with numerous disease states, raising the possibility that manipulation of these communities could be used to treat disease. This common inflammatory root is now connecting once disparate diseases. One such observation correlates low bacterial diversity in the gut to obesity and inflammatory bowel disease (IBD).[308]

Connections run deep. Recent evidence suggests that people who suffer from inflammatory bowel disease are more likely to have significant complications from a heart attack, including a significantly longer hospital stay. Indeed, merely the diagnosis of inflammatory bowel disease now confers additional risk for cardiovascular disease, and several different types of gastrointestinal cancer including certain kinds of lymphoma.[309, 310]

Irritable Bowel Syndrome (IBS) affects about 10 to 20 percent of the population worldwide, predominately in industrialized nations. It is associated with increased neuronal activity, often in response to stress. The symptoms of abdominal discomfort, irregular bowel movements, flatulence, and constipation or diarrhea that accompany IBS activate the brainstem, thalamus, insula cortex, anterior cingulate cortex, and the frontal cortex. There is no denying the gut-brain bidirectional connection.[311]

In patients suffering from IBS, there is dysregulation of the gut-brain axis. Research has also demonstrated a disorder of the gut microbiota in IBS. Although at this juncture a causal role cannot yet be confirmed, there are clear alterations in both community stability and diversity. Moreover, it has been reliably demonstrated that manipulation of the microbiota can influence the key symptoms, including abdominal pain and bowel habit, and other prominent features of IBS. Such research firmly establishes the gut microbiome as a critical node in the gut-brain axis and one which may be amenable to therapeutic interventions.[312]

Such chronic, continuous low-level inflammation originating in the gut is the mechanism by which disease with far more serious sequelae may manifest: atherosclerosis, diabetes, metabolic syndrome, rheumatoid arthritis, IBD, and other metabolic diseases and injuries are believed to potentially originate within the gut and involve the gut microbiota.[313, 314] These origins may hold clues in the prevention and treatment of certain malignancies. Research has demonstrated unique microbial signatures that correlate with different stages of esophageal cancer. The increased presence of *Fusiobacteria* species is associated with the development of colorectal cancer.[315]

Real world insights can be gleaned from the animal kingdom with stories that resemble *Tales from the Dark Side.* Toxoplasmosis is a parasitic organism that replicates only in the intestines of domestic cats. The new parasites are excreted in the feline feces where they can be communicated to a number of species including humans and rodents. However, what is fascinating is what happens when they are ingested by mice, a known prey animal of the domestic cat. What occurs is that the mice appear to lose all sense of fear. Some research actually suggests that the mice develop a sexual attraction to cats.

The consummation of such an exchange is that the mice are devoured. This of course brings the toxoplasmosis parasite back home to complete its circle of life and create another generation of miniature murine mind controllers.[316] While the behavior alterations have only been documented to occur in mice, this would explain a lot of crazy cat lady stories.

Work done by Professor Stephen Collins from McMaster University suggests that even a healthy, normal gut microbiome is influencing behavior. Germ-free mice are a type of research mouse that is born without a microbiome and is raised in a sterile environment so they are completely free of any commensal organisms. One of the interesting traits of these mice is that they exhibit abnormal behavior. Simply exposing these mice to a cocktail that allows them to generate a normal collection of gut microbiota changes their behavior profoundly. They now behave as completely normal mice.

Another breed of mouse, known as the Swiss mouse, has genetics which cause it to behave much more aggressively.

Add in a normal gut microbiome and the behavior becomes much less violent. Conversely, change the gut microbiome of the normally passive mice to that which is found in the Swiss mouse, and they become demonstrably more vicious.[317, 318]

There are even heftier implications than attitude alone when looking at the potential impact of the gut microbiome. As an example, the mice without a gut microbiome, germ free mice (GFM), are leaner than conventional, wild type (WT), mice when fed the same chow. In identical living conditions, with identical caloric expenditure, and eating the identical isocaloric chow, GFM are thinner.

WT mice can be made obese by feeding them the equivalent of the modern Western diet. Mice can also be genetically bred to develop obesity. Germ-free mice fed a Western diet (WD) have reduced adiposity compared to conventionally raised animals fed a WD, despite increased caloric consumption and decreased energy expenditure. Without a gut microbiome, GFM stay thin even eating a WD.

Given these findings, an ingenious experiment was devised (as shown in Figure 2). Germ-free mice which are naturally thinner than both obese- and wild-type mice were given fecal transplants. They were exposed to either the poop from normal WT mice or obese mice. This created two groups that differed only in the composition and character of the gut microbiome. What happened next was a "Holy Scheisse!" moment. The GFM colonized with the gut microbiome of the WT mice achieved a normal weight. The GFM colonized with the gut microbiome of the obese mice gained twice the body weight.

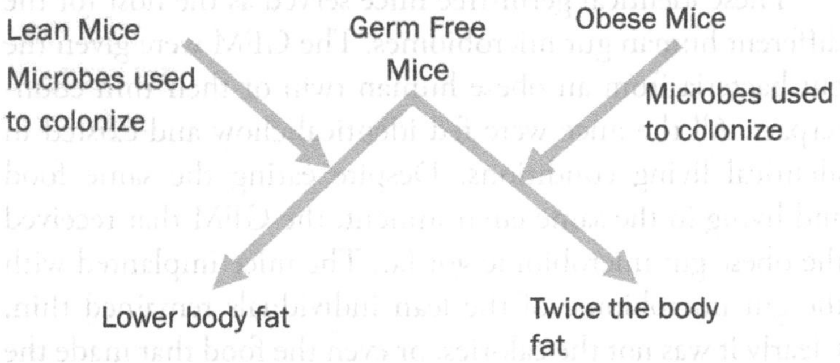

Lean Mice   Germ Free   Obese Mice

Microbes used   Mice
to colonize   Microbes used
                                              to colonize

Lower body fat   Twice the body
                                              fat

Figure 2

The obese mice, whether by diet (WD) or genetics, can transfer obesity to germ free mice through their poop.[319, 320] After colonization of germ-free mice with fecal content from conventional mice (WT), the originally germ-free mice rapidly gain weight and increase fat mass without any change in caloric ingestion. Such a phenomenon suggests crosstalk between the gut microbiota and host tissue homeostasis. Critically, this demonstrates the gut microbial ecosystem is transmissible.[321] As further verification, additional research has shown that gut bacteria can activate a mouse gene that burns fat.[322] The bacteria of the gut microbiome have the ability to turn on and turn off host genes.

These effects are not limited to rodents. Microbiota were obtained from four sets of identical twins. Because they are identical, the twins have the same genome; they are genetically identical. However, for this experiment identical twins were chosen that were phenotypically very different. One twin was normal weight and the other twin was obese. Since they are omnivores like us, the intestines of mice can readily support a human gut microbiome.

These identical germ-free mice served as the host for the different human gut microbiomes. The GFM were given the gut bacteria from an obese human twin or their thin counterpart. All the mice were fed identical chow and existed in identical living conditions. Despite eating the same food and living in the same environment, the GFM that received the obese gut microbiome got fat. The mice implanted with the gut microbiome of the lean individuals remained thin. Clearly it was not the calories, or even the food that made the mice fat or lean. It was the composition of the bacteria that grew in their gut.[323] (See appendix C1)

That would be scale-shattering if the story ended there, but it doesn't. Since mice have the useful laboratory trait of coprophagia—they like to eat each other's poo—the researchers put all the mice together. After a short time, all the mice shared the same gut microbiome. All the mice now exhibited a normal weight. Obesity was reversed by changing the gut flora. That is one golden colon.[324] (See appendix C2)

Much of the previous dogma regarding food, health, and nutrition that was felt to be set in stone is beginning to crumble like Ozymandias.[325] This even applies to the belief that obesity is simply more calories in then out. It is clearly a combination of genetics, behavior, the gut microbiome, and the quality and character of the foods we eat. It is not just calories, if it ever truly was.

Development of the inflammatory disease Type II diabetes mellitus (T2DM) is associated with the obesity seen in the mouse and twin experiments. Specific gut bacterial anomalies have been observed in patients with T2DM. *Faecalibacterium prausnitzii* (*F. prausnitzii*) is one of the most abundant types of bacterium in the human gut microbiota, comprising over 5 percent of the total population. These bacteria mainly produce butyrate and other short-chain fatty acids through the fermentation of dietary fiber. (See appendix C3)

T2DM is associated with gut dysbiosis and a reduction of *F. prausnitzii*. The characteristics of the T2DM gut microbiome are an increased level of bacteria involved in sulphate reduction, decreased resistance against oxidative stress, and a decrease in butyrate-producing bacteria compared to those of euglycemic individuals.

But since nature abhors a vacuum, less of one bacteria means more of another. In patients with T2DM there is an increase in *Proteobacteria*. An experiment with human volunteers that mimicked the mouse/twin experiment gave participants with T2DM a poop transfer from themselves or healthy subjects. After six weeks, those receiving trans-fecal transference from healthy folks had improved hepatic and peripheral insulin sensitivity by 119 percent and 176 percent, respectively. [326] This was accompanied by an increase in the butyrate-producing bacteria, such as *Roseburia*. [327] (See appendix C4)

At the complete other end of the spectrum is the iatrogenic (Latin for *your doctor did this to you*) condition of hospital acquired, antibiotic resistant diarrhea. Hospital acquired infections with the bacteria known as *Clostridium difficile* can be extremely hard to eradicate and is recurrent in up to 30 percent of patients. In severe cases, the infection can be life-threatening. Poo-power has been known in medical circles as the ultimate colonic tonic for many years. First used in the 1950s and then relatively reserved for the most severe and refractory cases, fecal microbiota transplantation (FMT) is quickly becoming a frontline therapy due to its over 90 percent initial success rate. [328] (See appendix C5)

Bacteria may not only serve as a cure, but may serve as a warning indicator as well. The products produced by certain gut bacteria have been shown to predict the risk of cardiovascular disease in humans.[329] When the atherosclerotic, cholesterol rich plaques associated with cardiovascular disease were examined, they were found to contain the DNA from gut bacteria. There was a direct correlation between the amount of inflammation and the amount of bacterial DNA in the plaque.[330] (See appendix C6)

Certain measurable bacterial products like Trimethylamine N-oxide (TMAO) are associated with increased CV risk. TMAO is derived from the gut microbiota. It is associated with poor cardiovascular outcomes in patients with cardiovascular disease. It is elevated in patients with chronic kidney disease (CKD), and T2DM. Increased levels of TMAO are correlated with the development of atherosclerosis, progression of heart failure, and increased early mortality.

Trimethylamine N-oxide is produced from the metabolism of dietary betaine, choline, carnitine, and phosphatidylcholine by commensal microbes.[331] Some of the most common dietary sources of phosphatidylcholine are meat, eggs, and fish. Betaine is found in wheat, shellfish, spinach, and beets.[332] These dietary constituents are hydrolyzed by trimethylamine lyase into tri-methylamine (TMA) by certain bacteria.

The TMA produced by the bacteria are then released into the bloodstream where they make their way to the liver. In the human liver, the enzyme flavin monooxygenase-3 (FMO3) converts TMA into circulating TMAO. (See appendix C7)

It is hypothesized that this compound can cause macrophages, normal infection fighting white blood cells, to form foam cells. Foam cells are one of the earliest markers and initiators of atherosclerotic disease. These macrophages ingest the oxidized LDL cholesterol in the walls of the arteries where they swell like an angry puffer fish. Here they become known as foam cells and are believed to instigate the inflammatory reaction that ultimately leads to cardiovascular atherosclerotic disease.

In one study, those with the highest levels of TMAO had over two and a half times the likelihood of having a serious cardiovascular event over a three-year period when compared to those with the lowest levels.[333] These increased TMAO concentrations were associated with not only an increased risk of major adverse cardiovascular events, but for increased risk of early death, even after adjustment for traditional cardiovascular risk factors.[334] (See appendix C8)

High concentrations of choline or betaine, which are dietary sources of TMAO, are associated with increased major adverse cardiac events, even after accounting for traditional cardiovascular risk factors, such as smoking, age, hypertension, dyslipidemia, and T2DM. However, this *only* applies when the TMAO levels are also elevated.

L-carnitine is another compound that can produce TMA. It is found in meat, poultry, and fish, although the concentration in red meat is significantly higher than other sources. It induces TMA production via the same pathways as phosphatidylcholine, and is associated with an increased risk of CVD and major adverse cardiac events. Modifications to the microbiota composition have been observed in mice and humans following L-carnitine supplementation. (See appendix C9)

This would seem to indicate a detrimental effect of L-carnitine consumption. But L-carnitine has multiple pathways and pleiotropic effects. It helps the body produce energy and is important for heart and brain function, muscle movement, and many other body processes. Clinical studies have observed that the results of consuming L-carnitine are the exact *opposite* of what one would expect based *only* on the potential TMAO effect. A meta-analysis of thirteen controlled trials indicated that L-carnitine supplementation after acute myocardial infarction compared to placebo treatment was associated with 27 percent reduction in all-cause mortality, 65 percent reduction in ventricular arrhythmias, and 40 percent reduction in symptoms of angina.[335] (See appendix C10)

When it comes to food, us, and the trillions of microorganisms indigenous to our gut, it is complicated to say the least. These microbes can express enzymes capable of interacting and interfering with the nutritional and pharmaceutical pathways of what we consume, ultimately impacting on their bioactivity. What we consume also impacts them. These microbial communities respond directly to the nutritional and pharmaceutical environment with which their host provides them. It is this synergy that largely dictates the ultimate hormonal and inflammatory tones.

As previously discussed in detail in *Ancient Eats*, the major interventions that have resulted in an overall increase in average life expectancy have been improvements in engineering and sanitation, reductions in childbirth mortality, childhood diseases, and infections, and success in mitigating the effects of disasters like droughts and famines.[336] It has not been, to a large extent, interventions that directly improve us. The maximum human life expectancy is little changed from the time of our most distant forebears.

When we consume certain foods, like those of the modern Western diet, we can negatively impact the character of the gut microbiome. We decrease the variety and number of beneficial bacteria and open the door for the influx of far less desirable players. In a recent study looking at human volunteers, a single typical fast food breakfast sandwich negatively altered the gut microbiome for several days.[337] These types of damaging alterations have been implicated in the development of obesity and in the possible modulation of human lipid metabolism itself.[338, 339]

Often underappreciated, and essentially unrecognized until recently, was the potential effect of the gut microbiome on nutraceuticals and pharmaceuticals. A review reportedly identified thirty common drugs which were open to metabolism by bacterial enzymes, through proteolysis, reduction, dehydroxylation, hydrolysis, and other reactions. It cuts both ways: drugs can impact the gut microbiome.[340]

Simvastatin (a kind of statin medication) is an example of such a drug which modulates gut microbiota composition. Interestingly, it appears the efficacy of such drugs may depend upon their ability to favorably alter the microbiome. Simvastatin has been shown to boost *Lactobacillus* populations.[341, 342] While clinical studies with simvastatin (Zocor) showed a reduction in adverse cardiovascular events, there was no demonstrable attenuation effect on atherogenic plaque development.[343] That is, the likelihood of a heart attack decreased but the blockages remained the same size, suggesting an anti-inflammatory mechanism.

Strong evidence continues to accumulate indicating that gut microbiota has the potential to modify, or be modified by, the drugs and nutritional interventions that we rely upon.[344] Plant sterol esters (PSE) in a mouse model have been shown to dampen the microbial production of TMA, the precursor to proatherogenic TMAO. (See appendix C11)

Oat β-glucan (OBG), the fiber found in oats, and the drug atorvastatin, a statin pharmaceutical known as Lipitor, were studied in the same experiment. OBG is a soluble dietary fiber that is found in the endosperm cell walls of oats, and is highly regarded due to its cholesterol-lowering properties. It is how the AHA justifies a heart healthy stamp of approval on breakfast cereals loaded with sugar and other additives.

Both the PSE and OBG reduced aortic plaque percentage. In other words, consuming certain plants or fiber reduced the likelihood of developing arterial blockages, but the statin did not. However, all three appeared to favorably alter the gut microbiome and enhance the production of certain short chain fatty acids (SCFAs)[345, 346, 347] (See appendix C12)

Metformin is another common pharmaceutical, widely used to treat T2DM. It is regarded as an insulin sensitizing agent. Its administration is associated with increased the levels of *Akkermansia muciniphila* (*A. muciniphila*). The increased levels of *A. muciniphila* are associated with an improved glycemic profile, and an increased number of mucin-producing intestinal goblet cells in mice fed a Western diet. (See appendix C13)

In a revealing insight into the power of our minions, oral gavage of *A. muciniphila* alone was able to recreate the beneficial effects of metformin on the glycemic profile and number of goblet cells. Administration of both metformin and *A. muciniphila* by oral gavage induced beneficial modifications on visceral adipose tissue inflammatory tone. It controlled blood sugars and addressed belly fat. These findings suggest a link between the gut microbiota and host metabolic biology and a role for the gut microbiota in the etiology, prevention, and treatment of insulin resistance and T2DM.[348]

Altered composition of the gut microbiota is associated with overweight and obese populations. In these populations, changes in the gut microbiome parallel weight-loss, which is known to improve cardiometabolic risk. Individuals from populations in Denmark and France who had low microbiota richness and a disturbed metabolic profile, including insulin-resistance, dyslipidemia, and systemic and adipose tissue inflammation were examined.[349]

Unsurprisingly, those individuals with high levels of *A. muciniphila* had a better metabolic profile with improved insulin sensitivity, less dyslipidemia, and better metabolic outcomes upon weight loss intervention compared to those with lower levels of *A. muciniphila*.[350] It is not only quantity, but quality that is important. (See appendix C14)

It is exactly like the considerations we make when we choose our food. Our inner world reflects what we populate it with from the external environment. Character counts for a lot; as without, so within. This is the Food Shaman working and functioning within the natural order of things.

Science agrees it is likely that such functional food ingredients act through manipulation of the indigenous microbiome.[351]

The disabilities and diseases associated with the MWD are increasingly being revealed not to be simple, single insults like a laceration, but complex multisystem disorders. Congestive heart failure (CHF) is just such a pathology. There are changes in intestinal morphology, permeability, and adsorption. There are alterations to the bacterial biofilm. These are potential contributors to chronic inflammation and malnutrition. CHF involves cardiovascular, musculoskeletal, neuroendocrine, metabolic, and immune systems.

A hallmark of CHF is increased chronic inflammation, reflected in increased levels of cytokines like TNF-α. The entire nervous system is amped up and there is increased sympathetic activity. Increased sympathetic activity means decreased parasympathetic activity, and this directly involves the gut and therefore affects the gut microbiome.

There is increased intestinal permeability. The normal structures in the gut are damaged in CHF. The bowel thickness in CHF correlates to leukocyte or white blood cell counts. Similar to IBD patients, there are changes to the mucosal bacteria such as an increase in adherent invasive *E.coli* strains. (See appendix C15)

It appears that the pathogenesis of systemic inflammation seen in CHF follows the pathway for many of the modern disabilities and diseases we confront. The experimental evidence suggests bacterial translocation from gut to bloodstream triggers body-wide inflammation. CHF patients have substantial quantities of pathogenic bacteria compared to controls. These bacteria include the pathogens *Candida* (fungal), *Campylobacter, Shigella, Salmonella,* and *Yersinia enterocolitica.* The bacterial changes correlated with markers of disease severity, increased markers of intestinal permeability (IP), right atrial pressure (RAP), and inflammation as measured by C-reactive protein (CRP).[352]

Such bacterial changes may result in the development of a chronic, continuous, pro-inflammatory state. The pro-inflammatory state exerts its effects both locally and systemically. A negative cyclic feedback ensues with increasing inflammation fueling hyperadrenergic responses. Cardiac depression may occur not because there are any blockages in the heart arteries, but as a direct result of toxins and cytokines.[353]

Such metabolites that are derived from the gut microbiota, like trimethylamine N-oxide (TMAO), are associated with poor cardiovascular outcomes in patients with cardiovascular disease. However, TMAO is also increased in patients with chronic kidney disease (CKD) before hemodialysis, and notably, it decreases after kidney transplantation.

A link between dietary choline exposure, systemic TMAO concentrations, CVD, and CKD has been demonstrated in humans and mice. TMAO is cleared by the kidney, and levels are therefore increased in patients with CKD compared to levels in healthy controls. Increased levels of TMAO have been shown to be predictive of an increased risk of all-cause mortality in patients with CKD as well as those with CVD.[354]

CKD belongs to a family of diseases collectively known as cardiometabolic diseases (CMDs). These are chronic coronary associated diseases. CMDs include obesity, metabolic syndrome, type 2 diabetes mellitus (T2DM), cardiovascular disease (CVD), and chronic kidney disease (CKD).

CMDs have been associated with changes in the composition of the gut microbiota. Patients with CMDs frequently exhibit enrichment or depletion of certain bacterial groups in their resident microbiota compared to healthy individuals. This microbial imbalance results in a CMD-associated dysbiosis.

Marked differences in the composition of the microbiota were found between the microbiota of healthy controls and those of patients with critical CKD or end-stage renal disease (ESRD).[355] This is a huge healthcare problem not only for the vast number of patients, but the global financial burden of CMDs is estimated cost over 12.5 trillion dollars by 2030.[356] (See appendix C16)

Previous discussion detailed how certain bacteria in the gut transform some of the foods we eat into a compound called tri-methylamine (TMA). *Proteus mirabilis*, a particular human commensal organism, is one of the bacterium known to cleave choline to produce TMA. Betaine is processed by the gut microbiome and can yield TMA.[357] TMA, in and of itself, is of little consequence until it is transformed in the liver to tri-methylamine N-oxide (TMAO). This occurs not only in humans, but also in mice, which makes them a convenient surrogate in the lab.[358]

So what is the typical Western solution to approaching this problem?

Simply make a drug that blocks our liver from converting TMA to TMAO. This might seem analogous to the popular statin drugs, which inhibit an enzyme and prevent cholesterol formation in the liver. However, like we are coming to expect from food and the gut microbiome, it is more complicated. Inhibition of the major enzyme involved in this process, hepatic flavin mono-oxygenase 3 (FMO3), does in fact reduce TMAO levels and atherosclerosis in mouse models.

However, it can cause hepatic inflammation, or hepatitis. This is a nasty side effect. Another side effect is observable in people with a genetic defect in FMO3, which prevents their livers from making TMAO. The side effects are pungently clear, the build-up in their bodies of trimethylamine makes them smell like three-day old fish.[359] This is the cause of the clinical condition known as fish-odor syndrome,[360] or as seen on *Bob's Burgers*, Mr. Calvin Fischoeder.

Instead of aiming at blocking our natural pathways, some smart scientists looked at targeting the bacteria by using a compound that is naturally found in food. A potent phytochemical was identified that occurs in some balsamic vinegars, some cold first pressed virgin olive oil, grapeseed oil, and red wines.[361]

It is likely no small coincidence that such foods are frequently encountered in the Mediterranean diet. The Mediterranean dietary approach with its emphasis on fresh, wholesome, authentic foods, continually shows the power of dietary choices in preventing, treating, and even reversing the curse of the modern Western diet. This particular substance, 3,3-dimethyl-1-butanol (DMB), acts as an antagonist to the naturally occurring substrate for the production of TMAO, choline.

DMB acts as a competitive inhibitor to choline. This suppresses TMA production with a subsequent decrease in TMAO accumulation and its effects. All this occurs without any changes in blood lipid levels. There is no impact on LDL or HDL cholesterol. Studies in humans demonstrated that some, but not all, TMA production is inhibited.[362]

The use of DMB in a mouse model significantly reduced aortic atherosclerotic lesions by working on this pathway. DMB lowered plasma levels of TMAO. DMB only worked when administered orally. If administered subcutaneously or by an intraperitoneal route it was ineffective. This strongly suggests that the pathway *must* include the gut microbiome for measurable effect. (See appendix C17)

Impressively, the aortic lesions showed significantly less foam cell formation and reduction of aortic atherosclerosis with DMB. As mentioned, this occurred without impacting blood lipid levels. Consuming the natural product DMB reduced artery blockages without changing blood cholesterol levels at all.[363]

The gut microbiota not only metabolizes ingested food, but is itself shaped by the mode of food consumption and the general environment. Differences in microbiota composition at the phylum level have been identified between populations residing in different geographic regions.[364]

Higher abundance of *Bacteroidetes* and a decreased abundance of *Firmicutes* and *Proteobacteria* were observed in African children compared to children living in Western Europe. The bacteria found in African children were more efficient at metabolizing fiber and could subsequently produce greater amounts of SCFAs.

The increased consumption of carbohydrates and fiber in the African diet might explain these differences and promote richness and diversity of gut microbiota. Differences in the richness of gut microbiota have been observed between American, Malawi, and American-Indian populations.[365, 366]

The healthy diet of other food cultures is associated with increased microbiota diversity whereas the MWD is associated with reduced microbiota diversity. The lack of microbial diversity in our gut tracks potently with other markers of health and disease.[367] The lack of diversity is specifically associated with reduced levels of *Faecalibacterium spp.* and worse systemic inflammation, compared to individuals with greater diversity.[368] (See appendix C18)

The ideas and discoveries surrounding the gut microbiome have yielded new concepts. It has been proposed that there is a continuum or gradient of bacterial species with functional properties rather than discontinuous segregated enterotypes. This composition of the microbiota is quite resilient over an individual's life span. Variations as a result of dietary modification may be observed at finer taxonomic levels for specific phylotypes such as *Roseburia spp.* and *Eubacterium rectale*, which are known to have a role in the digestion of dietary carbohydrates. Even with acute insults of dietary discretion, balance can be restored relatively quickly. Nevertheless, prolonged abuse can lead to the development of the disabilities and diseases associated with the MWD and irreparable harm. (See appendix C19)

The development of these maladies is portended by a measurable effect after eating a meal known as post-prandial dietary endotoxemia. Dietary or metabolic endotoxemia occurs when one's dietary consumption causes disruption in either GI permeability, the microbiota profile, or both. Levels of bacterial endotoxin, or LPS, can be measured in the blood.

Bacterial lipopolysaccharides (LPS) are the major outer surface membrane components present in almost all gram-negative bacteria. They are extremely strong stimulators of innate or natural immunity in humans. They are the endotoxins connected to the severe health consequences associated with gram negative bacterial sepsis. (See appendix C20)

In small doses, they trigger numerous physiological, beneficial immunostimulatory effects in mammalian organisms. In higher doses, they lead to pathological reactions such as septic shock and potentially death.[369] It is that medical truism once again; the poison is in the dose. When you eat the SAD, your body (and gut microbiome) gets mad. You agitate your gut microbiome and crank up the immune system.

Turns out, you don't need much. A study looked at fast food industrial pizza consumption on otherwise healthy college age volunteers. Markers of inflammation were measured including bacterial endotoxin, triglycerides, IL-12, IL-1β, IL-6, MCP-1, and ghrelin. In roughly 50 percent of those studied labeled "responders," there was a 500 percent increase in inflammatory markers after one meal.[370]

Part of the obesity seen with consumption of the MWD is associated with such a gut bacteria change. Human observational studies have suggested that abdominal obesity is associated with increased visceral permeability.[371] Bacterial translocation in the blood is increased at the onset of WD. As soon as mice are fed a WD, bacteria and bacterial products rise in the circulating blood, meaning the inflammatory instigators are deploying throughout the organism. This is followed shortly thereafter with insulin resistance. (See appendix C21)

The essential role played by the gut microbiome is clearly demarcated when antibiotics are administered. In genetically obese mice and mice fed a WD like the aforementioned, antibiotics that affect both metabolic endotoxemia and gut microbiota composition improve insulin resistance, decrease systemic inflammation, and reduce weight gain. Metabolic alteration induced by a WD involve a disruption of the gut barrier, as demonstrated by increased intestinal permeability in the mice, which can be reversed in part by antibiotic treatment, although the direct effects of antibiotics on the host cannot be excluded.[372]

This type of data suggests we can modify the gut microbiome with antibiotics or probiotics. The pathways are difficult to define because of the complexity of the living system. The previous methods used by nutritionists and researchers to discern effects, the method of investigating one action from one molecule, is impossible.

The living system is an organism defined by events in which the components cannot be viewed in isolation. All is interwoven, all is relational. We can describe this relation with the very words used to describe the universe: it "is a network of granular events. The dynamic that connects them is probabilistic; between one event and another, space, time, matter, and energy melt into a cloud of probability."[373]

That does not mean we cannot shift the probabilities in our favor. One potential area of positive intervention is in the emerging science of probiotics. Probiotics are collections of presumed beneficial gut bacteria. The idea is that by ingesting them we can help maintain a healthy composition within our gut microbiome and thus a healthy gut.

Preliminary studies in certain conditions have shown significant benefit. In the study of college students, those "responders" were then randomized to a probiotic or placebo. Thirty days of probiotic treatment reduced (but did not eliminate) the endotoxin response to such foods by 42 percent. The placebo group had a 36 percent *increase* over the same time period.[374]

However, since many preparations vary by bacterial species, bioavailability, and counts, it is extremely important to research individual brands in consideration of taking these formulations. Even when taking probiotics, it is important to consume healthful foods so that your inner garden can continue to grow. Like sea monkeys, once you have the wee beasties, you have to feed them. Foods that help maintain a healthy gut microbiome are known as prebiotics. There are available options that package both together, these are known as synbiotics.

Prebiotics modify the gut microbiota composition and subsequently host biology by selectively stimulating the growth and/or activity of a number of helpful bacteria. Obese mice treated with prebiotics displayed reduced metabolic endotoxemia, lower fasting glucose levels, reduced insulin-resistance, decreased fat mass, increased fat-free mass, and improved intestinal permeability and integrity compared to untreated obese mice.[375]

A shift in the microbiota composition was observed in the animals that received prebiotics, and this shift was associated with an improved metabolic phenotype. An increase in *Bacteroidetes* and a decrease in *Firmicutes* was observed at the phylum level. An increase in the abundance of *Akkermansia muciniphila* was noted at the species level.

When *A. muciniphila* was added as a probiotic to mice receiving a WD, the mice were protected from developing insulin resistance, had reduced metabolic endotoxemia, reduced adipose tissue, and less inflammation. Their guts were less leaky as reflected by improvements in gut integrity compared to those fed a WD without added *A. muciniphila*. Heat-killed *A. muciniphila* was inefficient in eliciting these protective effects. This intimates that it is the *living* bacteria that are necessary. (See appendix C22)

A study performed on infants born with cyanotic congenital heart disease demonstrates the incredibly powerful systemic effects of a healthy gut microbiome and the potential power of probiotics. These babies are born with life-threatening heart defects and require complex and immediate surgery. As a result, they suffer a high mortality rate from a number of complications.

A group of these high-risk babies was given a specified probiotic cocktail. Those who received the beneficial gut bacteria had an over 35 percent reduction in death.[376] A healthy gut with a healthy gut microbiome helped more of these critically ill infants survive even when the cause of their high mortality was critical heart disease and operative stress.

At variance, the SAD is known to have detrimental effects on cognition and the gut microbiota. A rat study investigated whether a probiotic could prevent diet-induced memory deficits. As expected, gut microbial diversity was dramatically decreased by a WD. For the rats consuming a WD, probiotics were shown to be beneficial in situations of gut dysbiosis associated memory deficits. With probiotic administration, affected brain areas recovered normal function.[377] When you affect the brain, you affect emotional state. In humans, probiotics delivered in the form of yogurt have reduced environmental stress in women.[378] (See appendix C23)

There are many things in our daily lives that can put us off kilter emotionally, physically, and spiritually. The food we eat should return us in power to our center. Stress, antibiotics, and particularly poor food choices can all cause unwanted changes in the character and composition of our gut microbiome. As mentioned, a study demonstrated that a *single* typical fast food breakfast sandwich can cause an alteration of the healthy bacteria in your gut that can last for almost a week.[379] Such artificial and highly processed foods are relatively new additions to our diet. The effects of these comestibles appear to be universally unfavorable.

Recent studies performed over the last five years have demonstrated that certain processed, ultra-processed foods, and additives, while they may not affect human cells directly, can have profound effects on the bacteria within us. Unfortunately, it appears the majority of such effects are detrimental.

An example briefly mentioned earlier includes certain types of zero calorie artificial sweeteners. These compounds are not absorbed or processed by our human gastrointestinal tract. Thus, in theory, since they would pass through our bowels unabsorbed and unaltered they would add sweetness but no caloric value. It turns out that the Law of Unintended Consequences is everywhere, even inside of us.

A majority of these compounds have not been tested, but instead are released under what is known as GRAS—the Generally Recognized As Safe program. As per the FDA:

> *The GRAS notification program provides a voluntary mechanism whereby a person may inform FDA of a determination that the use of a substance is GRAS, rather than petition FDA to affirm that the use of a substance is GRAS...For a substance to be GRAS, the scientific data and information about the use of a substance must be widely known and there must be a consensus among qualified experts that those data and infor-*

mation establish that the substance is safe under the conditions of its intended use.[380]

There are over ten thousand food additives currently in use, with a majority of them released under the GRAS program which has been around since 1958. "We simply do not have the information to vouch for the safety of many of these chemicals," Michael Taylor, former FDA deputy commissioner for foods, admitted.[381]

The regular, long-term consumption of the aforesaid low or zero calorie sweeteners can adversely influence the gut microbiota in susceptible individuals and lead to insulin resistance and T2DM. This disruption predisposes to the development of obesity. Low-calorie or zero calorie artificial sweeteners like sucralose, aspartame, and saccharin disrupt the balance and diversity of gut microbiota. Fecal transplant experiments, wherein microbiota from low calorie sweetener consuming hosts are transferred into germ-free mice, show that this disruption is transferable and results in impaired glucose tolerance, a well-known risk factor toward the development of a number of metabolic disease states.[382]

Other types of additives like dietary emulsifiers impact the mouse gut microbiota, promoting colitis and metabolic syndrome. A primary means by which the human intestine is protected from environmental dangers is via multi-layered mucus structures that cover the intestinal surface. This forms a "safe zone," keeping bacteria at a safe distance from epithelial cells that line the intestine. Thus, anything that disrupts this mucus "no-go zone" has the potential to promote dysfunction and subsequent dysbiosis associated with gut inflammation.

Emulsifiers are chemically similar to detergent. They bring compounds which may not normally combine, like oil and water, together into a suspended and dispersed state.

Emulsifiers are ubiquitous components of processed and ultra-processed foods and have been demonstrated to increase bacterial translocation across epithelia *in vitro*.

This raises the concern that such common and widely used additives may be actively contributing to the increase in inflammatory bowel disease observed since the mid-twentieth century. A study with mice was performed using common emulsifiers at relatively low concentrations. Two commonly used emulsifiers, carboxymethylcellulose and polysorbate-80, did in fact induce intestinal inflammation and initiate obesity and metabolic syndrome in mice. In susceptible mouse strains, severe colitis was precipitated.

Emulsifier-induced metabolic syndrome was associated with microbiota encroachment, altered species composition, and inflammation. These studies continue to accrue evidence that ongoing continuous, chronic low-grade inflammation initiates adiposity and metabolic syndrome with all its attendant sequelae. Moreover, it is possible that specific components of the MWD such as emulsifying agents might be contributing to an increased incidence of diverse and widespread chronic inflammatory diseases.[383]

Recent research has shown that "consumption of commonly used GRAS formulations drives the development of glucose intolerance through induction of compositional and functional alterations to the intestinal microbiota."[384] In other words, what was billed as inert apparently alters the very fibers of our being. Add to this that such compounds are among the most widely used food additives worldwide, and the magnitude of the issue becomes immediately apparent.

In examining the gut microbiome in its entirety as well as in the details of bacterial components, diseases like obesity, once attributed to poor willpower, simple overconsumption, and laziness, now begin to fit Koch's postulates for infectious disease:

- the microorganism or other pathogen must be present in all cases of the disease
- the pathogen can be isolated from the diseased host and grown in pure culture
- the pathogen from the pure culture must cause the disease when inoculated into a healthy, susceptible laboratory animal
- the pathogen must be re-isolated from the new host and shown to be the same as the originally inoculated pathogen.

Disability and disease develop or do not as a result of the interplay between our genetics and our environment. As we age, our environment can exert an ever-increasing impact. Our individual gut microbiome is arguably the most intimate, important, and influential interface between ourselves and the environment. Although for many years the gut microbiome received little or no recognition for its contribution to the efficacy of certain functional food ingredients, we are now beginning to appreciate its true influence.[385]

Our diet is the single most important determinant in the composition of our intestinal microbiota. They may be the single most important determinant in how our genetics are ultimately expressed within the environment in which we live.

Therefore, it is essential to maintain a healthy gut microbiome. A healthy functioning gut microbiome helps keep our immune system in perfect balance. Our wellbeing is not an isolated endeavor, nor a completely genetically prescribed phenomenon. We are fundamentally and critically dependent on our gut microbiome. They in turn are dependent upon what internal environment we create for them. The cornerstone of our internal environment is the food we choose to eat. A proper diet leads to internal balance, harmony, and health, both figuratively and literally. The Food Shaman first masters the internal. As within, so without.

Our inner gut microbiome is not unlike growing a garden outside. When we consume the foods of the modern Western diet we change our inner soil from a rich patch of heartland loam into a homestead at Fukushima. Yet for all the potentially dismal news, there is hope. This new knowledge can help us appreciate what our ancestors understood intuitively. Because we understand with the power of modern science, we open the door for scenarios of effective disease prevention through targeting the intestine by means of diet, probiotics, prebiotics, antibiotics, or even transplantation of gut microbes.[386]

The fact remains that we still have choice in what we choose to consume. For now.

All things are connected. This is becoming evident through new information about the gut microbiome and overall health. The ancients recognized that, "As above, so below; as outside, so inside." In the ecosystem that is us, there is continuity, and no separation of biological activity. We are like a wave on the ocean, a continuum of being. The gut microbiome is in a very real sense the living link to our "ancestors'" they are that remnant and connection to who and what we were and what and how we are. The human gut is among the most concentrated and complex ecosystems on the planet. We are not alone, and we need not look to the stars for company. The stuff of stars, Nature, dwells within us.

DOUBLE, DOUBLE, TOIL AND TROUBLE: UNDERSTANDING FOOD CHOICES

"Fillet of a fenny snake,
In the caldron boil and bake;
Eye of newt, and toe of frog,
Wool of bat, and tongue of dog,
Adder's fork, and blind-worm's sting,
Lizard's leg, and owlet's wing,—
For a charm of powerful trouble,
Like a hell-broth boil and bubble."
—*Shakespeare, Macbeth Act 4, scene 1, 13-20*

Food Value: Quality versus Quantity

How do we determine the value of food?

What is and wherein lies the true meaning of the food experience?

Are our measures all wrong?

When we make the choice to buy or not to buy something, we are inherently making a value determination. Is what I am exchanging my money for worth the cost? Is the value of what I am receiving in the transaction worth what I must sacrifice?

We utilize the exact same algorithm when we decide to consume an item or to take a pass.

Yet, when we look at how the experts confer food value for us, we often find that the emphasis solely on certain variables, or the complete exclusion of others, leaves us hungering for more. In our modern Western culture, serious discussion of food value tends to be defined solely by the nutritional sustenance that it provides. The worth of a particular comestible becomes nothing more than the aggregate of the various proteins, carbohydrates, fats, vitamins, minerals, and other necessities required to keep the human machine comfortably cruising along at the frenetic pace that is our modern society.

In the current scientific and medical analysis, this is the "food as fuel" approach. It reflects the prevailing attitude and forms the basis of current conventional wisdom. Its practice predominates and colors perceptions in both approach and recommendation. The result is a rather bland and sterile dissection, narrowly focused, and by its very nature objectively isolationist in its concern.

At the complete other end of the spectrum, others might argue that the value of food lies in the social aspects and individual interactions. As usual, the inimitable Tony Bourdain sums up this position quite succinctly in his debate with Alice Waters. She discusses her health concerns regarding consumption of industrial sausage. Bourdain returns a Mjolnir-like hammer blow in response:

> *Is it a good hot dog? That's all I want to know...I don't think the personal health and purity of my colon is that important*

compared to pleasure. As a chef, I'm not your dietitian or your ethicist. I'm in the pleasure business…My responsibility is to give you the most delicious tomato that I can afford, given the circumstances, and maybe increase the likelihood that you get laid after dinner.[387]

Therein lies the dilemma. The value of food is dependent upon both the completely objective nutritive properties *and* the completely subjective experiential attributes. This is the true reality of food as it exists within the realm of human experience.

If we temporarily table the business of subjective experience for now, and before we concentrate on the objective former, we first must characterize the term "food value." The value of anything, in broad terms, can be defined by the sum of two frequently opposing variables. The value of any object, X, is dependent on both the *quantity* received and the *quality* of the item. Simply expressed another way, the value of an object X (V_x) is the summation of the quantity received (N_x) and the item's inherent quality (Q_x):

$$V_x = N_x + Q_x.$$

A simple experiment highlights the theorem in practice. Suppose you were to offer one hundred people the following choice. They could have either one of the latest, cutting-edge, 80-inch, 3D, internet and Wi-Fi ready, ultimately tricked out super hi-res UHD televisions, or twenty-five black-and-white six-inch televisions from 1960 with no modern capabilities and rabbit ear antennas that might or might not get you a few stations if you are lucky and Mars is in the house of

Sagittarius. Most everyone would agree that the overwhelming majority, if not the entire one hundred, would choose the one big screen HD television.

The reason is simple. In the determination of value, the superior quality offered by the modern HD television clearly outweighs the increased quantity, but significant lower quality, associated with the black and white televisions. Twenty-five old and nearly useless black and white televisions are not as valuable as one big screen modern appliance. This is the type of calculation we make every day, sometimes unconsciously, whenever we purchase a product, a service or make some form of transaction or contract.

Except, it seems, when it comes to food.

When it comes to food we tend to focus on the quantitative measurements exclusively as a surrogate for food *value*. For example, we may make comparisons of worthiness based solely on the caloric values.[388] This is not only misguided, but it is a dangerous approach. We may focus on the nutrition labels and the percentage of various RDAs to the exclusion of how the food was produced and processed. We may become blind to not only what it contains, but what it doesn't.

If this simply quantitative approach was correct, even in the least, we would not witness the endless litany of superfood fails as they continue to parade before us, hearkening back to their origin in the days of snake oil salesmen. We've all heard the siren song of the latest miracle pill or supplement bar containing this extract or that ultimate antioxidant. We have watched them fade away into the late-night infomercial ether without ever making a mark of dietary difference.

Sometimes we address our quantifiable cravings in a more direct manner. We assign value based on economics. If a regular *Casket Crunch* snack bar costs a dollar and twenty-nine cents and we can supersize and get six more for only thirty-nine cents, that must be a bargain! A bargain means value, so we skip that brief pause of refection reflection and pony up the additional change. If we are only paying thirty-nine cents more for half a dozen, and they are still making a profit selling it to us, what sort of synthetic neo-slime are we being peddled?

And there's the chipotle-flavored rub.

We oversimplify.

In the strictly quantitative approach, for example, all red meat tends to be lumped together. An ounce of beef is presumed to be an ounce of beef in much the same way a pint is a pound all the world around. But the data shows a single one-pound ribeye from heritage breed, pastured, grass fed and finished cattle is a far cry from 16 ounces of the latest recombinant, massively processed disc of sheet-meat.

The origin, the breed, the variety, the growing and rearing method, all the little intangibles are what the French term the *terroir* when describing why two bottles of Bordeaux separated in time and space by only a hillside can be so vastly different on the palate. The method of finishing, degree of refinement, preservation, and packaging add additional layers of increasingly complex nuance for us to savor.

The changes to our food and food pathways, particularly since World War II, are why the strictly quantitative approach no longer applies. There was a day not that long ago when a chicken was a chicken. In this scenario where there is an equivalence of quality, quantity becomes the driving force. Since every one-dollar bill is worth one dollar, the *value* lies strictly in the *quantity* of dollars you can accumulate—or chickens, as the case may be.

But today a piece of chicken may range from a delectable Bresse chicken breast from France to a reconstruction of poultry scraps, commonly known as a nugget. We are only a few short steps away from complete reassembly utilizing 3-D food printers. Just for reference, yes, it's already been done, though not yet commercialized.

With the advent of modern global agribusiness and an ever-burgeoning fast food/convenience food industry, it has become an issue of quality versus quantity. To survive in the prehistoric world, we needed the skills to hunt and gather. As civilization progressed, we learned agriculture, farming, and animal husbandry. Eventually these survival skills became superfluous in our instant access world. We have lost all concept and connection to sourcing and preparing our food. When the current Q&A on the web is, "Why do hunters like to kill animals? Why don't they buy store meat where no animals were hurt to make it?"[389] we all weep for the future.

Ironically, our modern convenience culture has so divorced us from the reality of harvesting our food outside of a mega-mart that these survival skills have come full circle, and are now exactly what we do require. In our contemporary world, the circle is complete; we must return to hunting and gathering. We must utilize all our faculties to sleuth, search, and deduce.

Once again, we must learn how to properly source our food. It is not because as it was in a prehistoric world that failure to do so would result in starvation and death. It is precisely the opposite; that because we live in a world of excess and have the luxury of choice, we must learn to choose wisely. It is a failure of choice, not a failure of acquisition. Such failure, regardless of etiology, reaps the same consequence. Failure to properly source our food carries the same consequence today as it did in the times of our ancestors; disability, disease, and death.

To add insult to the proverbial injury is the fact that within the last decade, that variable of quality has become ever more complicated. Only recently have we begun to appreciate that a direct remnant of those prehistoric times plays a critical role in mediating us between health and wellness or disability and disease.

The human gut microbiome is our ancestral link to the power of our food choices. In fact, anything we choose to consume first interacts with the microbiome before it ever reaches our own cells. Therefore, what we choose to eat has a tremendous impact on the character of our gut microbiota, as was earlier discoursed. According to some studies, in as little as a day or even with a single meal we can significantly alter the bacterial composition of our alimentary associates.[390, 391] We are in charge of the condition of our own internal garden.

Many of our modern food products and additives, like artificial sweeteners and emulsifiers to name a few, were felt to be totally inert with respect to our metabolic pathways following ingestion. While it may be true that they do not directly interact with us, research has now shown that they can have a significantly detrimental effect upon our gut microbiome. The end result is a disturbance in our symbiotic organ that has coevolved to co-metabolize our food with us, and maintain the homeostatic point of health and wellness. The foodstuffs of the MWD cause organ failure of this mission critical component.

It now becomes incumbent based on this relatively new data that we further expand our definitions. In our original definition of food value, where we defined value of some food X as dependent upon both quantity and quality, we now further define objective food quality. The original equation,

FOOD SHAMAN

$$Vx = Nx + Qx,$$

now becomes more precise. There is an aspect of quality that can be objectively quantified as it relates to the "food as fuel" nutritional approach. This is the objective nutritional quality of food X: Q_{ONX}.

The objective nutritional quality of food X with respect to its direct impact on humans can be determined to some extent; these are the guidelines with reference to intake of proteins, carbohydrates, fats, and RDAs for vitamins, minerals, trace elements, and the like.

This measure of objective nutritional quality must now by extension be applied to the human gut microbiome. In this arena, we currently have limited insight into the needs of this symbiotic organism when compared to ourselves. It is not even clear if there is a singular human gut microbiome or as is more likely, that each individual's baseline healthy gut microbiota is as unique as that person's set of fingerprints.

So our objective measure of nutritional quality,

$$Q_{ONX},$$

is comprised of one variable in which we have some understanding,

$$Q_{Human\ Nutrition},$$

and one which is essentially a relative unknown,

$$Q_{Gut\ Microbiome\ Nutrition}.$$

To recap, the objective value of some food X can be expressed as the quantity and the objective measure of nutritional quality both in terms of known human nutrition and in terms of the nutritional status of the gut microbiome, which is a comparative unknown;

$$Vx = Nx + (Q_{\text{Human Nutrition}} + Q_{\text{Gut Microbiome Nutrition}})$$

All of these exist in the realm of absolute numbers. There are measurable quantities of food; we can count the hot dogs or weigh the radishes. There are percentages of RDAs and milligrams of sodium. It is, in one form or another, all ultimately a definable number.

Definable, completely objective quantities by their very structure imply limits. They are measurable and devoid of subjective bias. It is a dimension devoid of humanity. Ken Wilber elucidates:

> *Mumford called this the disqualified universe. It-language is essentially value-free, neutral. It has quantity, but no quality. So, if you describe everything in terms of quantities and objective exteriors and network processes and systems variables, then you get no qualitative distinctions whatsoever—you get the disqualified universe...extension—orders of magnitude replace orders of significance.*[392]

But there is one more critical aspect to quality that was briefly touched upon when we first broached this topic. It is a variable that is not so easily objectively quantified. That is the completely *subjective* variable of the food experience.

This is to Tony Bourdain's point, the pleasure principle. It is food and sex, it is a powerful aspect of the food experience. In conjunction with an avoidance of suffering, it is the pleasure principle that drives our behavior. Between the two, the pleasure principle fuels our long game. We like to feel good. This is the human element. It is at once personal and societal.

Ken Wilber details how such a personal subjective encounter affects the larger community through social interaction.

> Each individual action exists against a vast background of cultural practices and languages and meanings, culture itself is not simply disembodied, hanging in idealistic mid-air. It has material components, much as my own individual thoughts have material brain components. All cultural events have social correlates.[393]

Our individual actions undulate upon the fabric of society as a pebble thrown upon the surface of a still pond. Our life can be characterized as a series of such tosses. The collection of which, some would argue, is all we get to take with us at the end of days, that our lives constitute one long recorded, rippling memory.

Food affects us so deeply and primally because it is so fundamentally bound to taste and smell. As previously explained, of all our senses, only taste and smell are directly plugged into the base of our brain. As we listen, see, touch, and feel, the food component is unconsciously branding the entire experience into our hippocampus; that area of the brain where memory and emotion, pleasure and pain, dwell.

These memories live. The moment is ever alive in that complex reality that exists between the observer and the observed, the taster and the tasted. This is why the wholistic *food experience*, wrapped in the DNA of our social experiment called civilization, is so powerful.

How do we define such a potent value?

The total Value of the Food Experience, V_{FE}, is equal to the subjective quality of the experience; its human element, V_s, plus the objective nutritional value of the food, V_o:

$$V_{FE} = V_s + V_o.$$

The objective value, V_o, is the sum total of the objective nutritive value of all the individual meal components;

$$V_o = SUM\ M_{Vx};$$

where M is each individual component of the meal and V_x represents the quantity of each individual component, N_x, and its qualitative healthful effects on the human, $Q_{Human\ Nutrition}$, and gut microbiome, $Q_{Gut\ Microbiome\ Nutrition}$;

$$V_x = [N_x + (Q_{Human\ NutritionX} + Q_{Gut\ Microbiome\ NutritionX})]$$

This yields an objective value for all the components that are part of any meal as

$$V_o = SUM\ M_{[Nx + (QHuman\ Nutritionx + QGut\ Microbiome\ Nutritionx)]}.$$

The objective nutritive value of any meal is how much you consume of each component and its relative nutritional value to both you and your gut microbiome. Unfortunately, current approaches *only* focus on these objective measures. There is no input into consciousness, emotions, feelings, values, intentions, hopes, and fears. And yet it is the subjective quality of the food experience that is arguably the most powerful of all the variables. A complete definition of the *value* of any food experience is:

$$V_{FE} = V_s + SUM \ M_{[Nx + (QHuman\ Nutritionx + QGut\ Microbiome\ Nutritionx)]}$$

The import of the subjective quality cannot be understated. It is what elevates the value of mere sustenance into the food experience and thus transforms the simple act of eating into a uniquely human-defining endeavor.

A meal made with sumptuous farm to table ingredients and perfectly crafted by a Michelin star chef makes for a fine experience as part of a business dinner. Those hot dogs Anthony Bourdain chows down on with his buddies during a midnight midtown escapade make for fond memories, even if the morning after is a bit rougher. A perfect meal of meticulously prepared and wholesome produce enjoyed in spectacular ambiance with those most dear is sublime beyond description. It is why food, and particularly food of love, is an integral part of those memories we call life.

So forget the supersizing. That's not value. Life's memories are not sold by the pound; they are graded by the experience. Strive to make your meals like your life—wholesome, natural, authentic and satisfying. If you follow the proper form, healthful function will follow.

The Art of Source-ry

"It is the quality of your consciousness
at this moment that is the main determinant of
what kind of future you will experience."
—*Eckhart Tolle*

The difference between good and great can often be measured in degrees. Indeed, it often comes down to less than degrees. Measurements in minutes, and even seconds, can draw a clear demarcation between the penultimate and the simply average. In the world of food, this can all come down to proper sourcing. You can't make chicken fricassee from chicken feces.

In simple terms, sourcing is merely the acquisition of ingredients, produce, and product that make up the meal. In practical application, it is everything that happens to the ingredient you will use, before you use it. Understanding the intricacies of proper sourcing and taking the time to execute this preparatory task well gives you great control not only over the taste and texture, the composition and craft of any dish, but also upon its healthful characteristics, or lack thereof.

As you seek to acquire your ingredients, just asking these three simple questions of every comestible you seek to purchase is guaranteed to step up your sourcing game.

- How was it bred?
- What was it fed?
- Where was it led?

"How was it bred?" concerns itself with origins. Is this particular foodstuff an heirloom, heritage, conventional, or GMO product? Is it 100 percent natural, artificial or synthetic, or a combination? It answers the basic question: What is it and where did it come from?

"What was it fed?" concerns itself with where, when, and how the item was raised or grown. Was it produced locally or shipped from halfway across the globe in a country or region in which consumer regulatory protections may be much

laxer than our own? Or even worse, not exist at all? Was it cultivated or raised sustainably, organically, conventionally, or industrially? Was it wild harvested or farmed? When was it harvested and what is the remaining shelf life? It answers the basic question: How was it grown or raised?

"Where was it led?" concerns the nature of post-harvesting processing. Was it processed? If it was processed, how was it processed? Was it inspected or certified by any agencies or organizations? It answers the basic question: What happened between harvest and here?

There are other subtleties of sourcing that are worthy of consideration. Understanding the influence of rhythm is a great example. Nature, and thus food, has cycles and variations. Like the slowly unwinding change of perspective on a merry-go-round, nature unfolds a yearly precession of seasonality.

Watch the undressing of the darkness. It starts with a false dawn. That time at the end of night when the sky starts to lighten with milky tones. The sun hasn't risen yet, but it's coming. Truly that veil between the end of the evening and a new dawn. A very brief instance when one thing is ending, but the other has not yet quite begun. As the dimness eases, the stillness retreats. The breeze picks up ever so slightly, a few leaves fall. It is so quiet you can actually hear it happen.

Everywhere the seasons change, in some places the changes are much subtler, but they are changed nonetheless. Nature alters not only her bearing, but also her voice. Sometimes she shouts, sometimes she whispers, sometimes she sings, and other times she screams. But she is always talking if we choose to take the time and listen. The shaman is first and foremost a keen observer of experience. The Food Shaman is a good listener.

Learn to recognize the time of the year. Many of our modern observances correlate to such shifts because the roots of the story that connect us to Nature and the Earth are as unconscious as they are deep and strong. Memorial Day weekend is the Beltane of the grilling season, welcoming the spring, fresh bounty, and char-grilled patties of pleasure. Labor Day weekend signals the yielding of summer and the backyard grill. There will still be days to cook and enjoy as the weather cools, but there is no mistaking the message; those days are numbered.

As you sip some of your way too early coffee, allow yourself to settle into the gentle turning of Earth-time. It is a not a time of seconds and appointments and meetings, nor even a time of minutes or hours or days. It is a time of seasons, and rhythms, centuries and millennia. It is at once very personal and very ancient. It feels very good. Allow yourself the space to embrace the gentle nudge of change.

In this space-time, if everything seems to slow and time ceases, enjoy the reality of the Universe. For, according to loop quantum gravity theory, time does not really exist anyway. It is a human construct. There is no "absolute simultaneity...there is no collection of events in the Universe that exist now."[394] What exists, what constitutes time, is the existence and unfolding of events and relations. Time exists as experiences that are measured in their passing relative to each other and to us. Reality, and thus time, is a function of perspective.

As fall colors the landscape our thoughts and cravings will drift away from the summer feasts. All those tomatoes from the garden were delicious, and we may have more for a time. But now a crispness in the morning air and the loamy perfume of autumn bring about different desires. It's much more primal than a Starbucks pumpkin spice latte; it's about some spice marinated pork, tender and seasoned to perfection. It's about some roasted apples, all wood smoke and cinnamon.

To cook food greatly requires observance and restraint. Let the rhythm of the season reveal itself to you, expose what is fresh, and right. Always allow the ingredients to whisper to you the little techniques, seasonings, and methods they need from you to shine. Always take a little time for yourself, to listen—to the food, the season, the very harmony of Earth-time. It is not always about get-up-and-go, rat races, and deadlines. They say the early bird gets the worm, but that means the early worm gets eaten. Nature, and a great meal, are all about balance and proper timing.

While different species are certainly subject to differing rules of engagement, deer provide an extreme example of the perils of eating out of time and out of harmony with the natural cycles. The food that deer consumes, particularly in the northern climes, changes with the seasons. Like all mammals, the deer process food in conjunction with their own unique gut microbiota that has coevolved to co-metabolize what they consume, exactly as the human gut microbiota has coevolved along with us.

As the deer adjust to the available food sources, their gut microbiota undergoes a change in its character and composition. The bacteria and other constituents of their gut microbiota shift from those that process summer grasses and similar foods to those that can handle the rough barks, twigs, and other lean bits that are served at winter's table. During these long, cold, dark winter months, many well-intentioned people try to help the deer by laying out some of their favorite summer staples. Among these are hay, and particularly corn.[395, 396]

As wildlife expert Jim Knight warns though,

> *Feeding deer hay or corn can kill them,*
> *because they cannot always digest it. Deer*
> *digestion involves protozoa and bacteria that*
> *help break down food. Different micro-or-*
> *ganisms help digest different types of vege-*
> *tation. If a deer has been feeding on aspen*
> *or willows, it has built up the micro-organ-*
> *isms that digest only this kind of vegetation.*
> *If this same deer suddenly fills its stomach*
> *with corn or hay, it may not have enough of*
> *the corn- and hay-digesting microorganisms*
> *in its stomach to digest the food. A deer can*
> *starve to death with a full stomach.*[397]

As one might suspect by simple observation, is not just the animal kingdom that is in tune with the rhythms of the seasons. Plants help us forecast the change as their growth and decay serve as harbingers of the future. Yet it's even more remarkable than that. Plants respond and adapt on a daily basis. In other words, not only can they can drive it to the green, they have a helluva short game.

The circadian rhythm of plants is a well-known and well accepted scientific fact. However, what has recently been shown is that this biological attunement can actually continue after plants are harvested. While in the grocery store, freshly harvested cabbage responds to the ambient light. While growing in the field, the plants will vary the production of certain phytochemicals according to the time of day.

They maximize their production of naturally occurring pesticides (yes, plants produce their own pesticides because like all living things they prefer not to be eaten) during the times they are most likely to be assailed by hungry bugs. Many of these phytochemicals are of the varieties that have been shown to be extremely beneficial to humans, including anticancer compounds. The further removed plants are from their time of harvest, the longer they sit in the bin, the less vigorous the response and the level of these types of phytochemicals correspondingly drops.[398]

Professor Janet Braam explains,

> So when the crops are growing in the field, they respond to the light-dark cycles, and they—all plants have a circadian rhythm, so they have patterns of behavior that they control or that are under the influence of their circadian clock. And when you harvest vegetables and fruits, these vegetables and fruits really stay very much alive even though they've been removed from the whole plant. But then when we store them under constant conditions like in constant light in the grocery store, their circadian rhythms begin to dampen. And so then they lose the ability to show these rhythmic behaviors…. We know from basic plant biology research that plants have these circadian clocks, and we know that they use them in part to respond or to prepare for seasonal changes. But in addition, we recently found that these circadian clocks are also very important for plant defense against insect attack. So plants are able to turn on their defenses at a time when insects are most likely to seed [sic]. So in that way, they can

*prepare for attack before it actually happens.
And this is clearly advantageous. Plants are
much more resistant to insects if their clocks
are functioning properly....
...because these chemicals taste bad or
make the insects sick. But these same chemicals that are in our model plants are also
in things like cabbages and broccoli, cauliflower. And what we've shown is that those
chemicals accumulate with circadian peri-
odicity in these post-harvest vegetables just
like they do in our model plant. But in—
for us, eating these vegetables like cabbage,
those chemical compounds are—have been
found to be potent anti-cancer compounds.
So they have anti-cancer activities....it
might make a difference at what time of
day you actually eat your vegetables. You
could plan to eat it at the time of day when
those chemicals are at their optimal level.*[399]

Therefore, proper sourcing involves not only detailing
the what, where, and how, but the when. Freshness does matter, both in terms of flavor and texture as well as health and
nutrition. When it comes to filling your larder, approach it in
the same way all the great chefs do. Be nosy. Ask questions.
If the answers are suspect or not forthcoming, then take your
business elsewhere. One of the great things about our modern age is that the ability to procure the product we need is
almost always available. If you live in the city and don't have
access to heritage breed, pastured, and grass-fed beef, with a
few clicks of the button the Internet can often reveal a suit-
able choice both in terms of the protein and the economics.

Utilizing a network of like-minded individuals and chatting with chefs and other culinary and food professionals can reveal many hidden local gems. The more people who shop this way, the greater the financial drivers to supply that need. As a response to the growing demand for this sourcing knowledge, there is a growing availability to the average consumer to procure local ingredients and organic ingredients.

When buying your comestibles, remember that these labels are not always synonymous, although they may be. You will have to decide, based on your budget, which are more cost effective, and which you prefer. Both local and organic are often labeled under the umbrella term "green," but the two sourcing strategies are different. Organic food is regulated by the United States Department of Agriculture (USDA), and concerns how the food is grown and processed. It meets strict regulation and inspection to be able to place the organic seal on the product.

This increased cost of certification is passed along to the consumers in the form of higher prices. According to the USDA, the average premium for organic ingredients is as much as 100 percent for vegetables, 200 percent for chicken, and 300 percent for eggs. It is somewhat of a sad commentary that in our modern world we must pay extra to certify that our food is produced in accordance with the ways nature intended and the ways that humankind has consumed it for thousands of years.

Conversely, the definition of local food is not something that is regulated. Local can mean the food comes from around the corner or across the state. Among culinary professionals, the rule of thumb adopted for local ingredients is that they come from within a one hundred and fifty-mile radius. That is hardly set in stone, however, and is subject to misperception and misrepresentation by unscrupulous peddlers.

Just because something is sold at a farmer's market does not guarantee it is local or organic. And even if it is local, many local producers often falsely tack on the term "organic" to nonorganic food items because it is a buzzword. Here again, there is no substitute for conducting your own research and fact checking. With that being said, many suppliers of local produce and other products often meet or exceed organic standards. These may not be labeled as such because small-scale producers often cannot bear the financial burden of attaining such certification.

Another advantage of acquiring your ingredients locally and seasonally is simple dollars and cents. When all the farms are harvesting strawberries and zucchinis, the price drops. Quite often, a local farmers' market of the products in season is substantially cheaper than buying similar items at a megamart where they may have been shipped in from halfway around the globe. Local often translates into fresher, tastier, and ultimately, more healthful.[400]

One of the other advantages of getting your supplies from such outlets is that they tend to have undergone significantly less post processing manipulations. Because many minimally processed foods are healthful, and many more highly ultra-processed foods are not, this can serve as a useful general rule, although it is not absolute. Therefore, when sourcing, be wary of both the type of food and its processing. Look for foods that are both innately healthful and less processed, and try to avoid foods rich in refined grains, starch, added sugars, and harmful additives.

Regardless of organic or local (ideally both!), the USDA organic regulations assure that the food is produced according to specific guidelines that require environmentally friendly practices that are better for the Earth. Local ingredients travel shorter distances, which mean a smaller carbon footprint, all the while infusing dollars into the local economy.

It is important that you know the story of your food. That story becomes your story, those pages become your pages. Food is our fountainhead, and from there we step forward and engage in the Art of Source-ry. We commune with Nature through consumption, and in doing so we become The Source.[401]

Meat and Poultry

Guidelines for consumption of foods like meat and poultry have been historically based on minimally adjusted ecological comparisons and theorized effects of isolated nutrient content (e.g., saturated fat, dietary cholesterol). What is often ignored are the neutral cardiovascular effects of certain saturated fats and dietary cholesterol and the potentially more relevant effects of other compounds in meats, such as heme iron, sodium, and other additives and preservatives. We lump all meat together and label it "bad" because of fat and cholesterol content. Yet recent data including many individual studies and meta-analyses support a much stronger negative health effect that seems to correlate solely with processed meats, including low-fat deli meats.[402, 403, 404, 405, 406, 407]

Newsflash: not all meat is the same.

Processed meats are approximately 400 percent higher in sodium because of the alterations they undergo in their manufacture. Importantly, there is a vast skewing and reversal of the sodium to potassium ratio in the unfavorable direction. A risk for diabetes mellitus may be linked to iron content[408, 409] and possibly lipid and amino acid metabolites, advanced glycation end products, trimethylamine N-oxide, and nitrates/nitrites found in these highly ultra-processed food products.[410, 411]

Regardless, there is little support for the current conventional guidelines to choose meats based on fat content, i.e. to focus on selecting lower-fat or lean meats. Rather, it would be prudent to consume reasonable amounts of unprocessed red meats several times a week to obtain readily bioavailable iron and zinc, while minimizing or entirely avoiding highly processed meats such as industrial bacon, sausage, salami, and low-fat processed deli meats engineered from chicken, turkey, pork, or beef.[412]

Before anything is ever processed or not, a large determinant of value depends on from whence it came. Genetic modification uses biotechnology to alter crop or livestock genes to improve insect or virus resistance, herbicide tolerance, nutritional qualities, or resistance to environmental stressors. Based on first principles (*a priori*), genetic modification should be considered a tool, not an end point. Its potential effects on human health (positive, neutral, negative) will relate to the *specific compositional changes in the food*, not to the method itself.[413] When it comes to sourcing food, this means knowing how it was bred.

The next question is equally important. What was it fed? Differences in bovine feeding systems can influence nutrient contents of meats. For example, in comparison with grain, grass feeding results in less intramuscular fat and therefore, when visible (extramuscular) fat is trimmed away, higher contents of omega-3 polyunsaturated fats, conjugated linoleic acid, and vitamins A and E, and lower contents of saturated, monounsaturated, and trans-18:1 fats.[414, 415] Not to mention a deeper, richer flavor. Know what it was fed.

Not all fat is bad. In fact, a majority of it is not once you exclude artificially produced TFAs. A great example of a natural luxury food, imbued with fatty goodness, is foie gras. Foie gras is fatty duck or goose liver, delicious in its myriad forms of presentation. It has been demonized. Like Polanski's *Tess of the d'Urbervilles*, a 'victim of her own provocative beauty'[416]; foie gras is a victim of its own provocative tastiness.

Foie gras is natural fat. A natural fat does not contain things like trans-fats (TFAs), with a narrow few exceptions already covered. Many people are unaware that trans-fats are a class of compounds principally created by man primarily to unnaturally extend the shelf life of other fat containing products. As mentioned, the few pure natural TFAs exist only in trace amounts in meat and dairy, mostly as vaccenic acid, known as octadec-11-enoic acid. While TFAs are unsaturated fats, unlike many other unsaturated fats, they behave badly. They are associated with increases in inflammation and LDL ("bad cholesterol"), lowering of HDL ("good cholesterol"), and they are most definitely not essential. Nature put an expiration date on things for a reason.

Some fats are essential. Some fat is necessary. Ever wonder why old people look old? In addition to the breakdown of elastin and collagen as we age there is thinning and loss of the layer of subcutaneous fat under our skin. That little layer of fat keeps us looking young. More importantly, fat is used as:

- An energy source,
- A transport for fat-soluble necessary vitamins such as A, D, E and K,
- A source of raw materials that are used in maintaining normal healthy cellular function,
- An essential starting block for hormone production.

Additionally, several fatty acids (fats) are considered essential, meaning we cannot exist healthfully-or at all-without them. Finally, food cooked in natural fat tastes scrumptious.

Foie gras is such a natural source of fat. It has been around since at least 3000BC in ancient Egypt. The geese there naturally fatten their livers in preparation for their annual migratory journey. The ancient Egyptians discovered these remarkable delicacies. Foie gras may have even helped build the pyramids, or at least some of the ancient Egyptian monuments, because contrary to popular misconception, foie gras is very healthful.

In the original "French Paradox" study by Doctor Serge Renaud back in 1991, he noticed the area within France with the lowest cardiovascular mortality and highest life expectancy was Toulouse in the Gascony region. In Toulouse, the capital of foie gras production, they consume insane amounts of foie gras several times a week. In the study, the rate of death for middle aged men from heart attack in the U.S. at that time was 315/100,000, in France as whole it was 145/100,000, in Toulouse it was 80/100,000.[417]

Roughly 65 percent of foie gras is unsaturated oleic acid, the same oil that constitutes 68 percent of olive oil. It contains omega-3 and omega-6 essential fatty acids. To quote Doctor Renaud, *"Goose and duck fat is closer in chemical composition to olive oil than it is to butter or lard."*

The approach to consuming foie gras is as essential as the ingredient itself. Too much of anything, even water, can be detrimental. Within the natural rhythms we must seek stability. A native of Gascony, Robert Jacquerez, who lived into his late 90s, remarked that balance is the key. "Always have a salad with your cassoulet, bread with your foie gras. Always drink as much mineral water as wine."

The story told of meat, especially red meat, has never focused on being balanced. It is a story of protein and fat, particularly saturated fat. The "cornerstone of dietary advice for generations has been that the saturated fats in butter, cheese, and red meat should be avoided because they clog our arteries,"[418] according to the mainstream media. It is time the true tale was told.

That story begins before any human being cooked anything. This account starts back beyond the origins of modern humankind. It was a time where we need to dispel what is oft portrayed as "the vegan myth." It was a time where, according to those seeking to claim both dietary and moral superiority, our ancestors existed in contemporary harmony with all other lifeforms, eating and sharing the abundant plant life. They had an idyllic existence among the trees eating fruit and leaves and frolicking with the unicorns.

The truth of the matter is that our distant forebears existed in a violent Pleistocene world. It was much more like *Planet of the Apes* than *Curious George*. Along with fruits, vegetables, and insects, they consumed fish and meat. In fact, the desire to procure meat proactively can be seen in our close relatives, the chimps, today. There is well recorded evidence of chimps actively hunting smaller primates for meat. The historical reality is we ate meat and we liked it. As omnivores, our ancestors ate whatever they could get and that included meat.

Our digestive systems are unique and reflect our very unique human diet. Carnivores generally have shorter digestive tracts and colons that we somewhat mirror. Unlike carnivores, our stomachs tend to be on the small side and we have a shorter gastric transit time. But we have a greater short intestine to long intestine ratio which makes us overall more akin to carnivores than herbivores. In the spectrum of omnivores, our digestive system is built more in the carnivorous style than that of a true herbivore.[419, 420]

Even compared to other primates we have less colonic length and therefore less colonic transit time. This is important because it affects the gut microbiome. Affecting the microbiome will affect fermentation, energy extraction, and a host of regulatory and immune functions.[421]

As a species, *Homo sapiens* has significantly reduced tolerance to many plant toxins and tannins. When we eat plants, we ingest these compounds. They are produced by plants because they, like all living things, prefer not to be eaten. Therefore, they have developed over millions of years an array of biochemical defenses that we are much less adroit at dealing with than our more "primitive" primarily vegetarian relatives.[422] Even within the world of primates, our digestive tract is unique.

We have developed an exceptional physiology to adapt to *our* omnivorous diet. A diet that is extraordinary in its utilization of *cooked* food. The result is a distinctively human gut microbiome that has co-evolved to co-metabolize such a diet in concert with us. The result of the interplay of these forces is...evolution!

Our evolutionary success is fueled on the tripod of fire, fat, and protein. Fatty acids are necessary for life. There are essential fatty acids. We need protein to provide us with essential amino acids. We see the necessity of these nutrients by their absence. Deficiency syndromes like essential fatty acid deficiency (a very creative and original descriptor), Kwashiorkor (adequate energy in terms of carbohydrates but inadequate protein) and both energy and protein deficits like marasmus, one of the protein energy malnutrition syndromes, or PEMs.

Conversely, carbohydrates are not essential for life if one acquires the needed nutrients from other sources.[423] There is no evidence of any known human carbohydrate deficiency syndrome. To repeat Harold Draper: "There are no essential foods—only essential nutrients."[424] In theory, all the essential nutrients needed can be had without ever consuming a carbohydrate. The aforementioned Inuit diet is probably as close as humans have come to carb-free dining, and the population's health speaks for itself.

Fire is a critical component of the fat-fire-protein triad, because it really changed the equation. Unlike any other animal species, we use fire to cook our food. For the first time ever, an animal species processed food, even if initially by thermal means only. Processing and refining food leads to greater energy extraction.

The caloric value of food is misleading because it does not account for the efficiency of extraction. For example, an experiment fed mice raw food or highly processed food. Some was thermally processed, some highly refined. Both groups got the same components and caloric values. Mice consuming processed foods gained more weight.[425, 426]

The result of this triumvirate is that we became much more efficient biological machines. We had energy (due to fire and energy dense fat) *and* the raw materials (due to protein and fat consumption from foods like red meat) in place to develop the brainpower and make us the dominant species on Earth.[427, 428]

We need fats to maintain that edge. We may be intelligent, but we are in truth fat-heads. About 25 percent of the body's cholesterol, required for the proper functioning of each individual cell, is located in our brains where it plays a critical role in the composition of the myelin sheaths that allow rapid neuronal communication. Indeed, remove the 75 percent water and you will find that the entire brain is about 60 percent fat—the fattest organ we have!

Behind all the cerebral success that made us the smartest guys and gals on the planet was carnivory.

The consumption of red meat, along with marine food sources, was one of the primary drivers for our success as a species. So it is interesting that in our modern age we wind up even questioning whether or not we should be consuming it at all. How did we find ourselves at this intersection of contradiction, looking for directions on a road to nowhere, hundreds of thousands of years later?

It was because after eons of evolution fueled by fire, fat, and protein, a problem was identified. Enter again Ancel Benjamin Keys, he of the 1961 *Time Magazine* cover, who received widespread praise for categorizing fat, saturated fat, and cholesterol as a significant health problem, a specific cause of cardiovascular disease—the so-called "cholesterol hypothesis." It took over fifty years for butter to again grace the cover of *Time Magazine* making us question whether he (and by extension we) had gotten that all wrong.

Following World War II, the point of introduction of the modern Western diet, Ancel Keys observed a previously unseen rise in cardiovascular morbidity and mortality in the United States. He noticed a dearth of such phenomenon in Europe. He hypothesized that the cause of disease in the US was the result of increased consumption of cholesterol and saturated fat. The so called "cholesterol hypothesis" was first presented in 1955 at a conference in Naples where it was not well received.

Never one to give up when he was sure he was right, Keys went back and refined his data into the seminal Seven

Countries Study, eventually published in 1970 (see Figure 3). This study of nearly thirteen thousand men from Japan, the US, and Europe demonstrated compelling evidence between increasing saturated fat consumption, blood cholesterol levels, and cardiovascular morbidity and mortality in seven countries: Greece, Italy, Spain, South Africa, Japan, Finland, and the United States.

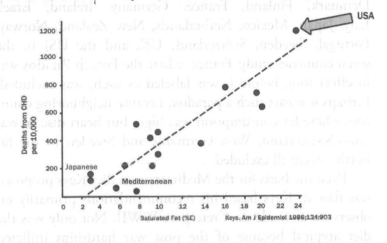

Figure 3; Keys (1970)

Look who is number 1 on the charts. The United States! Yeah us!

There were multiple cohorts from seven countries and it is obvious to any and all who examine that data that it is impressive, powerful, and definitive. Maybe a little too definitive. We'll never know the answers for sure because Keys took these answers to the grave. Because, you see, there were more than seven countries studied at the time.

Keys apparently did not let the data get in the way when he was sure he was right, either. Countries in which the data did not fit the hypothesis were left out. Norway, where the saturated fat consumption was high but there was little cardiovascular disease, was not included. Neither was Chile, where the converse was true; cardiovascular disease was high but saturated fat consumption was low.

All in all, there were actually twenty-two countries (Australia, Austria, Canada, Ceylon {Sri Lanka}, Chile, Denmark, Finland, France, Germany, Ireland, Israel, Italy, Japan, Mexico, Netherlands, New Zealand, Norway, Portugal, Sweden, Switzerland, UK, and the US) in the seven countries study. France, where the French Paradox was in effect long before it was labeled as such, was excluded. Perhaps it wasn't such a paradox, because neighboring countries where fat consumption was high, but heart disease was not—Switzerland, West Germany, and Sweden to the far north—were all excluded.

Even the basis for the Mediterranean diet Keys proposed was flawed. Keys based his recommendations primarily on observations made on Crete post WWII. Not only was the diet atypical because of the post war hardships inflicted upon the island and its population, but dietary recordings were made during Lent, which seriously biased the findings. When all the data is analyzed, the findings and conclusions are much less convincing.[429]

Starting in 1961, Keys held a prominent position on the American Heart Association nutrition committee, which issued the country's first ever guidelines addressing saturated fat intake. During the 1970s, there was a huge political movement to establish national dietary guidelines driven by presidential candidate and then senator George McGovern.

What was eventually approved and put forth in 1977 were recommendations for sodium, salt, cholesterol, and fat, among others. This resulted in the infamous food pyramid. There were now instituted regimens of approaching food. These called for 55 to 60 percent of daily energy (calories) in the form of carbohydrates. The recommended intake of carbs exceeded that of fresh fruits and vegetables. Fat was limited to 30 percent with 10 percent saturated fat.

Cholesterol intake was limited at 300mg. per day (one egg is 175 to 200mg). Sugar was limited to 15 percent of daily energy, and sodium intake was set at 3g/day. The rationale behind such sanctions on certain groups of foods was not, as Harvard nutrition professor Mark Hegsted said in 1977, a question of why we should do this thing, but *why not?* "People will reap important benefits," he argued. And the risks? "None can be identified," he said.[430] We were advised to base our diet on healthy choices like refined Wonder Bread and sugar-coated Frosted Flakes. Talk about cereal killers.

Not everyone was aboard. These guidelines were subject to contentious debate, particularly from certain corners of the medical community. Professor Yudkin implored the powers that be that the evidence pointed to sugar and refined carbohydrates as the culprits. Professor Olson, who was chairman of the dietary committee, addressed Senator McGovern during the hearings and recounted that he "pleaded in my report and will plead again orally here for more research on the problem before we make announcements to the American public." The Senator replied, "Senators don't have the luxury that the research scientist does of waiting until every last shred of evidence is in." What a philosophy to have when implementing public health policy that affects every single individual in the country, and affects their health.[431]

MICHAEL S. FENSTER, MD

The following figure highlights the results of said policy implementation. The graphic charts the prevalence of obesity in the US from the 1960s and the red arrow marks the time of the dietary guideline implementation. It is easy to track the change in the rate of rise, the slope of the curve, and the inset shows that this is independent of age group, generating parallel curves irrespective of age or sex.

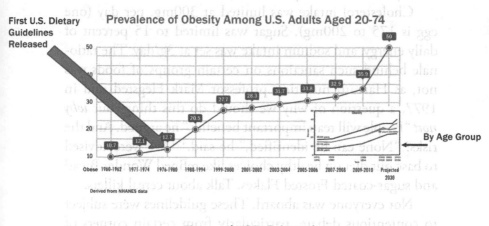

First U.S. Dietary Guidelines Released

Prevalence of Obesity Among U.S. Adults Aged 20-74

By Age Group

Derived from NHANES data

Figure 4; CDC (2009)

Along similar lines of logic as Senator McGovern, the NIH Consensus Development Conference proclaimed in 1985 that, "It has been established beyond a reasonable doubt that lowering definitely elevated blood cholesterol levels (specifically, blood levels of low-density lipoprotein (LDL) cholesterol) will reduce the risk of heart attacks caused by coronary heart disease..."

Yet in going back to the future in 2016, the evidence that verdict was built on was as reported in *Time Magazine* on January 8, 2016 was flawed: *"Experts Say Lobbying Skewed the U.S. Dietary Guidelines."* Marion Nestle, PhD and former chair of the Department of Nutrition, Food Studies, and Public Health at New York University expounded further in the article:

> *Throughout the 1980s and 1990s, the USDA treated fat as the primary harm in the American diet. Along with its anti-fat stance—a stance researchers say was never grounded in science—the guidelines also encouraged Americans to eat hefty amounts of carbohydrates. The new dietary guidelines at least acknowledge past errors. As Professor Nestle opines, "in the previous decades we treated fat as the primary harm. This anti-fat stance was never grounded in science. The reality is that fat doesn't make you fat or diabetic."*[432]

Not only is the advice erroneous; it is detrimental. "This advice to eat more carbs and avoid fat is exactly backward if you want to improve health and lower body weight," according to Doctor Robert Lustig, Professor of Pediatrics in the Division of Endocrinology at the University of California, San Francisco.[433] And while there is a tip of the hat as the new guidelines specifically *avoid* a cap on the overall fat in the diet, it still calls for a limit to 10 percent saturated fat.

What's the evidence for that?

The trail again goes back again to Keys. He noted that heart disease "tended to be related" to serum cholesterol that in turn "tended to be related" to the proportion of saturated fat in the diet. But as any good scientist knows, correlation is not causation.

The 10 percent saturated fat recommendation was adopted in the US in 1977 and in the UK in 1983. It was based on six trials, five of them secondary prevention, consisting of 2,467 participants, mostly middle-aged Caucasian males. Not one trial actually tested the recommendations as proposed. In the trials studied, there was no significant difference in absolute mortality or cardiovascular mortality between the groups. The intervention groups, however, did have statistically significant lower cholesterol levels. So in essence, the data used to promote the low fat (30-percent total) and low saturated fat (10 percent) showed the opposite, that lowering the cholesterol through dietary restriction did *not* impact overall or cardiovascular survival.[434]

Despite no documented efficacy and no trials that actually tested the recommendations as proposed, dietary policy was put forth affecting two hundred and twenty million Americans and fifty-six million UK citizens based on at best specious results from less than two thousand and five hundred mostly ill, middle-aged white guys. Despite this lack of vetting, Americans listened. From the 1970s through the 2000s Americans significantly decreased their percentage intake of fat and in particular, saturated fat.

How did that work out for us?

From 1971-2000 obesity more than doubled from 14.5 percent to 30.9 percent. Total fat consumption decreased from 36.9 percent to 32.8 percent for men and from 36.1 percent to 32.8 percent in women. Saturated fat consumption decreased from 13.5 percent to 10.9 percent for men and from thirteen percent to eleven percent for women. All of these are statistically significant reductions.[435] Americans have continued to eat less food derived from animals, as advised. Whole milk consumption is down 79 percent; red meat by 28 percent, and beef by 35 percent; egg consumption is down by 13 percent, and animal fats are down by 27 percent. Consumption of fruits is up by 35 percent and vegetables by 20 percent.[436]

This obsession with fat resulted in what can only be termed the lipid distraction. Since the aforementioned guidelines were instituted in the late 70s, Americans have decreased their consumption of both total fat and saturated fat. However, in response to that we've seen a rise in obesity, as measured and defined by the body mass index (BMI), and conditions like diabetes and their associated morbidities and mortalities.[437]

Because of the initial push to implicate fat and saturated fat in the genesis of cardiovascular disease, many fats were only studied in terms of the relationship to their effect upon blood lipid levels. As we focused on fat, the rise in diabetes and other inflammatory disabilities and diseases has continued to increase. The role of fats was confined to focusing on a test tube and their impact on a lipid profile. Little effort was made to elucidate or understand their physiological role and importance. What is important is the effect as a result of the relationship.

For example, it was little appreciated that the primary reduction of low density lipoprotein, LDL, cholesterol that accompanies a reduction in dietary saturated fat tends to be a decrease in the large, buoyant, or type A LDL pattern. Consuming saturated fat correlates with a reduction in small, dense (sdLDL) or type B LDL pattern. When we refer to LDL cholesterol we are referencing the total cholesterol amount in the LDL layer.

When we give a number associated with LDL, or "bad" cholesterol, we are speaking only of the quantity of material, not the quality. Like everything food related, it is about both quantity *and* quality. A pound of plastic can be used to make a few beach balls or a lot of ping-pong balls. From a given quantity of cholesterol, the body can fashion a lot of smaller, denser type B LDL particles or fewer, larger type A LDL molecules.

The difference in particle type is critical. It is the small, dense LDL pattern that is associated with the development of cardiovascular disease and seen in metabolic abnormalities like metabolic syndrome and diabetes. It is believed that the risk associated with a higher sdLDL is because the egress of the molecules from the bloodstream into the vascular wall occurs in a gradient driven fashion. [438, 439]

There are any number of studies that have failed to show a correlation between saturated fat intake and the risk of developing cardiovascular disease. This makes perfect sense if we remember that the increase in LDL associated with fat consumption is type A LDL, often with a corresponding reduction in the atherogenic type B LDL.

A meta-analysis performed by Siri-Tarino examined twenty-one studies consisting of almost three hundred and fifty thousand people. The meta-analysis found that "there is no significant evidence for concluding that dietary saturated fat is associated with an increased risk of CHD or CVD." [440] Their analysis showed that as the percentage of the diet consisting of carbohydrates increased, so did the percentage of sdLDL or type B versus type A LDL. Because when you remove the fat from the diet, you have to replace it with something; it is a zero-sum game.

A more recent meta-analysis examined over half a million people in thirty-two different trials and concluded that "current evidence does not clearly support cardiovascular guidelines that encourage high consumption of polyunsaturated fatty acids and low consumption of total saturated fats."[441] What people replaced the saturated fat in their diet with when it wasn't refined carbs tended to be vegetable oils like safflower, corn, sunflower, and soy that are predominately pro-inflammatory omega-6 polyunsaturated fatty acids (PUFAs).[442] Replacing saturated fat with vegetable oils rich in omega-6 PUFA, essential fatty acids like linoleic acid (LA), according to several studies and a meta-analysis, can result in an increased risk of death. Omega-6 PUFAs provide substrates for the generally pro-inflammatory pathway.

Over the last several decades, the single largest change in terms of consumption of any individual food type is the increase in the intake of vegetable oils. Baked goods, along with condiments and salad dressings, now account for the highest contribution to fat in the Western diet. Meat and poultry are second. In 1900, consumption of such vegetable oils was approximately zero. Currently about 8 percent of all energy in the modern Western diet is now derived from vegetable oils.[443] This is the largest increase in any food type over the last century.

Such consumptive patterns are associated with an increased risk of cancer, increased oxidized LDL, reduced HDL levels, and increased cardiovascular events. As an interesting aside, in studies looking at such a replacement strategy; those with higher omega-6 PUFA intake had a higher rate of death from violent accidents and suicides. Alarmed by these findings, the National Institutes of Health convened researchers several times in the early 1980s to try to explain these "side effects." Experts now speculate that certain psychological problems might be related to changes in brain chemistry caused by diet, such as fatty-acid imbalances or the depletion of cholesterol.[444]

Exposing such vegetable oils to high temperatures causes their oxidation. Remember, it is the oxidized LDL that is involved in the inflammatory aspects of atherosclerosis. Exposure to high temperatures results in the production of compounds like monochloropropane diols (MCPD) and glycidol esters.

According to the European Food Information Council, no limit on 3-MCPD (3-monochloropropane-1,2-diol or 3-chloropropane-1,2-diol) esters have been set. They have only recently been discovered "in all refined vegetable oils, and all manufactured products containing those oils. The compound 3-MCPD is released from 3-MCPD esters by regular digestion in the human digestive tract. The 3-MCPD esters are therefore considered to have the same toxicological profile as 3-MCPD." [445] The 3-MCPD molecule is an organic chemical compound which is carcinogenic and highly suspected to be genotoxic in humans.

Glycidyl esters are compounds formed independently from 3-MCPD esters during the processing of all oils and fats. They are likely formed from the diglycerides during the deodorization step in the refining process of processed oils, and therefore occur in almost all refined edible oils. naturally present in all oils when heated to temperatures greater than two hundred and twenty degrees Celsius. They are consequently found in foods that contain such refined oils and fats. When consumed, glycidyl esters are converted into free glycidol. Free glycidol itself is categorized as "probably carcinogenic to humans." These are not issues with naturally occurring animal fats like butter, lard, and tallow.

Replacing saturated fat with carbohydrates, especially refined carbohydrates, likewise results in worse outcomes. There is an increase in the type B or sdLDL pattern, lower

HDL, and an increase in obesity, diabetes and associated complications. There is a shift to an overall atherogenic lipid profile, lower HDL-C, increase in triglycerides, and an increase in the ApoB/ApoA-1 ratio; smaller improvements in glucose tolerance, body fatness, weight, inflammation and thrombogenic markers; and an increased incidence of diabetes and obesity.[446] The substitution of fats in the diet with refined carbohydrates correlates with obesity and other inflammatory mediated pathophysiologies like diabetes. These conditions are reaching epidemic proportions. In the United States, two people die of diabetes-related causes every five minutes, and fourteen adults are newly diagnosed.[447]

Over the last forty-plus years, Americans have decreased their percentage of fat, and saturated fat intake. But in looking at diets, including the low-fat approach popularized for so many years, it is clear that eating fat does not make you fat. Compared to low-fat diets, fat sparing (isocaloric) approaches yield greater weight loss, improved lipid profiles, and improved insulin resistance.[448] A study of more than three thousand and five hundred people found consumption of fats like those found in whole-fat dairy decreased the risk of developing T2DM by 60 percent.[449] (See appendix D1)

In light of these findings, is it really a surprise then that when we look closely, we find that 75 percent of patients admitted with acute myocardial infarction, a heart attack, have LDL cholesterol in the desirable range (100-130 mg/dL)? Even if we apply a more rigorous standard of less than 100 mg/dL, about half still fall into the goal range. Regardless of LDL level, about one third of these patients have concomitant diabetes, underscoring the importance of metabolic abnormalities in the pathophysiology of CVD.[450]

This lipid distraction has culminated in the dietary cholesterol fallacy. This is the commonly held, but wrongly assumed idea that the cholesterol consumed as part of the diet is directly related to blood lipid profiles. Cholesterol comes from three pools; each a complex interconnected web within the body. Cholesterol consumed in the diet must undergo modification in the gut as the bulk of such esterified cholesterol is poorly absorbed. Cholesterol is recycled through reclamation in the gastrointestinal tract. Finally, cholesterol is produced through de novo hepatic synthesis.[451]

If we could easily alter cholesterol through diet and dietary modification had the purported effects, we wouldn't need statins to the tune of almost twenty billion dollars per year worldwide (2012 data).[452] (See appendix D2)

In short, the cholesterol you eat has little to no impact on your blood lipid profile. The 2015 dietary guidelines acknowledge this fact by removing dietary cholesterol restrictions. But as recently as 1999, the AHA was still advising Americans to reach for "soft drinks," and in 2001, the group was still recommending snacks of "gum-drops" and "hard candies made primarily with sugar" to avoid fatty foods.[453] The AHA freshly warned the public to avoid coconut oil because it is a saturated fat. In June of 2017 they doubled down on this approach, recommending even stricter avoidance of saturated fat with a president's advisory:

> *The American Heart Association recommends reducing saturated fat to no more than five to 6 percent of total daily calories...*[454] *We conclude strongly that lowering intake of saturated fat and replacing it with unsaturated fats, especially polyunsaturated fats, will lower the incidence of CVD.*[455]

Here is the meat of the evidence to date:

- The original recommendations, as mentioned, (1973 in the US, 1983 in the UK) had no basis in *any* scientific evidence derived from randomized, controlled clinical trials—the recognized gold standard in such matters. The analysis examining the approval of these guidelines concluded that "The dietary fat guidelines were not supported by RCT [randomized controlled trials] or epidemiological evidence available at the time of their introduction."[456]

- A study which systematically reviewed saturated, not just total, fat had mortality as the end point. They found that "Saturated fats are not associated with all cause mortality, CVD [cardiovascular disease], CHD [coronary heart disease], ischemic stroke, or type 2 diabetes."[457]

- Another meta-analysis also looked at saturated, not just total fat, with disease as the end point. The researchers concluded that "Meta-analysis of prospective epidemiologic studies showed that there is no significant evidence for concluding that dietary saturated fat is associated with an increased risk of CHD or CVD."[458]

- Yet another group of scientists examined the saturated fat question, concentrating on saturated, not total fat, and its relationship with the risk for CAD. They looked in detail at saturated, monounsaturated, polyunsaturated, and trans-fatty acids (TFAs). They also examined the specific long chain saturated fatty acids, palmitic (C16:0) and margaric (C17:0); because even among classes of fats (like long chain saturated fatty acids), the body is built to utilize many fats uniquely according to their individual characteristics. The conclusion of their analysis was that "Current evidence does not clearly support cardiovascular guidelines that encourage high consumption of polyunsaturated fatty acids and low consumption of total saturated fats." [459]

- A 2009 meta-analysis conducted a systematic review and meta-analysis of randomized controlled trials and prospective cohort studies looking at total and saturated fat and the risk of CHD and mortality. The take-away was that "Intake of total fat was not significantly associated with CHD mortality. Intake of total fat was also unrelated to CHD events." [460]

- The most recent investigation published in 2017 "Finds that the epidemiological evidence currently available does not support the dietary fat guidelines.... The conclusion of the four systematic reviews and three meta-analyses is that there was no evidence to support the dietary fat guidelines being introduced and there is no evidence currently available to support them. Not one review has found evidence to support [current] public health dietary fat guidelines." [461]

And yet per the AHA and their disseminated mouthpieces, the egg white omelette made with hydrogenated vegetable oil is the "healthy choice."

Is it any wonder the public remains confused?

Despite the ineffectual changes that occur in trying to limit cholesterol intake, or replace saturated fat, and the confusion swirling about the recommendations, the fact remains that dietary choices *are* powerful.

Comparing an isocaloric low-fat versus a low-carb diet, reducing carbohydrates was associated with less body fat, less triglycerides, better glucose tolerance, and reduced insulin resistance. Importantly, there was a significant reduction of markers of inflammation like TNF-α, IL-6, Il-8, monocyte chemotactic protein-1, E-selectins, intercellular adhesion molecule-1, and markers of thrombogenic activity like PAI-1 (tissue plasminogen activator-1). There was an increase in HDL and a reduction, as has been discussed, in sdLDL.[462, 463] All this *and* you get to eat more fat, and that means more flavor.

The Mediterranean diet and the Mediterranean approach have been examined in a number of trials. The PREDIMED group showed that compared to a traditional "low fat" approach there was a 30 percent reduction in CV endpoints following a Mediterranean diet. This was so powerful the trial was stopped early and is on par, if not in excess, of the outcomes seen with statin therapy.[464]

Additionally, following a Mediterranean approach as compared to the modern Western diet has been shown to prevent diabetes and even reverse it in certain individuals. All this while consuming *more* fat than is found in the standard American diet.

One of the cornerstones of the Mediterranean approach as mentioned is its emphasis on fresh, wholesome, seasonal, and local foods. One of the main differentiators between diets supporting healthy populations and the disability and disease seen with consumption of the modern Western diet has to do with the *quality* of the comestibles. Clearly there is a need to move beyond the popular misconception that simply focuses on caloric comparisons. Simply put, a calorie is not a calorie. In fact, to assume such is to violate the Second

Law of Thermodynamics.[465] Likewise, a piece of meat is not a piece of meat, once again breaking the news that not all meat is created equal.

This is particularly true when it comes to red meat. As previously mentioned, a meta-analysis done at Harvard in 2010 examined twenty studies comprising over 1.2 million people across the globe. This was one of the first studies to look in depth, in a detailed way, at the difference between fresh, unprocessed red meat and processed meat-like products. Consuming four ounces per day of beef, pork, or lamb yielded *no* increased risk of cardiovascular disease or diabetes. Conversely, only two ounces per day of processed meat products increased the risk of diabetes by almost 20 percent and the risk of cardiovascular disease by 42 percent.[466]

Of note, in the study analysis there was a *higher* cholesterol content in the fresh meat versus the processed meat products. As an aside, it was clearly not the nitrates/nitrites in the processed meats that were responsible for the increased risk with these options. The levels of nitrates and nitrates were not substantially different between the two groups, and this included an analysis including nitrosamines. Anywhere from ninety to 95 percent of dietary intake of nitrates/nitrites actually comes from vegetables, and it is clear we need to eat more of these.

The other previously mentioned trial, the EPIC Trial, was a prospective trial involving almost half a million people in ten European countries. They were followed for over a decade. They found *no* increased risk for cancer, CVD, or early mortality at any level of fresh red meat consumption. However, they found that for every 50g of processed meat there was a 22 percent increased risk of early mortality, a 30 percent increased risk of CVD, and an 11 percent increased risk of cancer.[467] In the Japan Collaborative Cohort Study, meat consumption up to 100g/day was not related to increased mortality from cardiovascular disease.[468]

The largest study so far, the National Institutes of Health-American Association of Retired Persons (NIHAARP) cohort in the US, reported positive associations of both red and processed meat consumption with risk for all-cause mortality. In that cohort, the association was stronger for red meat than for processed meat intake, which might be due to the fact that red meat in that US cohort also *included* processed meat. This type of confounding continues to confuse the issue. It is like comparing apples and oranges and then drawing the conclusion to stay away from cabbage.

Speaking of vegetables, a meat-free diet may not necessarily be the healthiest. The EPIC results do not show the lowest relative risks (RRs) for subjects in the lowest meat intake category, but a slight J-shaped association with the lowest risk among subjects with low to-moderate meat consumption. This was observed for red meat and poultry.

Taking into account the results from the studies that evaluated vegetarian and low-meat diets, it likewise appears that a zero consumption of meat is not necessarily the most beneficial for health. This is in agreement with many studies that examine dietary and health related relationships including subjects as diverse as sodium intake and BMI, both J-shaped mortality curves. There is a threshold below which mortality increases. More is not necessarily better nor is less necessarily best.

Based on this type of data, the WHO recently labeled processed red meat a group 1 carcinogen. Such was not the case for unprocessed red meat. Do note, the IARC labeled the herbicide Round-Up as a probable human carcinogen, even though there have been numerous claims to its safety toward humans. Plants like soy, corn, and canola are exposed to high levels of this herbicide through the use of GMO variants.[469, 470] Many of these are then used in animal feed, ultimately making their way to our table.

How did we get here? From carnivory and red meat propelling us from the treetops into our modern technological age to face-planting us on crumbling feet of ground beef?

We changed the equation.

With the onset of the industrial revolution, and particularly over the last fifty to seventy-five years, post-World War II there have been huge changes to our food and food pathways. The result is our modern Western diet with components like processed red meat. Remember, you *never* dine alone. The gut microbiome with a hundred trillion bacteria is there with you at every meal. Everything you eat is subject to co-metabolism. Every bite is a dinner party. Yet the success or failure of the dinner party is as much about the guests as the food. The interaction of the gut microbiome is so profound as to render it a symbiotic endocrine organ.[471]

What changes is the quantitative and qualitative components of the gut microbiome. In essence, when we consume natural, wholesome, and authentic foods, we create a microenvironment through a process of natural selection in which beneficial bacteria thrive and pathogenic bacteria decline. When we choose industrial and ultra-processed meats we are creating a toxic dung heap. Our internal landscape is a proverbial mirror to the environmental one. When we preserve and work with nature, life flourishes. When we dump toxic by-products into the waters, pollute the air with lethal fumes, and pile undegradable refuse across the landscape, we reap despair. "As without, so within."

Evolution supports our red meat cravings.[472] It was carnivory and fire that propelled our species to its current dominant status. As a reflection of that contribution and its importance, we can take some small solace in the current guidelines which finally begin to acknowledge that along with total fat, dietary cholesterol does not correlate to disease risk. The 2015 guidelines eliminated dietary restriction on cholesterol consumption. You *can* have a real omelette, with yolks, and made with butter.

Saturated fats are a broad class with many categories and constituents, and thus broad effects. Fats, like people, will need to be evaluated on an individual basis and per-haps observed in the company they keep. Unprocessed red meat consumption does not translate into CVD, cancer, or increased mortality risk. However, it appears refined and highly processed meat-like offerings do carry a risk. Such a diet like the modern Western diet built on the expedient use of such compounds clearly does correlate with inflammation and associated disease states.

It is not only the quantity of a broad food category, but the food *quality* that has a major effect on us and our gut microbiome. When it comes to meat, there are myr-iad factors that affect the quality parameter. For livestock, this involves the breed, feed, and rearing method.[473] Often unappreciated is the significant impact the method of har-vesting the animal can have on the quality of the meat. This harvest includes the time periods both immediately prior to the actual harvest as well as the immediate time periods fol-lowing the event. The harvest and butchery are critical steps in assuring a quality comestible.[474]

The simple takeaway is that all meat is not equal. While breed certainly does contribute to the quality of the meat, the method of rearing is of perhaps the most serious import in determining the overall healthful or unhealthful qualities of the product.[475] But there is a question often unasked and thus as yet mostly unanswered in many of these studies. The meat that has been studied thus far, while fresh and unprocessed was, for the most part in the United States, the result of Concentrated Animal Feeding Operations (CAFOs). CAFOs involve the production of foodstuffs through industrial manufacturing techniques, applications, and pathways. These products are often referred to as conventionally produced.

Conventional can be defined as that "which is concerned with what is generally held to be acceptable at the expense of individuality and sincerity, based on or in accordance with what is generally done or believed."[476]

Within the conventional wisdom, red meat is unfairly maligned as a uniformly unhealthful choice. Yet, the term red meat consists of a diverse group of protein sources: beef, lamb, bison, goat, and any number of wild game sources such as deer, elk, and moose. Pork can intermittently be found included in these studies that seek to explore the health ramifications of such comestibles in the diet.

As the most commonly eaten meat on the planet, pork accounts for approximately 40 percent of all such protein consumed worldwide, and therefore deserves significant consideration.[477] Careful and thoughtful contemplation of the risks and benefits of the many different choices available should be *de rigueur*. Yet our porcine predilections are driven by forces that favor profit over palate. Once again, the engines of eatery that supply the modern Western diet offer us up a singularly industrially manufactured adulteration of the original and seek to persuade us that this is convention. They proclaim that this singularity is our only choice.

All the while, they ignore the fact that how the animal is bred, and what it is fed, makes a world of difference. Our concerns should focus on the underlying *quality* of the product that speaks to its true value in a much greater way than its price per pound. It's about the character of the comestible; about the personality more than the price.

Most of the commercially produced meat in the US is industrially produced utilizing CAFOs. The U.S. Environmental Protection Agency (EPA) defines Animal Feeding Operations (AFOs) as agricultural enterprises where animals are kept and raised in confined situations. AFOs congregate animals, feed, manure and urine, dead animals, and production operations on a small land area. Feed is brought to the animals rather than the animals grazing or otherwise seeking feed in pastures, fields, or on rangeland. There are approximately four hundred and fifty thousand AFOs in the United States.

A CAFO is another EPA term for a large concentrated AFO. A CAFO is an AFO with more than one thousand animal units (an animal unit is defined as an animal equivalent of one thousand pounds live weight and equates to one thousand head of beef cattle, seven hundred dairy cows, two thousand and five hundred swine weighing more than fifty-five pounds, one hundred and twenty-five thousand broiler chickens, or eighty-two thousand laying hens or pullets) confined on site for more than forty-five days during the year.[478]

These factory farm raised animals are often fed a mixture of genetically modified (GMO) corn, GMO soy, chicken manure, hormones, antibiotics, and ground up parts of other animals. Additionally, the animal varieties selected are picked with an emphasis on quick maturity, large size, and weight. Additional processing adds another potential layer of adulteration. There is little, if any, accounting for flavor or healthful benefits in the conventional approach.[479]

Such "conventional" animal husbandry is in truth the opposite of what occurs naturally. Heritage breeds are generally longer maturing, genetically distinct varieties less uniform in size and shape. They are often pasture raised in accordance with environmentally sound and organic production principles.

While heritage breeds raised in organic and humane manners have been prized by chefs for decades for their unique tastes and textures, only now is science beginning to reveal their nutritional superiority. Firstly, breeding matters. This is evident, particularly in the character and composition of the different fats.

As all chefs know, fat is flavor. Therefore, it comes as no surprise that the different tastes and textures reflect *quantitative* and *qualitative* differences in the fats of various heritage breeds compared to conventional industrial species. Such heritage breeds tend to be distinctly lower in certain types of saturated fats and higher in omega-3 polyunsaturated fats, lending a healthful boost to the accentuated flavor. The way the specific breed is then reared only acts to enhance beneficial attributes or to amplify potential negativities. Not only are we what we eat, we are whatever has been eaten by what we eat.

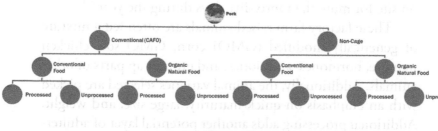

Figure 5

As reflected in Figure 5, for each seemingly single meat choice there are at least eight different possibilities. Each of these decision points before dinner reaches the table affects the flavor and texture of the final product. Chefs have understood for millennia that how it is bred, what it is fed, and where it was led have critical implications for the gastronomic properties of the final product. This is why so many great young chefs are obsessive and near maniacal in their sourcing of ingredients. This attention to detail is one of the key traits that separate great from good; that separate delicious and nutritious from mediocre and malignant.

Science is now discovering in the wake set by these self-same cutting-edge chefs, ones engaging in slow food, farm to table, and other similar practices, that such variables are key determinants in the healthful or unhealthful impact of consuming such foods.

If we expand our horizon beyond the conventional and include, in the case of pork, such heritage breeds as the Berkshire (Kurobuta in Japanese), Red Wattle, Gloucestershire Old Spot, Tamworth, Duroc, *Pata negra*, and Large Black, we see that the potential choices explode in terms of variety and number.

Compare a pork chop from such an animal or a comparable cut of beef to an industrially CAFO produced poultry reconstructed chicken nugget or ground turkey. Often today, the reflex is that the bird is the word and a more healthful choice because it tends to be marketed as "lower in saturated fat." Clearly from the previous discussion, this is simply not the reality in terms of healthful, or flavorful, comestibles.

Industrial poultry breeds are built for rapid maturation, not flavor or healthful attributes. They live stressed lives and are fed with industrially sourced products that alter their health and affect their internal gut microbiome. The mass abattoir processing and packing does nothing to redeem this paltry poultry. Yet for the masses, this becomes the ideal of a smart healthy selection versus a grass-fed and finished, pastured filet mignon or a free ranged Berkshire chop raised on fall apples and forest mast. The first inquiries are finally being made and showing significant differences in the nutritional profile and components of meat based on breed and method of rearing.[480, 481, 482, 483]

The checklist is as follows:

- *How was it bred?* Heritage breed for flavor versus conventional for rapid maturity and rapid weight gain
- *What was it fed?* Natural organic diet supportive of the animal and its gut microbiome health versus potential mix of antibiotics, hormones, and/or GMO industrial feeds
- *Where was it led?* Craft butchery versus CAFO.

The next time you're sourcing a protein, think like a chef and not a recipe collector. Step beyond the conventional and put personality over price. Procure the unconventional. Focus on freshness and flavor; function will follow. Make it personal.

Fish and Seafood

Similar to the approach with meat and poultry, when it comes to fish and seafood, it is not only the food type but the food *quality* that has a major effect on the gut microbiome. For seafood, it may be substantial differences in farmed versus wild caught. For all comestibles, it is reflected in the processing, the preserving, and the final preparatory methods. A deep-fried square of cobbled together piscine parts on an industrially refined bun is not a smarter, tastier, or healthier choice than a grass-finished, grilled beef burger on a fresh baked ancient grains roll.

Real seafood and fish is not only yummy; it is good for us. In comparison with little or no consumption, moderate consumption of fish which translates as approximately two or more servings per week, and regular consumption of long-chain omega-3 PUFAs which translates as approximately 250 mg/day, associates with a lower risk of fatal CHD.[484, 485] Regular fish consumption has weaker, but still significant associations with reductions in nonfatal cardiac events and stroke.[486, 487] Consumption of fish and seafood can deliver adequate omega-3 PUFAs that reduce inflammatory bio-markers, reduce myocardial oxygen use, and enhance cardiac function. But you cannot just supplement the benefits with a magic pill. Fish oils have not shown the same degree of healthful benefit.[488]

Alternatively, because the dose-response effect of omega-3 PUFAs for fatal CHD appears nonlinear, higher background intakes of fish among subjects enrolled in more recent trials may have diminished the ability to detect any benefits of adding fish oil.[489, 490, 491] Which is to say that if you eat some fish and seafood regularly, you'll get the benefits and additional supplementation likely yields little. Spend your money on a quality filet, not pills, and you need not worry.

The types of fish consumed and preparation methods may influence cardiometabolic effects, with greatest benefits perhaps obtained from non-fried, dark-meat or oily fish. These sources can contain up to tenfold higher omega-3 fatty acids than white-meat fish like the ubiquitous tilapia.[492] The importation of tilapia from certain countries has resulted in a potentially dangerously unhealthy product of poor quality and worse taste.

Such a stinker of a dining experience with fish is a shame, for what drove our ancestors to plunder the oceans, seas, rivers, and lakes was the not just the availability, but the taste of the final product. It was not only the world's very first chefs birthing the art of cooking, a feat that remains un-replicated by any species on the planet save our own, but the choice of comestibles that gave rise to intellect and ultimately planetary domination. Among the protein sources that supplied the building blocks for superior brainpower, the evidence suggests that marine sources provided a critical foundation. When your mother told you that fish was brain food, as usual, she was right.

At that time in prehistory when we first discovered the bounty of the sea, and for many millennia to come, all such food was wholesome, organic, and authentic. It is only within very recent memory that we have tried to correct our adulterations to the naturally occurring food and food pathways through supplementation.

Omega-3 polyunsaturated fatty acid supplementation, primarily through the use of fish oil processing, is a prime example. Lovaza, the prescription FDA approved fish oil supplement, has recorded over one billion dollars' worth of sales. That is even though the only FDA approved indication to take fish oil is to treat hypertriglyceridemia or high blood levels of triglycerides. Real health starts and ends with real food. Despite millions of dollars and years of studies to prove the efficacy of a single magic bullet, a pill-borne substitution approach to health, the waters remain murky.[493]

Recent studies like the previously discussed MESA study have revealed insight into why in many situations a varied diet rich in one particular compound or nutrient yields healthful benefits while supplementation with mega doses of the same compounds or nutrients fail to yield any demonstrable advantage. Subgroup analysis of the MESA study found that calcium supplementation combined with a calcium poor diet increased the risk of developing CAD by almost 30 percent. However, consumption of a calcium rich diet without any adjunct of calcium supplementation was found to confer an over 20 percent *reduction* in the likelihood of developing CAD.[494] That is almost a 50 percent swing in differential! With that being said, fish oil supplementation has uncertain benefits, but an excellent safety profile to date and may be considered for people who do not, or cannot, eat fish.

There is clearly a time and a place, and a potentially beneficial role, for supplementation. What is truly remarkable, although it shouldn't be, is that despite the inability to identify a singular super food isolate, the results with real whole food have been consistent and impressive. Fish and seafood consumption follows this pattern.

A recent study examined the connection between omega-3 polyunsaturated fatty acids and the development and risk of coronary heart disease. Unlike some previous analyses which used methods like dietary recall questionnaires to measure consumption—an understandably inaccurate measure—this analysis examined nineteen studies that measured fatty acid biomarkers to accurately reflect the levels of omega-3PUFA intake.

The combined studies comprised sixteen countries and over forty-five thousand individuals. There were four specific omega-3 polyunsaturated fatty acids that were identified. Three came from marine sources; eicosapentaenoic acid (EPA), docosapentaenoic acid (DPA), and docosahexaenoic acid (DHA). One was derived from plant sources: alpha linolenic acid (ALA).

Higher levels of the seafood derived omega-3 PUFAs was associated with an approximately 11 percent reduction in the risk of developing fatal coronary heart disease. In other words, regular consumption of seafood reduces your risk of dying from heart disease by over 10 percent. Higher levels of docosapentaenoic acid (DPA) were associated with an approximately 6 percent reduction in the risk of developing CHD at all.

Naturally occurring sources of DPA include fat-rich fish like salmon or tuna, and grass-fed beef. In addition to reducing platelet aggregation, the cause of heart attacks, DPA improves endothelial function. Abnormal endothelial function is abnormal functioning of the lining of the blood vessels. This is one of the earliest signs of atherosclerosis. DPA appears to improve neural health and reduce overall chronic inflammation. It is interesting to note that DPA is a prominent constituent, in terms of omega-3 PUFAs, in human breast milk, suggesting an important role in the healthy development of babies.

It appears that adequate levels of DPA, as well as EPA and DHA, are best achieved through direct consumption. Eating plants high in the essential fatty acid ALA does not yield increased levels of EPA, DHA or DPA. This is because in the human body the conversion of ALA to EPA, DHA, or DPA is minimal to absent. Healthy young women can convert over 20 percent of plant derived LA to EPA, but only 9 percent to DHA and even less at about 6 percent to DPA.

Men fare even worse, being able to convert only about 8 percent of ALA to EPA and DPA, and lack the ability to convert any ALA to DHA. Strikingly, these amounts are reduced even further by about 40 percent when the diets are high in the pro-inflammatory omega-six fatty acids, a characteristic component of the modern Western diet. This is because omega-6 PUFAs compete with omega-3 PUFAs for the same enzymatic pathways. Genetic variations can result in even less efficacy.

Increased consumption of the plant-derived alpha linolenic acid was associated with an approximately 9 percent lower risk of fatal coronary heart disease. However, it did not appear to reduce the risk for developing coronary heart disease or suffering a nonfatal myocardial infarction. Nevertheless, a diet rich in both plant and animal derived omega-3 polyunsaturated fatty acids impacts not only the development of cardiovascular disease but attenuates such risk factors as triglyceride levels, blood pressure, heart rate, heart rate variability, endothelial function, and myocardial oxygen demand. Along with the animal derived omega-3 PUFAs, plant derived ALA appears to act in concert by reducing overall inflammation. Chronic inflammation is the common root to many of the modern maladies we suffer.

In contradistinction to whole foods, the experience with supplementation has been a mixed bag. So instead of spending time and money in an attempt to supplement your way to good health, why not simply eat deliciously? Fresh fish like salmon, tuna, mackerel, herring, and sardines make savory and scrumptious meals. The consumption of just twelve ounces of salmon would provide up to 1,336 mg DPA per week. A serving of grass fed beef or lamb with fresh garden vegetables is a tremendous source of these potent anti-inflammatory omega-3 polyunsaturated fatty acids as well.

But the most important reason to eat seafood and fish is because they taste great. When we see food, it makes us hunger for the simple natural pleasures we were born to consume. By indulging in such whole, natural, and authentic comestibles we achieve satisfaction in both body and soul. Epicurean enlightenment is there for the taking. Simply expand your vision and reward your taste buds.

But beware!

Just when you've picked the perfect prize, the devious chimera emerges to challenge your source-ry. When you go shopping, what exactly confronts you there, lounging lazily upon the ice in the fresh seafood case?

What do you see, what do you hear?

There under harsh fluorescence, she calls to you, cool and tempting.

Her flesh is the soft orange glow of a setting sun, her scent speaks of seafoam. You touch and feel her firm, gentle curves that bespeak a streamlined grace. You bring her closer and she whispers tantalizing images of succulence yet to come.

The siren song is irresistible.

You lay down your dollars and buy the filet.

The label reads "Fresh Atlantic Salmon."

What exactly have you bought?

If it says Atlantic salmon, it is not wild. Since true Atlantic salmon is critically endangered, the Atlantic salmon sold in the United States is farmed. It may also be genetically modified (GMO), because current labeling laws do not require any disclosure on that front.

If it is not wild caught, then what exactly have you bought?

It is farmed, but the real question is it pharm'd?

Population pressures and consumer predilections continue to drive farming aquaculture. China is currently the world leader and produces about 70 percent of the world's aquaculture. Initially, the bulk of farmed fish were fed a diet of wild caught smaller fish, following the natural law that big fish eat little fish. Approximately one third of all small wild fish caught are used to produce fish meal and fish oil, which is used not only to support aquaculture, but is used in the pursuit of terrestrial animal husbandry.

However, since approximately 50 percent of the world's seafood is now the product of aquaculture, producers are looking to cheaper alternatives. This has caused a shift in the feeding practices from the traditional diets of these animals to one that is based on more plant based material and cheaper, commercial feeds.

These feeds are predominately manufactured from major crops such as soy and corn. The fish oils that have been replaced are the industrially processed vegetable oils primarily made from soy, canola, palm, and sunflower sources. The top five crops used in commercial aquaculture feeds are canola, soybean, corn, nuts, and wheat. Canola and soy alone account for over 50 percent of all the oils used.[495]

This practice brings to the forefront two important considerations. Firstly, by replacing the natural fish oils with plant based alternatives, the balance of critically important polyunsaturated fatty acids (PUFAs) is thrown askew. The result is a product that is often deficient in eicosapentaenoic acid (EPA) and docosahexaenoic acid (DHA) compared to its wild-based alternative. Such PUFAs are responsible for many of the health benefits associated with seafood consumption.

These practices serve to lower the absolute amounts of omega-3 PUFAs that contribute to the healthful benefits we observe in diets rich in marine sourced comestibles. The result is a food source that is significantly higher in its omega 6:3 ratio. This is a characteristic of the many adulterated and processed foods found in the modern Western diet. There is evidence that this favors the development of a pro-inflammatory environment from which disabilities and diseases associated with the standard American diet are linked.

The final consideration is the raw ingredients used in the creation of the commercial feeds. Almost 99 percent of the soy grown, and approximately 90 percent of the corn and canola raised, are GMO varieties. These GMO variants have been produced to be resistant to the herbicide Round-Up. The finale in your filet is accumulation of a recognized potential carcinogen (recent World Health Organization declaration, 2015) in the fish.[496] Forget the tarragon Hollandaise—you just got a free side of glyphosate.

The fish and seafood checklist is as follows:

- *How was it bred?* Is it wild or farmed? If it is farmed can you identify the source country and the method of production? Is it GMO?
- *What was it fed?* Wild fed? Farm raised on a natural organic diet supportive of the animal and its gut microbiome health or a potential mix of antibiotics, hormones, and/or GMO industrial feeds? If farm raised, were the methods sustainable or not?
- *Where was it led?* Was it processed locally, or regionally? In the US or overseas? If overseas was it industrially or overseen by other methods? If overseas, under what conditions? If it was wild caught, sustainable methods or not?

These differences present themselves in the most prominent way possible, in the taste and presentation of the fish. Compare the preparation of farm raised versus wild salmon. Farm raised salmon tends to contain on average about four times more fat than wild salmon. As previously mentioned, because of breeding, rearing, and feeding methods, this does not necessarily translate into health or taste benefits. But it does mean that for a perfectly cooked fillet the temperature should be around 125 degrees F. Serve a wild salmon at this temperature and because of the relatively less fat and higher collagen composition, you will get overcooked, dry and unpalatable. Wild salmon needs to be no more than around 120 degrees F. All of which serves to highlight the critical importance of proper sourcing of ingredients. What on the surface may appear to be succulently, tastefully, tempting, and healthful beyond measure may prove to be a siren song of obfuscation and illusion. Approach with trepidation and a weather eye the labels accompanying our sea-kissed comestibles. For as Odysseus himself observed, "Skepticism is as much the result of knowledge, as knowledge is of skepticism."

Grains and Seeds

Contrary to the current Paleo and low-carb craze, carbohydrates have constituted an important food class since the dawning of the human species. Even today, carbohydrate-rich foods comprise more than half of all calories in most diets globally. Much like caloric consumption, *total* carbohydrate consumption has little relation to cardiometabolic health. It is the *quality* of carbohydrate-rich foods that is directly linked to risk.[497, 498, 499, 500, 501, 502, 503, 504, 505]

Conventional, chemistry-based classification of simple carbohydrates defines them as sugars and complex carbohydrates. Meanings such as starches has, in truth, little physiological relevance. This is because saccharide chain length, the basis of such arbitrary distinction, has little influence on the digestion rate or the metabolic effects of different carbohydrates.

It is more meaningful to examine characteristics that include dietary fiber content, glycemic responses to digestion, and whole-grain content. The degree of processing that carbohydrates undergo before we consume them is extremely important. Grains and seeds may range in form from raw and intact, to partially milled, to fully milled, or highly processed into liquid form.[506]

When a seed or grain enters the mouth without its natural armor of whole-grain or fiber-rich packaging, our enzymes, including oral amylase, promptly initiate the breakdown of the plant product into free glucose. This is a process that is rapidly completed in the upper small intestine. The free glucose is absorbed and causes a brisk rise in blood glucose with insulin release. The rapidity at which this occurs is known as the glycemic index or, when multiplied by portion size, the glycemic load of a carbohydrate. (See appendix D3)

High glycemic load diets may paradoxically act to reduce total energy expenditure.[507] Despite eating more, your body acts as if it is in "starvation" mode. It acts to conserve fuel, turning down our internal thermostat. By expending less energy, the process of obesity is accelerated. The magnitude of such potential harms, for reasons not entirely clear, appear to be larger in women,[508] and others predisposed to insulin resistance and atherogenic dyslipidemia. They seem to be of a lesser magnitude in men and in younger, lean individuals with high levels of physical activity.

There are multiple independent characteristics that influence carbohydrate quality; fiber content and character, glycemic response, processing, whole-grain content, to name just a few. Currently, there is not a single criterion that appears perfect for distinguishing and classifying carbohydrate-rich foods. This is part of the confusion surrounding this group, which includes fruits and vegetables that will be discussed separately.

Precisely because the foods that are classified as carbohydrates include fruits and vegetables, for decades they served as the foundation of a healthful diet. One need look no further than the placement of grain products at the base of the 1992 Food Guide Pyramid. Since that time, it has become clear that, although total carbohydrate has little influence on cardiometabolic health, the types and *quality* of carbohydrate do have a major impact.

Certain carbohydrates like fruits, legumes, vegetables, and minimally processed whole grains appear to function in a protective role against the development of the disabilities and diseases of the MWD. Other carbohydrates composed primarily of refined grains, *e.g.*, modern white bread, crackers, cereals, bakery desserts, and added food stuffs composed primarily of sugars, *e.g.*, SSBs and candy, encourage the development of such pathologies. Therefore, any conversation regarding carbohydrates and their ingestion is moot without further delineation and classification.

The added sugars found in the majority of the dietary constituents compromising the SAD are often composed of table sugar. This is a natural sugar, so don't be fooled by labels touting "naturally sweetened." Table sugar is chemically identified as sucrose and is a disaccharide composed of one molecule of glucose and fructose. It is refined into the white crystalline powder we refer to as "sugar." Natural sources often find it keeping company with vitamins, minerals, or other redeeming compounds.

These naturally occurring springs of sweetness include honey, sugar beets, sugar cane, maple syrup, and other various originations. These unprocessed wellsprings are associated with some form of nutritional benefit beyond that derived from simple sucrose consumption. They often add distinct textures and tastes which can increase the complexity of crafted foods. The man-made derivatives of sucrose include primarily iterations of high fructose corn syrup (HFCS).

High fructose corn syrup contains differing amounts of fructose and glucose. There are important metabolic differences between glucose and fructose. In particular, high doses of rapidly digested glucose induce postprandial hyperglycemia, hyperinsulinemia, and related metabolic disturbances.

Fructose metabolism is antithetical. High doses of rapidly digested fructose have little influence on blood glucose or insulin levels. Yet perhaps even more dramatically in terms of long term pathology, fructose acts to directly stimulate hepatic *de novo* lipogenesis, hepatic and visceral adiposity, and uric acid production. Thus, high doses of rapidly digested glucose and fructose are each harmful, with such effects occurring via both separate and partly overlapping pathways.[509, 510, 511, 512, 513, 514] Together they represent an insidious scourge that acts slowly over time and at multiple levels to initiate and maintain chronic, continuous, low-level systemic inflammation.

In addition to sugar type and content, another important consideration when sourcing seeds and grains relates to gluten content, or lack thereof. This is currently a huge area of marketing focus. In 2015, the gluten-free market passed twenty-three billion dollars in annual sales. Four years earlier, that market stood at just over eleven billion dollars per year. That is a growth curve that fosters extended shelf space and lighter wallets for consumers. But is the price worth a leaner purse? Are there any health benefits demonstrable for the dollars cast?

The allure of easy profits can prove too tempting to some disingenuous marketers. They are willing to employ sales tactics that entice the susceptible among us (and who isn't when it comes to cure-alls for health and weight?) to purchase more expensive, but potentially less useful, products.

For those with a true type of immunologic reaction to ingestion of gluten, known as celiac disease, the incidence holds to its historic precedent—about 1 percent of the population. There is perhaps another roughly 6 percent of the population that may suffer from some form of gluten intolerance. Given those numbers that at most, only about 7 percent of the population demonstrates any gluten-free needs, over 30 percent of adults in the US strive to avoid gluten in their belief that it leads to better health. Is it worth it, as Zooey Deschanel opines, "To be a gluten-free vegan," because as she explains, "(it) is, like, the most difficult thing you can possibly be."[515]

While Gwyneth and friends may not shed a tear over dishing out eleven hundred dollars for an Aquaovo ruby water filter, the average Joe can quickly appreciate the irony that getting less gluten costs more cash.[516] Sometimes a lot more cash. Gluten-free foods can be significantly costlier than their wheat-ier contemporaries.

That extra expense and loss of the comforting, bready aroma and texture of such baked goods might be justified in light of powerful and undeniable healthful outcomes. Perhaps one could argue the worth of giving up a meal of that crusty loaf of freshly baked French bread and creamy, foot-funky smelling cheese for significant health gains. At least then you might be able to rationalize it amongst the tears of such loss and sacrifice (not really).

But alas, *Zut alors!*

Gluten-free options are often not only more expensive, but may be *worse* for overall health. They often contain many artificial flavors, additives, stabilizers and the like. Additionally, their base may be corn or rice flour. That brings discussions on GMO corn and arsenic in rice flour to the table.[517]

There is recent evidence suggesting that eating foods the way nature originally packaged them is healthier; less adulteration is more flavor and more health benefit. Diets higher in gluten are associated with a lower risk of developing type II diabetes mellitus (T2DM). A recent study found that research participants who ate less gluten tended to eat less cereal fiber, a known protective factor for reducing the risk of developing T2DM.[518]

Gluten is a protein found in wheat, rye, spelt, triticale, and barley. It is not found in other grains and seeds, which is why oats and corn can never yield you a baguette. Labels may state possibly containing gluten in products containing oats, for example, if there is a risk of cross-contamination during processing, but oats, corn, and rice do not inherently contain gluten.

It is gluten that gives bread and other baked goods elasticity during the baking process and the final chew and crumb texture in finished products. While avoidance may be necessary for that small percentage of the population that cannot tolerate gluten due to celiac disease or gluten sensitivity, there is lack of evidence that reducing gluten consumption provides long-term health benefits for the majority.

Because these products are often highly refined and processed, there can be a loss of micronutrients along with naturally derived fiber. Micronutrients are dietary components such as vitamins and minerals. Unfortunately, for those that do consume gluten, it is most often in a highly processed form like pastas, cereals, pizza, muffins, pretzels, and bread, which can result in a loss of the same.[519] Nonetheless, for some, an exclusionary approach to some natural foods is an example of food faddism without scientific grounding. It can result in inciting inflammation and subsequent disease. Such approaches are a double-edged dinner knife; they may not only cost more for no benefit, they may actually participate in pathology.

It is easier to sell someone a loaf of manufactured pseudo-bread if they have no idea what gluten is. For if we know what gluten is, we become an educated consumer. It becomes much easier to make an informed decision. A well-educated and well-informed consumer is the most powerful medicine available to counteract and prevent the disabilities and disease of the MWD. For the Food Shaman, knowledge is power.

It is collections of proteins like gluten that make such cereals as wheat, barley, and rye ideal for bread making. The dough depends on the quality and the quantity of these proteins, and two in particular: gliadin and glutenin. Both are what are known as prolamin-type seed storage proteins. These two proteins combine to form strands of gluten.

Gliadin and glutenin vary in composition between the different cereals, and thus yield different types of glutens, much the way a Fiat and a Ferrari are different cars. They are both automobiles with the same basic construction of parts, but the details of those parts and how they are assembled yield very different beasts; or in the case of cereal grains, different breads.

In fact, the gliadin and glutenin can vary between different species of wheat so that the bread produced from a dough made from an ancient grain like durum wheat can be significantly different from a bread produced from modern bread wheat, even though they both come from wheat. Ford manufactured both the iconic and enduring F-250 four-wheel drive truck and the self-immolating Pinto.

Gliadins are smaller proteins known as monomers and come in four types: alpha (α), beta (β), gamma (γ), and omega (ω). Gliadins contribute to the viscosity of bread dough. Glutenins are large protein molecules known as polymers and are divided into low molecular weight (LMW) or high molecular weight (HMW). Glutenins have the ability to form some of the largest and most complex protein polymers in nature. HMW glutenins may have molecular weights in excess of ten million. Glutenins contribute to the elasticity of bread dough.

In flour, these protein molecules remain separated. When water is added and the dough is kneaded, gliadin molecules and glutenin molecules begin to cross link together through disulfide, ionic, and hydrogen bonds. None of this occurs before water is added to the mix. It is why you can work your pie or biscuit dough with the shortening (butter or lard) without fear of it getting tough. Once the water is added, manipulation is kept to a minimum or lots of gluten will develop and render it chewy. Chewy is great for bread but lousy for pies, where the goal is tender and flaky.

The glutenin and gliadins from the different varieties and species of cereals will yield different glutens. These glutens have varying properties. It is why a loaf of rye bread is different from a loaf of Wonder Bread. Flour mixes reflect this as well; cake flour is low-protein so there is less gluten formed and the cake is tender. Bread flour is the exact opposite; rich in protein and thus glutenins and gliadins for chewy, flavorful artisanal loaves.

Ancient grains produce gluten distinctly different from that found in modern bread wheat (*Triticum aestivum*), which accounts for 90 to 95 percent of the wheat-based products available on US shelves today.[520] These differences have huge impacts on not only the taste, texture, flavor, and form of baked goods, but their nutritional and healthful or unhealthful considerations as well. Suffice to say, you should not be spending more to get less gluten. For better health and better flavor, you may merely need an appointment with Doctor John Barleycorn.

Ancient grains like barley exert their healthful effects via multiple pathways. Fiber does exert a healthful effect simply through physical principles. Fiber is important for normal laxation. Increased fiber results in increased stool weight due to the physical presence of fiber, increased water content, and increased bacterial mass from fermentation. This results in decreased intestinal transit time. Fiber makes you poop. (See appendix D4)

However, some fiber types may not exert their beneficial properties through their physical properties. Inulin, while extensively fermented, has little effect on stool weight and thus transit time. Bulking up on fiber sources such as fructo-oligosaccharides can cause GI intolerance at low doses, as little as 10g in some persons. Other starches such as polydextrose and resistant starch have been consumed upwards of 50g without issue.

Some fiber components, such as beta-glucans found in oats and barley, can affect human health as discussed by interacting directly with immune cells. It is clear that adequate fiber intake lowers CVD risk and CHD as it lowers cardiovascular risk factors like LDL, apolipoprotein levels, and blood pressure. Water soluble fibers including beta-glucan, psyllium, pectin, and guar gum are very effective in lowering LDL.

Other soluble fibers in addition to pectins, such as glucans, can lower lipids. Since the soluble and viscous fibers found in cereal are among the most effective in reducing these cardiovascular risk factors, the US FDA currently allows such health claims for oats, barley, and psyllium. The overall health benefits associated with increased fiber intake is reflected in a reduced CRP which correlates to less stress and a reduction in systemic inflammation.

Not surprisingly, a reduction in systemic inflammation seen with increased fiber consumption means less T2DM. Regular fiber consumption attenuates the glucose absorption rate. It subsequently acts to help prevent weight gain, all the while increasing delivery of important nutrients and antioxidants. At 15g fiber per day, there is a significantly lower risk of developing T2DM. Insoluble fiber at 17g per day or cereal fiber at 8g per day lowered the T2DM risk.

Higher fiber diets are correlated with diets that are lower in energy density regardless of fiber source. As one would expect, this higher fiber intake results in lower body weight. Increased fiber consumption tracks with decreased obesity and with less disability and disease, particularly CVD. However, mechanisms appear markedly less straightforward than the previously assumed simple binding hypothesis.

Although it was previously thought that fiber may bind dietary cholesterol and by reducing cholesterol absorption from the GI tract and reduce CVD, with the failure to demonstrate a cause and effect with ingestion of dietary cholesterol or saturated fat and CVD events, this explanation became less plausible. Such pharmaceutical agents like fibrates that act in this manner have been dropped from front-line medical recommendations precisely because of their underwhelming performance in reducing events in those suffering from cardiovascular disease.

A principal area of action for plant fiber, the β-glucan soluble fiber component in the case of barley, is to "favorably alter the composition of gut microbiota and this altered microbiota profile associates with a reduction of CVD risk markers."[521] Other types of beneficial plant fiber include oligosaccharides. These are considered dietary fiber (DF) because of physiological effects, and this group includes inulin and fructo-oligosaccharides. The benefits of fiber were appreciated at least as far back as Hippocrates in 430 BC. He observed the superior laxative effects of coarse wheat compared to the ingestion of the more refined soft, white wheat.[522]

It is estimated that prehistoric hunter-gatherers may have consumed as much as 135g/day of fiber. The current dietary recommendations are for at least 25g fiber per day. The typical US/European diet provides only several grams per day, often not even reaching half the recommended amount on a daily basis.

One very important way that fiber exerts an effect through the gut microbiome is in the role of prebiotics. While supplements of probiotics may be useful, eating four gallons of live culture yogurt per day does no good if it is followed with six cartons of flatline fries and a half-dozen colas. Gut bacteria are like sea-monkeys; you have to feed them to keep them active and amazing.

Prebiotics are that food source. All research thus far has shown that all prebiotics are carbohydrates. These carbohydrates consist primarily of oligosaccharides; these include inulin, oligofructose (OF), lactulose, and resistant starch (RS). Inulin is a not very digestible carbohydrate and associated with impaired gastrointestinal tolerance at higher doses. Asparagus, leeks, onions, bananas, wheat, Jerusalem artichokes, and garlic are potent sources of inulin.

Other prebiotics include galactooligosaccharides (GOS), transgalactooligosaccharides (TOS), polydextrose, wheat dextrin, acacia gum, guar gum, psyllium, banana, whole grain wheat, and whole grain corn. Unlike inulin, prebiotics like wheat dextrin and polydextrose are tolerable at upwards of 30–45g/day. All of these various prebiotics are known to stimulate beneficial bacteria like *Bifidobacterium* and *Lactobacilli*. Soluble, viscous fiber may be particularly useful in alleviating conditions such as IBS, especially guar gum.

Prebiotic benefits include, among others, improved gut barrier function, improved host immunity, and reduction of pathogenic bacteria. To be classified a prebiotic requires (at present) that a compound meet three criteria. The constituent:

* Resists gastric acidity, hydrolysis by mammalian enzymes, and absorption in the upper GI tract;
* Is fermented by intestinal microflora; and
* Selectively stimulates the growth and/or activity of intestinal bacteria potentially associated with health and well-being.

Many of the bacteria in the gut microbiome metabolize these indigestible bits of our diet by fermentation. This is a biological process that occurs within the colon. Sources for bacterial fermentation include mucus, dietary carbohydrates like resistant starch, non-starch polysaccharides (cellulose, hemicellulose, pectins, and gums), non-digestible oligosaccharides, and sugar alcohols.

The colon is diversely colonized with over one thousand known bacterial species and populations 10^{11} to 10^{12} CFU/g. In addition to bacterial composition, the metabolic activity of the gut microbiome can vary substantially due to transit time, available nutrients, and pH. Other factors that affect the gut microbiome include host age, stress, genetics, health status, diet, and environmental circumstances like concomitant antibiotic therapy.

There are bacteria to help us digest both carbohydrates and proteins; saccharolytic versus proteolytic. Significant healthful benefits seem to correlate to saccharolytic metabolism. Chief among this beneficial group is *lactobacilli* and *bifidobacteria*. Reflecting a pro-inflammatory state, obese people tend to have lower populations in their gut microbiome of *Bacteroidetes* and more *Firmicutes*. The character and composition of the gut microbiome is critical in determining our overall energy balance. Obesity is associated with phylum level changes in the gut microbiome, reduced diversity, and altered representation of genes and metabolic pathways

The beneficial saccharolytic bacteria utilize a fermentation pathway that generates pyruvate from hexoses in the undigested carbohydrates. These are the short chain fatty acids (SCFAs). SCFAs appear to improve human immune function. The predominant SCFAs produced are acetate, propionate, butyrate, and lactate. From every 100g of carbohydrates fermented, we generate 30g of bacteria.

The SCFAs produced by the bacteria are water soluble and absorbed into the bloodstream where they can then be transported throughout the body and can have long reaching effects. In effect, these bacterial products can function as hormones and energy sources. SCFAs contribute 7 to 10 percent of daily energy production.

Colonic epithelial cells utilize butyrate as a preferred energy source and may play a role in providing protection against colonic disorders. Acetate is metabolized by brain, muscles, and various other tissues. Propionate is cleared by liver and may lower cholesterol levels by interfering in cholesterol synthesis.

The very process of fermentation and the SCFAs produced inhibit pathogenic organisms by reducing luminal and fecal pH. The lower pH inhibits proteolytic degradation and thus formation of ammonia, amines, and certain phenols which can be detrimental to human physiology. These products inhibit certain competing bacterial enzyme pathways that could likewise be deleterious to us.

Research suggests that prebiotics reduce the prevalence and duration of infectious and antibiotic associated diarrhea, and reduce the inflammation and symptoms associated with IBD. The symptomatic reductions in the severity of IBS was associated with changes in the microflora of the gut. They appear to exert protective effects to help prevent colon cancer and also enhance the bioavailability and uptake of minerals, particularly calcium with fructans.

Modern-day foods which are rich sources of prebiotics include: leeks, asparagus, chicory, Jerusalem artichokes, garlic, onions, wheat, oats, and soybeans. Flour, grains, and potatoes are among the largest sources of fiber, while fruits, legumes, and nuts supply the least amount per serving. Fruits and legumes are, however, among the best sources of soluble fiber, which is particularly important in maintaining the health of the gut microbiome.

After Hippocrates, the import of fiber was basically ignored until it was briefly researched in the 1920s and 1930s by J. H. Kellogg. It was then forgotten again until the 1970s. Currently, good sources of fiber are considered those foods that provide 2.5g per serving. Excellent sources provide 5g or more per serving.

Increased fiber consumption two weeks prior and during travel (10g/day inulin or 5.5g/day GOS, mixture of inulin and FOS) reduced the severity and frequency of travelers' diarrhea.[523] All of this is from dietary components that within recent memory were felt to be irrelevant because humans could not digest them.

Such recent and rapid advancement is one of the reasons behind the continuing confusion. Different types of fiber are defined differently throughout the world. Therefore, working definitions have been proposed in an attempt to form a common vocabulary. A few working terms have been proposed, according to the Institute of Medicine:

- Dietary fiber: non-digestible carbohydrates and lignin that are intrinsic and intact in plants,
- Functional fiber: isolated, non-digestible carbohydrates that have beneficial physiological effects in humans,
- Viscous: exhibit gel-forming properties in the intestinal tract,
- Fermentable: can be metabolized by colonic bacteria,
- Added fiber: isolated, non-digestible carbohydrates that have beneficial physiological effects in humans, and
- Total Fiber is the sum of Dietary Fiber and Added Fiber.

Terms like soluble and insoluble are being phased out, but they have a long history and are still commonly used. Traditionally, soluble fibers had beneficial effects on lipids while insoluble fiber was linked with laxation benefit, yet this is quite variable. In general, soluble fibers tend to be more completely fermented with higher viscosity than insoluble fiber. However, not all soluble fibers are viscous (e.g. partially hydrolyzed guar gum and acacia gum) and some insoluble fibers are well fermented. Thus the confusion and need for a more directed and specific set of terms.[524] A more detailed classification of fiber types is provided in Table 1.

Table 1: Fiber Types and Classes

Fiber	Classification
Dietary Fiber	Lignin
	Cellulose
	Beta-glucans
	Hemicellulose
	Pectins
	Gums
	Resistant Starch
Soluble Fibers	Beta-glucans
	Gums
	Wheat Dextrin
	Psyllium
	Pectins

Fermentable Fibers	Wheat Dextrin
	Pectins
	Beta-glucans
	Guar Gum
	Inulin
Viscous Fibers	Pectins
	Beta-glucans
	Some gums (e.g. guar gum)
	Psyllium
Functional Fiber	Resistant dextrins
	Psyllium
	Fructooligosaccharides
	Polydextrose
	Isolated Gums
	Isolated Resistant Starch
Insoluble Fibers	Cellulose
	Lignin
	Some Pectins
	Some Hemicelluloses
Non-fermentable Fibers	Cellulose
	Lignin
Non-viscous Fibers	Polydextrose
	Inulin

In looking to sources of prebiotics and fiber, vegetables, fruits, legumes, seeds, and whole grains present themselves as important considerations. However, the category of whole grains, like the category and sub-categories of fiber, is fraught with potential pitfalls. Here in the confusing collection of carbohydrate conditions, definition makes a difference in being able to wade through the data and the distraction. Firstly, what exactly is a "whole grain?" According to the Whole Grains Council:

> *Whole grains or foods made from them contain all the essential parts and naturally-occurring nutrients of the entire grain seed in their original proportions. If the grain has been processed (e.g., cracked, crushed, rolled, extruded, and/or cooked), the food product should deliver the same rich balance of nutrients that are found in the original grain seed.*
>
> *This definition means that 100 percent of the original kernel—all of the bran, germ, and endosperm—must be present to qualify as a whole grain.*[525]

Whole grain is not the same thing as multi-grain or the ever misleadingly popular twelve-grain. These terms have no legal meaning and merely suggest the presence of more than one grain type, all of which may be refined flours. The same is true for the term "wheat flour," this is just a clever way to market refined white flour. Both "bleached" and "unbleached wheat flour" are refined white flour. If the package reads just "wheat bread," it is likely made from a majority, if not entirely, from refined wheat flour.

Likewise, the phrases "made with whole grains, 100 percent wheat, multi-grain, contains whole grain, 7 grains, cracked wheat, made with whole wheat, bran, and multi grain," may be manufactured predominately with refined white flour.[526] Products that carry the phrase "high in fiber," may have had fiber additives like carboxymethylcellulose (CMC), maltodextrin, or other compounds added during the manufacturing process. The phrase that means something (in the US at least, as it varies by country) is "100 percent whole wheat" or "whole grain whole wheat." This implies that you are receiving whole grain wheat products.

Refining is a process that normally removes the bran and the germ, leaving only the endosperm. Removing the bran and germ removes fatty acids, and thus significantly increases shelf life. However, without the bran and germ, about 25 percent of a grain's protein is lost, and the remaining product is greatly reduced in at least seventeen key nutrients.

Processors can add back some vitamins and minerals to supplement refined grains, so refined products labeled "enriched" can still contribute valuable nutrients. However, they often remain inferior to whole grains in terms of protein, fiber, and many important vitamins and minerals.

All grain products contain carbohydrates. Refined wheat flour products, since they contain mostly endosperm, are predominately carbohydrate in composition. Carbohydrates can be defined chemically as neutral compounds of carbon, hydrogen and oxygen. Carbohydrates come in simple forms such as sugars and in complex forms such as starches and fiber.

Whole grains may be eaten whole, cracked, split, or ground. They can be milled into flour or used to make breads, cereals, and other processed foods. If a food label states that the package contains whole grain, the "whole grain" part of the food inside the package is required to have the same proportions of bran, germ, and endosperm as the harvested kernel does before it is processed. Make sure you use this as a guide and look for this when sourcing your foods.

A recent study, a meta-analysis of over seven hundred and fifty thousand people drawn from over fourteen different studies, examined the role of whole grain consumption in maintaining health. Specifically, the researchers looked at the rates of total mortality, cardiovascular mortality (CVD), and cancer mortality with respect to consumption of whole grain servings. They compared those who consumed the most to those who consumed the least.[527]

The researchers conducted a whole grains meta-analysis and showed impressive benefit to including such comestibles as part of a healthful dietary tactic. Many indigenous diets and approaches like the Mediterranean diet emphasize these wholesome, authentic foods over highly processed ones. The group eating the most whole grains, compared to the group consuming the least, reduced their overall early mortality rate by 16 percent. They were 12 percent less likely to die from cancer and 18 percent less likely to die from cardiovascular disease.[528] Interestingly, another recent study looking at barley, a Mediterranean staple, and showed that it significantly reduced two different forms of LDL, or "bad" cholesterol.[529]

Each 16g/day serving of whole grains, an amount which is considered a daily serving, reduced total mortality by 7 percent, cancer mortality by 5 percent, and cardiovascular mortality by 9 percent. The highest consumers ate three or more servings per day.[530] In other studies, whole grains have been shown to significantly reduce the incidence of stroke and type II diabetes (T2DM).[531] Current Dietary Guidelines for Americans recommends at least three servings per day of whole grain intake.

Including such whole grains in the diet does not always require the consumption of gluten, either, since gluten, as previously noted, is only found in wheat, barley, rye, spelt,

and triticale (a rye/wheat hybrid). Other options that are gluten free include some seeds, but since they are prepared and
consumed like grains they are usually included with them.
Using sprouted flours or methods like sourdough fermentation can decrease the gluten content, although not completely eradicate it. But remember, the governmental standards for gluten-free do not require it be free of gluten in the
common-sense way that gluten-free would mean no gluten.
The government only requires that:

> *In general, foods may be labeled "gluten-free"
> if they meet the definition and otherwise
> comply with the final rule's requirements.
> More specifically, the final rule defines "glu-
> ten-free" as meaning that the food either is
> inherently gluten free, or does not contain
> an ingredient that is: 1) a gluten-contain-
> ing grain (spelt, wheat); 2) derived from a
> gluten-containing grain that has not been
> processed to remove gluten (wheat flour); or
> 3) derived from a gluten-containing grain
> that has been processed to remove gluten
> (wheat starch), if the use of that ingredient
> results in the presence of twenty parts per
> million (ppm) or more gluten in the food.
> Also, any unavoidable presence of gluten in
> the food must be less than twenty ppm."[532]*

Therefore gluten-free, a voluntary labeling, is less than
twenty ppm per serving, not zero. A partial gluten-free list
includes amaranth, buckwheat, corn, millet, quinoa, rice,
wild rice, sorghum, teff, and oats, although as previously
noted, many prepackaged and pre-prepared oat products

contain a gluten warning because there is possible cross contamination in the plants where they are manufactured.

Our diet, like our lives, needs balance. In the addition or
subtraction to make it so, remember to keep it forever delicious. At the end, it is the taste of the experience that lingers.
Eat fewer refined grains and more whole grains, changes the
latest research supports. Reduce the amount of added sugar
in your diet. Experts now correctly recommend the guidelines should be simplified to emphasize "real" foods, especially plants, over processed or packaged goods.[533]

"The guidelines should also remove talk of recommended
daily allowances (RDAs)...This focus on RDAs is confusing
and not helpful, since people do not eat nutrients one by
one but in combination, in the form of whole and processed
foods," says Doctor Walter Willett, chair of the Department
of Nutrition at Harvard School of Public Health.[534]

The seeds and grains checklist is as follows:

- *How was it bred?* Is it heirloom? Is it GMO? Is it wild
  harvested or farmed? If it is farmed can you identify
  the source country? If wild sourced, from where?
- *What was it fed?* Organically raised? Sustainable or
  commercial? Industrially produced? Artificial fertilizers? Pesticides? Industrial pesticides?
- *Where was it led?* Was it processed? If so, locally, or
  regionally? In the US or overseas? If overseas, was it
  industrially processed or overseen by other methods?
  If overseas, under what conditions? What was the
  processing method (e.g. stone ground versus industrial rolling and extraction)? Degree of processing—is
  it whole wheat whole grain, partial, or totally refined?

Eggs and Dairy

What is the dish on dairy?

The cardiometabolic effects of different dairy foods represent a major unanswered question of modern nutrition science. Most dietary guidelines simply group different types together (e.g., grouping milk, cheese, and yogurt as "dairy"), categorize these by fat content, and then recommend selection of low-fat products. Such recommendations largely derive from theoretical considerations about selected single nutrients (e.g., calcium, vitamin D, calories, saturated fat), rather than empirical evidence on health effects of the *actual* foods.[535]

Such a concept utilizing theoretical models is a common approach to the complexities of detailing the health effects of food consumption. However, very frequently, such an approach finds itself at odds with the observational data. While this should prompt a review of the underlying hypothesis, the retort is often to dismiss the empirical data. This folly has coalesced into the lump of confusion that currently surrounds public perception of salt, red meat, fat, saturated fat, alcohol, red wine, gluten, carbohydrates, and dairy to name but a few visible upon the tip of the expert opinion iceberg.

One particular area of misconception when it comes to dairy is the deception of full fat dairy. The dissemination of the myth that all fat, particularly saturated fat, is bad has led to the ostracization of dairy products in their full fat natural state. This has spawned complete industries manufacturing low fat, skim, fat-free, and other unnatural permutations of dairy foods.

It is all false.

In longitudinal studies evaluating habitual intakes of dairy foods, relationships with CVD and diabetes mellitus do not consistently differ by fat content, but appear more specific to food type: e.g., cheese, yogurt, milk, butter.[536, 537, 538, 539, 540, 541, 542] It matters *what* you eat and its *quality*, not how much fat or calories it contains. Think of real butter from pastured, grass-fed cows without recombinant bovine somatotropin (rBST) injections versus trans-fatty acid laden margarine and you get the idea.

It depends on what category of dairy you choose to eat. For example, the intake of yogurt, but not milk, is consistently associated with lower incidence of diabetes mellitus. It is clearly not fat or calorie content that is the driver. The intake of cheese, which has high caloric, fat, and saturated fat content, is associated with lower diabetes risk in several studies.

Although total milk intake is generally not associated with an increased risk for the development of diabetes mellitus and other diseases associated with the MWD[543], fermented milk products are clearly linked to lower risk. [544, 545, 546, 547, 548, 549, 550, 551, 552, 553, 554] These findings suggest that the health effects of dairy may depend on multiple complex characteristics (e.g., probiotics in yogurt, fermentation of cheese). In observations that examined the effects of dairy foods instead of drawing conclusions based on preconceived theories, researchers found that in cohorts using objective blood biomarkers, greater dairy fat consumption was associated with a lower incidence of diabetes mellitus and CHD.[555, 556, 557, 558, 559, 560, 561]

Despite evidence to the contrary, current United States dietary guidelines continue to recommend the consumption of low-fat dairy products for improved cardiovascular health. These recommendations continue even though documentation from many randomized controlled trials (RCTs), the gold standard of clinical data acquisition, contradict this conventional wisdom.

Such broad policies are traditionally focused on viewing isolated nutrients or components, often in the context of their effect on specific variables or components. In the case of cardiovascular disease, the focus is often on the effect of raising or reducing LDL or "bad" cholesterol. The logic behind promoting low-fat or fat-free dairy alternatives (often containing significant additives) is to avoid consumption of the potentially cholesterol raising saturated fatty acids (SFAs) that are found in traditional, unadulterated dairy products.

Interestingly, the Institute of Medicine recently observed that the beneficial cardiovascular effects associated with the class of prescription medication of cholesterol-lowering drugs known as statins should not be extrapolated to dietary induced changes. In other words, the cardiovascular benefit of such drugs as statins may have other mechanisms in addition to, or independent of, any LDL cholesterol lowering effect. Statin medications are known to have anti-inflammatory properties.

Thus, with respect to full fat dairy products, what does the dairy dossier reveal?

LDL cholesterol: The data from both meta-analyses and a number of RCTs suggest that increasing the consumption of dairy products (including high-fat) has no net effect on the LDL cholesterol concentration in otherwise healthy individuals. Even consuming such a paragon of full fat dairy evils as cheese with its high cholesterol and saturated fat content had no effect on LDL cholesterol concentrations in postmenopausal women. Consuming other fermented dairy products like yogurt likewise had no net effect on LDL cholesterol concentrations in otherwise healthy women compared to a *dairy-free* diet. Even when a high dairy fat was compared to a similar, but low dairy fat diet, there was no significant difference in the LDL cholesterol levels. The conclusion is that *fermented* dairy products like yogurt, irrespective of fat content, do not impact LDL cholesterol levels.

HDL-cholesterol: The comparison of a diet high in dairy versus a low dairy alternative yielded no difference in HDL, or "good" cholesterol levels. Likewise, there was no impact when comparing low dairy fat alternatives to more traditional high fat dairy foods. This data suggests that dairy fat *per se* has no impact on HDL cholesterol concentrations. This is important because by affecting neither the LDL nor HDL cholesterol level, the LDL to HDL cholesterol ratio remains unchanged. This ratio correlates well with overall likelihood of cardiovascular events and is used in assessing cardiovascular risk.

Triglycerides: Triglycerides are another blood lipid parameter used to assess cardiovascular health. A recent study found that a Mediterranean style dietary approach utilizing whole milk products and yogurt for three weeks significantly reduced the fasting triglyceride concentrations compared to a similar diet that replaced the whole fat products with skim versions of milk and yogurt. A study comparing a vegetarian diet to the Mediterranean diet found the Mediterranean diet more effective in lowering triglyceride levels and 15 percent more effective in significantly lowering thirteen markers of inflammation than the vegetarian approach.[562] Overall, the consumption of various types of dairy foods does not appear to significantly impact the fasting or postprandial triglyceride levels.

Inflammation: Many of the disabilities and diseases associated with consumption of the modern Western diet are associated with underlying inflammation. A recent meta-analysis looking at high risk individuals, overweight and obese adults, found no adverse risk from dairy consumption with respect to circulating biomarkers of inflammation. Other studies corroborate these findings. They have found that high dairy consumption compared to low dairy consumption had no impact on plasma C-reactive protein (CRP) concentrations. CRP levels are associated with generalized, systemic inflammation. Dairy consumption had no impact on other inflammatory biomarkers such as adiponectin, IL-1β, IL-6, monocyte chemoattractant protein 1 (MCP-1), and TNF-α.

Insulin resistance: Insulin resistance is the hallmark of type II diabetes mellitus, which has reached epidemic proportions in the United States and many other industrialized countries. A close examination of the meta-analysis and the RCTs gives some insight into some of the previously contradictory findings with respect to the consumption of dairy, insulin resistance, and T2DM.

Short-term studies reveal no significant negative impact on insulin resistance with dairy consumption. However, studies in which there was a longer period of dairy consumption (twelve weeks or greater) suggest that over the *long term* such dairy consumption is associated with *favorable* changes in glucose and insulin homeostasis. Such findings are in concordance with epidemiological studies which suggest that populations which have significant dairy intake are associated with a lower risk of T2D.

Thus, short term consumption of full fat dairy yields no increased danger of developing T2DM, as one might expect based on current evidence. However, with prolonged consumption a *beneficial* effect emerges. If the mechanism involves affecting the gut microbiome due to probiotic delivery from comestibles like yogurt and cheese; the tincture of time required for demonstrable change is in perfect concordance with this natural progression.

In the face of such data, one of the studies adroitly concludes:

> *The purported detrimental effects of SFAs [saturated fatty acids] on cardiometabolic health may in fact be nullified when they are consumed as part of complex food matrices such as those in cheese and other dairy foods. Thus, the focus on low-fat dairy products...in the current guidelines is not entirely supported by the existing literature, because no evidence currently supports a detrimental effect of regular or high-fat dairy products compared with low-fat dairy on a large spectrum of cardio-metabolic disease risk factors.*
>
> *No long-term studies support harms, and emerging evidence suggests some potential benefits, of dairy fat or high-fat dairy foods such as cheese. Together these findings provide little support for the prevailing recommendations for dairy intake that are based largely on calcium and vitamin D contents, rather than complete cardiometabolic effects; that emphasize low-fat dairy based on theorized influences on obesity and CHD, rather than empirical evidence, or that consider dairy as a single category rather than separately evaluating different dairy foods. Little evidence supports the opposing hypothesis, i.e., the superiority of*

low-fat dairy products for health, including
for risk of obesity.[563]

Long-term effects may vary by the type of dairy. For instance, children who drink more low-fat milk gain more weight over time, whereas those who drink more whole-fat milk gain less weight.[564] In longitudinal studies among adults, neither low-fat nor whole-fat milk are appreciably related to chronic weight gain.[565, 566, 567]

As previously intimated, both animal models and trials in humans suggest that probiotics and probiotic-microbiome interactions do play a key role in the protective effects seen with yogurt consumption, particularly with respect to the risk of developing obesity and related conditions such as gestational diabetes.[568, 569, 570, 571, 572, 573, 574, 575, 576] Naturally fermented foods of all types, nature's synbiotic, offer healthful benefits across a wide variety of tastes and textures. Almost every culture has a history of food fermentation, along with alcohol production, of some type or another. Many diary rich societies have some form of fermented milk, cheese, or butter.

In the discussion of specific dairy, there have been few foods in recent history as maligned and misunderstood as butter.

Butter has long been an important dietary staple of many societies around the globe. From the five thousand-year-old bog butter of Ireland to the sub-continent of India where *ghee* (a type of clarified butter) remains not only a cooking staple, but also a medicine, butter has been important nutritionally, culturally, religiously, and perhaps most pertinent in the present, tastefully.

Yet today butter is the poster child of fat shaming. Back in the day when everything was simpler and more confused, it was conventional wisdom that dietary cholesterol and fat, particularly saturated fat, would increase not only your waistline, but your cholesterol level. That meant an early death from cardiovascular disease.

Such an obvious and straightforward connection opened the door for replacements as butter went the way of lard and tallow; left on the floor of a culinary abattoir. So we invented things to look, cook, and taste like butter while not actually *being* butter. While we couldn't "Believe It's Not Butter," we chowed down on artificially created trans-fatty acids (TFAs) that detonated in our arterial walls like time delayed IEDs.

Now, over fifty years since the government delivered us unto the aisles of *low-fat, fat-free, less fat,* and a host of other tasteless substitutions, we're beginning to turn the massive ship of guidelines and recommendations onto a proper course. In the meantime, generations remain lost in a sea of misinformation. As Mark Bittman so succinctly comments:

> *the industry's idea of "low fat" became the emblematic SnackWell's and other highly processed "low-fat" carbs (a substitution that is probably the single most important factor in our overweight/obesity problem), as well as reduced fat and even fat-free dairy, on which it made billions of dollars. (How you could produce fat-free "sour cream" is something worth contemplating.)...And let's not think about the literally millions of people who are repelled by fat, not because it doesn't taste good (any chef will tell you that "fat is flavor") but because they have been brainwashed.*
>
> *Why would you buy a processed food that tastes worse than what it was designed*

to replace, doesn't exist in nature, and helps kill you? [577]

Why indeed?

Because of the "fat is bad" fallacy, butter, which is the dairy product highest in fat, became emblematic of all America's food-borne ills. It became the poster and practice of what was wrong with the American diet and what needed to be avoided at all costs.

Except the premise was wrong.

Remember the French Paradox? The French live longer (eighty-two versus seventy-eight years), have an obesity rate that is over 50 percent less than ours (14 percent versus 35 percent), and have healthier elder years (43 percent of those over sixty-five with ≥2 more chronic conditions versus 68 percent) compared to the U.S. [578] They also eat more butter than anyone else in the world, roughly 17.6 pounds per person per year. *Vive La France!*

A recent meta-analysis sought to examine this mystery, looking at "the evidence for the relationship between butter consumption and long-term health." Their analysis combined nine trials involving fifteen countries and over six hundred thousand people. Of significant interest was the fact that there was *not one* randomized, controlled clinical trial. [579] Despite the excommunication of an entire food source from the gastronomic pantheon, replete with warnings, guidelines, recommendations, and dire prophecy, not once did anyone ever look to compare the outcomes of butter consumption to what was being offered in its place.

In a large pooling project of European cohorts, individuals consuming any butter, in comparison with none, experienced a lower risk of diabetes mellitus. [580] Butter consumption is not significantly associated with incident CHD, stroke, or total mortality. [581, 582, 583]

What is the relationship between butter with all its evil saturated fat and the risk of developing cardiovascular disease (CVD)? Nothing, nada, zero. As the researchers concluded, "butter intake was not significantly associated with CVD."[584] Same for risk of stroke.

What about the risk of developing type 2 diabetes mellitus through the consumption of butter? Other recent research has suggested that those "with diabetes have a 50 percent increased risk of dying following an acute myocardial infarction (AMI) compared with those who've had a heart attack but don't have diabetes."[585] If fat makes you fat (as we have been led to believe), and obesity is a risk factor for developing diabetes, then butter clearly is the "die" in diabetes.

Except, once again, when we actually look at the data, it's not.

The investigators found that "butter consumption was associated with a *lower* incidence of type 2 diabetes, with 4 percent lower risk per daily 14g serving." They went on to note that:

> *Current dietary recommendations on butter and dairy fat are largely based upon predicted effects of specific individual nutrients (e.g., total saturated fat, calcium), rather than actual observed health effects. Our findings add to a growing body of evidence on long-term health effects of specific foods and types of fats. Conventional guidelines on dietary fats have not accounted for their diverse food sources nor the specific individual fatty acid profiles in such foods. Different*

*foods represent complex matrices of nutri-
ents, processing, and food structure, which
together influence net health effects.*[586]

This does not even begin to delve into the effects of different foods on our gut microbiome, our symbiotic organ of
environmental interface. Because the quality matters, sourcing is important. Milk fat, which butter is so rich in, contains extremely potent compounds like the anti-inflammatory
omega-3 fatty acids (ω-3FAs). It is rich in conjugated linoleic
acid (CLA), and a number of healthful vitamins and minerals. Additional research has correlated "dairy fat consumption
to diminished weight gain, attenuated markers of metabolic
syndrome, including waist circumference, and reduced risk of
CVD and colorectal cancer."[587] These are health benefits that are
associated with not only eating more dairy, but *more dairy fat*.

Yet there are important differences in our options even
when looking at the same food. This is one of the obsta-
cles when trying to determine the effects of foods and diet.
Within the same food choice, the options are not identical.
Industrial butter is produced in a manner that is reflective
of the highly processed nature of the modern Western diet.
Many such manufactured dairy products including butter
have an elevated omega-6 (ω-6) to omega-3 (ω-3) ratio.

There is increasing evidence that the dietary balance of
ω-3 and ω-6 FA is at least as important, and perhaps more
important, than the absolute amounts of saturated, monounsaturated, and total fat that obsess the current public narrative. While the ideal ratio is unknown, experts believe it
is somewhere in the 1:1 to 3:1 range. Current estimates put
the US diet at 15-17:1 and over 20:1 in some studies. Even
human breast milk has seen a dramatic increase in the ω-6:
ω-3 ratio as a result of changes in the maternal diet.

Milk, and thus butter, from cows allowed to consume their natural food like grass has higher concentrations of ω-3 FAs and CLA than that from cows lacking routine access to pasture and fed substantial quantities of grains, especially corn.[588] The balance of FAs in foods like butter depends on the animal's diet and on its digestive physiology. That digestive physiology, just like ours, is greatly dependent on the integrity of the natural gut microbiome. This can be radically affected by the living and rearing conditions as well as the feed. Feed made with GMO containing product has been shown to negatively alter the gut microbiome of livestock.

Organic milk, butter, and other milk derived products are not allowed to be produced from animals that consume GMO feed. The U.S. National Organic Program (NOP) stipulates that certified organic farms receive at least 30 percent of daily Dry Matter Intake (DMI) from pasture during that portion of the year when pasture grasses and legumes are actively growing, with a minimum of 120 days per year. Pasture and conserved, forage-based feeds account for most of the DMI year-round on a growing portion of organic dairy operations in the United States.

The same labeling laws apply to dairy products like cheese. Although they are perhaps not as necessary compared to a fresh dairy product like butter because of the way cheese is produced and the natural fermentation it undergoes. Until very recently, the prevailing conventional wisdom for healthy eating relegated consuming cheese to a failing of the ignorant, simple, or misguided. From the late 1940s through the 1970s and continuing to today, there remains a mandate from many so-called experts and powers that be to consume less fat and particularly saturated fat, principally those derived from animal sources such as meat, poultry, and dairy.

That admonishment has continued to echo and drive poor culinary choices over the ensuing half-century plus. This meant pass over the cheese.

An honest historical glance would reveal that a modest, living, fermented food like real cheese has helped sustain and advance humankind across civilizations and across the globe. While a large portion of the world's population is lactose intolerant and therefore unable to consume or potentially benefit from raw or fresh milk products, cheeses, particularly aged cheeses, are an exception.

The milk sugar, or lactose, is what causes the issue in those lacking the enzymatic machinery to process fresh dairy. This sugar is utilized by various beneficial bacteria, such as *Lactobacillus*, in the production of cheese. Along with the fats, most of which are saturated, and proteins, and through the process of fermentation, raw milk undergoes the transformation from raw milk product to cheese. As certain cheeses age, there is often less and less lactose present. Thus, for many, even those who are lactose intolerant and unable to tolerate fresh milk, such delicious pillows of probiotic loaded goodness as naturally fermented cheese can be enjoyed.

Until the most recent times real cheeses were often discounted as part of a healthful approach to eating primarily because of their saturated fat and cholesterol content. While the Mediterranean diet was promoted as an ideal dietary model, this misrepresented dairy aspect of that gastronomy was shoved into a corner where it lingered and moldered.

Often unappreciated is the historical fact that fermented dairy has a long and prominent place in ancient diets. This is because while fresh milk can be consumed, it is quite perishable and much more valuable as a raw material. Raw milk can be turned into several products like cream, butter, yogurts, kefir, whey, and cheese, all of which have a substantially longer shelf life.

Cheese reemerged from the shadows with the insights gleaned from the French paradox of the 1990s. The French, who drank wine and consumed butter, cream, and over one hundred different kinds of cheese, most of which are oh-so-stinky good, all these tasty bits that were *verboten* in the US at the time, had significantly less cardiovascular disease.[589] It turns out it was more than the wine.[590]

A dietary approach like Mediterranean style cuisine, rich in natural, wholesome, and fermented foods, has been shown to reduce generalized inflammation and stress. Oxidative stress and inflammation play major roles in the onset and development of diabetes and its precursor, metabolic syndrome. Metabolic syndrome is diagnosed by the presence of central obesity and at least two of the following four additional factors: high triglycerides, low HDL or "good" cholesterol, high blood pressure, or increased fasting plasma glucose concentration.

Sub-group data from the European Prospective Investigation into Cancer and Nutrition (EPIC) study examined sixteen thousand eight hundred and thirty-five healthy and twelve thousand four hundred and three diabetic participants from eight European nations. The researchers found an inverse association between cheese, fermented dairy consumption, and the incidence of diabetes. Eating only 55g/d total of cheese and/or yogurt was associated with a 12 percent reduction in the incidence of type 2 diabetes mellitus.[591]

Another study revealed that just thirty grams daily of a Parmesan-like Italian cheese, Grana Padano, lowered blood pressure as effectively as the typically prescribed antihypertensive pharmaceutical. This occurred, even though the cheese contained the equivalent amount of sodium that would be found in consuming a one ounce serving of potato chips.[592]

Previous studies had isolated some particular tripeptides in certain types of cheese and demonstrated a relationship to being able to lower blood pressure. These particular compounds are formed through the interaction of human gastrointestinal enzymes and the gut microbiota.

These peptide complexes have angiotensin-converting enzyme inhibiting properties. Such ACE inhibitors constitute an important class of medications that not only lower blood pressure, but are a foundation of therapy from those suffering from cardiomyopathy or congestive heart failure from a variety of causes.[593]

Another study examined almost twenty thousand participants. It examined the association between cheese consumption in various age groups and circulating concentrations of HDL or "good" cholesterol and triglycerides, negative and positive risk factors for cardiovascular disease, respectively. The more cheese consumed the higher the HDL and the lower the triglycerides. The researchers suggested that this was the result of the particular fatty acid composition of cheese and its inherent, probiotic, bacterial content.[594]

The high protein and probiotic content of cheese is believed to contribute to its almost neutral effect on plasma cholesterol. Even though cheese is high in cholesterol and saturated fat, like so many other such natural foodstuffs, its impact on blood lipids and total cholesterol is negligible. Some kinds of cheeses, namely those infected with *Penicillium* bacteria such as Roquefort, Stilton, or Gorgonzola, exhibit high concentrations of andrastins A, B, C, and D.[595] (See appendix D5)

Oligosaccharides, which are present in cheeses, are prebiotics. This is the food that sustains a healthy gut microbiota. It is what feeds the wee beasties. Cheeses, which contain both prebiotics and probiotics, become that penultimate gut microbiome inoculum: a synbiotic.

Another study demonstrated that cheese consumption directly altered the gut microbiome in an extremely favorable way.[596] Certain gut bacteria are associated with the production of a compound known as trimethylamine-N-oxide or TMAO; which was previously covered in detail. The bacteria produce this compound in response to the dietary ingestion of choline, among other compounds. Levels of TMAO have been found to correlate with and are directly predictive of, cardiovascular risk.

The consumption of cheese rapidly altered the composition of the gut microbiome. There was significantly less TMAO produced. The positive changes to the gut microbiome associated with the regular consumption of such a powerful, wholesome, naturally fermented, synbiotic food as cheese may explain the relatively low incidence of cardiovascular disease in high cheese consumption countries.[597]

When it comes to cheese, the stinkier the better. More funk correlates to longevity, at least in theory. A study published in *Nature* suggests that a particular compound found in stinky, aged cheese could be the key to longevity and cardiovascular health.

This compound is particularly prevalent in bleu cheeses, as well as other pungent, aged varieties of naturally fermented cheeses. The molecule is known as spermidine, because, well, it was discovered first in semen. The researchers used a murine model to compare cardiovascular endpoints in animals that received spermidine-infused water versus those that had not. The diet was otherwise identical. The mice consuming spermidine lived longer and were healthier than those that did not consume the compound. The researchers suggest that this compound may be involved in human longevity.[598] (See appendix D6)

Canned cheese doesn't cut it. For health, long life, and potent interludes, cut authentic, stinky cheese and serve it up. You simply cannot deny the power of authenticity.

Real whole eggs, like butter and cheese, received banishment from the culinary kingdom for perceived crimes: possession of fat, saturated fat, and cholesterol. Eggs are so rich in dietary cholesterol at roughly 275mg of cholesterol per yolk that they can serve as a dietary bellwether of cholesterol consumption. At the beginning of governmental edicts concerning diet in the 1970s, cholesterol consumption was about 600mg per day, or roughly two eggs.

Americans were admonished to abstain from the evil egg and salvation was instead to be found in whites only (talk about dietary discrimination), or syntho-egg-like creations poured from a carton. The population complied, egg consumption dropped, and daily cholesterol consumption fell to the then recommended guidelines of 300mg per day. Obesity, diabetes and their associated morbidities rose.

This type of all too common result from empirical edicts is one reason, among the others previously discussed, that dietary restrictions for cholesterol were abolished in 2016. The 2015 Dietary Guidelines Advisory Committee concluded that "dietary cholesterol is not a 'nutrient of concern for overconsumption,' based on low mean population cholesterol intake and no appreciable relationships between dietary cholesterol and serum cholesterol or clinical cardiovascular events in general populations."[599]

When such groups are studied, egg consumption has no significant association with incident CVD. [600, 601, 602] Whole eggs, including the yolk, are inexpensive, readily available, and contain high quality proteins, essential vitamins and minerals, as well as the antioxidant carotenoids lutein and zeaxanthin, lecithin, choline, and cholesterol.

Eggs remain the World Health Organization standard for complete dietary protein delivery, with one egg delivering 12 percent of daily protein needs. Eggs are considered a complete protein and supply leucine, isoleucine, valine, methionine, cysteine, lysine, tryptophan, and other essential amino acids.

Conjugated linoleic acid (CLA) has been shown to have antitumor activity. It also helps with glucose regulation and decreases body fat. CLA, like many of the important components of the egg, is found exclusively in the yolk. Chickens raised naturally and organically produce eggs significantly higher in CLA and omega-3 PUFAs like alpha linolenic acid (ALA) and docosahexaenoic acid (DHA).

Even examining patients among those at the highest risk for cardiovascular events, those with T2DM, egg consumption did not increase their risk profile. A study looked specifically at egg consumption, eating two eggs per day over six weeks, in those with T2DM. The researchers found that "(h) igh egg consumption did not have an adverse effect on the lipid profile of people with T2D in the context of increased MUFA and PUFA consumption. This study suggests that a high-egg diet can be included safely as part of the dietary management of T2D, and it may provide greater satiety."[603]

Contrary to expectations, no differences were shown for total cholesterol, low-density lipoprotein cholesterol, or triglycerides among those consuming eggs compared to those that do not. A meta-analysis of clinical trials looking at egg consumption and health effects found:

the majority of RCTs in individuals with diabetes or at risk for developing diabetes found

*that egg consumption (six to twelve eggs/week)
did not have a negative effect on major CVD
risk factors...(there is) currently no evidence
that consuming additional eggs increases
CVD risk in people with type 2 diabetes.*[604]

Other groups, like men who carry a genetic variant known as the ε4 allele (APOE4) in the apolipoprotein E gene (APOE), are at high risk of developing CVD. Researchers have likewise found that egg or cholesterol intake are not associated with increased CAD risk, even in in highly susceptible individuals like ApoE4 carriers.[605]

For the average person, the evidence suggests that eating just "one egg/d was sufficient to increase HDL function and large-LDL particle concentration; however, intake of two to three eggs/d supported greater improvements in HDL function as well as increased plasma carotenoids. Overall, intake of ≥ three eggs/d favored a less atherogenic LDL particle profile, improved HDL function, and increased plasma antioxidants in young, healthy adults."[606] In other words, eating up to *three eggs per day*, compared to not eating any eggs, increased the *favorability* of the blood lipid profile.

Despite this overwhelming evidence, organizations like the American Heart Association continue to recommend egg whites without the yolks as a heart-healthy source of protein.[607] Recent guidelines from the AHA in conjunction with the American College of Cardiology go further and recommend severe limitation on egg consumption.[608] This continues despite, as previously mentioned, the removal of the 300 mg/day limit of dietary cholesterol in the 2015-2020 Dietary Guidelines for Americans.

In fact, research suggests that consuming two eggs per day decreases ghrelin, the hunger causing gremlin, while having no effect on the LDL/HDL ratio (a powerful predictor of cardiovascular risk) compared to an oatmeal breakfast.[609] A reduction in ghrelin is significant because decreased levels of ghrelin have been related to decreased appetite and can increase weight loss. At least one egg per day reduces inflammation, as measured by blood levels of the inflammatory marker tumor necrosis factor alpha (TNF-α), when compared to oatmeal.[610]

These studies put eggs under the broiler. Eggs are being compared to the food *recommended* by the AHA and awarded the ability to claim it is heart healthy. Despite the evidence, these professional organizations are condemning the food that in some respects is superior to what they currently recommend.

If you look carefully, you will find the experts putting this document together as an expert consensus panel published in the *Journal of The American College of Cardiology*, have a lot of distractions from industry. There is a large paragraph of disclosures including involvement on the McDonald's Global Advisory and at least two of the authors have their own commercial, low fat dietary regimen and products.

When making dietary decisions, Mother Nature seems to be the best, and final, arbitrator.

The dairy checklist is as follows:

- *How was it bred?* Is it from heritage breeds? Is it from conventional breeds? Is it GMO? Where are the animals from (country of product origin)?
- *What was it fed?* Is it organically produced? Was it subjected to GMO feed? Were hormones like rBST or other agents used? Were animals pastured or CAFO? Grass fed or grains? Natural diets or commercial feed?

- *Where was it led?* Was it processed? If processed, locally, or regionally? In the US or overseas? If overseas was it industrially or overseen by other methods? If overseas, under what conditions? For fermented products are the cultures still alive? For fresh products, are they pasteurized, ultra-pasteurized?

The egg checklist is as follows:

- *How was it bred?* Is it from heritage breeds? Is it from conventional breeds? Is it GMO? Where are the animals from (country of product origin)?
- *What was it fed?* Is it organically produced? Was it subjected to GMO feed? Were hormones or other agents used? Were animals pastured/free ranged or CAFO? Natural diet or grains?
- *Where was it led?* Look for use by date on carton? Any post-harvest modifications besides simple packaging?

Vegetables and Fruit

Eat more fresh fruits and vegetables.

This is probably the one thing all diets, healthful approaches, expert guidelines, and recommendations can agree upon. The MWD has displaced vegetable and fruit consumption from the table in favor of processed, sugar, salt, and fat laden alternatives loaded with artificial flavors, preservatives, emulsifiers, and other industrial modifiers.

Minimally processed foods like fresh fruits and vegetables are consistently linked to better health outcomes. These are reinforced with long term outcomes.[611, 612, 613, 614] Foods like berries and nuts are particularly rich in phytochemicals and particularly potent with benefit. Potatoes contain fiber, potassium, vitamins C and B_6, and other trace minerals. Organically grown plants, on average, have higher concentrations of antioxidants, lower concentrations of cadmium, and a lower incidence of pesticide residues than the non-organic comparators across regions and production seasons.[615]

Bioactive polyphenols such as flavonols can be found in onions, broccoli, tea, and various fruits. Parsley, celery, and chamomile tea are great sources of flavones. Other polyphenol antioxidants like flavanones are found in citrus fruits, flavanols (flavan-3-ols) such as catechins and procyanidins are abundant in cocoa, apples, grapes, red wine, and tea. Purple colored vegetables and fruits like berries are rich in anthocyanidins. Soy supplies potent isoflavones. The remarkable heterogeneity of different flavonoids and their plant derived dietary sources inspires wonder and excitement at such a tasteful, delicious, and vibrant cornucopia of pharmacopeia. These vegetables and fruits continue to demonstrate evidence for cardiometabolic benefits and overall benefit in the prevention and treatment of the disabilities and diseases associated with the SAD.[616, 617, 618, 619]

However, the topic of fruits and vegetables invariably raises the specter of genetically modified organisms (GMOs) in short order.

What exactly are GMOs and how are they used?

Ever since the agricultural revolution thousands of years ago, humankind has been selecting plants and animals on the basis of certain traits. You might select a certain animal to breed because it is more docile and easier to manage or sow a certain plant because it produces a tastier or more abundant crop. In any case, you bring to the forefront naturally occurring traits. However, no matter what traits you select, the DNA of that blackberry is 100 percent blackberry as nature designed it.

A GMO is a manmade product. A genetically modified corn like NK603 GM, manufactured by Monsanto, is engineered to overexpress the modified version of the *Agrobacterium tumefaciens* 5-enolpyruvylshikimate-3-phosphate synthase (EPSPS-CP4).[620] This makes the maize resistant to the effects of the herbicide Roundup.

Agrobacterium tumefaciens is a rod-shaped, gram-negative soil bacterium also known as *Rhizobium radiobacter*. It causes crown gall disease, which affects a number of plant species. The gene from this bacterium is introduced into the DNA of the corn so the plant produces the bacterial product itself, rendering it immune to the effects of the herbicide.

Currently there is a vehement debate about the potential effects of such manipulations. Particularly, there is concern over the potential health effects of the chronic consumption of such GMOs. As remarkable as it may seem, currently no regulatory agency requires any mandatory chronic animal feeding studies to be performed for GMOs destined for human consumption.[621] Given the fact that the full formulations of herbicides and pesticides are not required to undergo such studies, this should not surprise us.

With respect to herbicides and pesticides, only the active component is required to undergo testing. For example, in the case of Roundup, only the active agent, glyphosate, was subject to toxicity studies.[622] This is important because there are possible direct biological effects from the other chemicals utilized in the formulation. Additionally, there may be indirect effects as the other constituents can affect the absorption and metabolism of the active component. Several pesticides have demonstrated significantly increased toxicity when the full formulations are studied as compared to the active principle alone.[623] The full formulations are how these agents are applied in agricultural practice.

Nonetheless, in an effort to demonstrate safety, the agricultural biotechnology industry has conducted several ninety-day rat feeding trials primarily utilizing genetically modified soy and maize. The vast majority of the genetically modified plants have been constructed to be resistant to the effects of the herbicide Roundup, or to produce a modified *Bacillus thuringiensis* (Bt) toxin, insecticide, or both. Such studies form the basis of the agribusiness claims as to the safety of genetically modified foodstuffs.[624, 625]

Bacillus thuringiensis is a spore forming bacterium that produces crystals protein (cry proteins), which are toxic to many species of insects. It is often used in organic farming as a natural pesticide. In genetically modified plants, the bacterial gene that produces the cry proteins is transferred into the DNA of the plant. The plant is now directly able to produce the insecticide.

In the case of the Roundup resistant genetically modified plants, the ability of the cash crop to be resistant to the herbicide allows for liberal application. This can result in the presence of herbicide in food that is eaten and for potential accumulation and concentration when it is used as feed for animal products. As a result, some countries have developed maximum residue levels (MRL) for these compounds. Unfortunately, these levels are often determined by toxicity studies that once again only target the active principle, not the compound at it as it is utilized in agricultural application.

The original study aimed at documenting the safety of Roundup resistant genetically modified maize demonstrated statistically significant differences in the liver and kidney function between the rats fed the GMO versus the non-GMO.[626, 627] The Monsanto sponsored authors explain this finding as not "biologically meaningful."[628] As in all such cases to date, the governmental regulatory agencies have accepted such explanations at face value.[629]

However, a published study examining the effects of the *chronic* consumption of Roundup resistant, Monsanto NK603 genetically modified maize represents contradictory and potentially landmark findings.[630] It was the first study to look at the chronic effects on mammalian physiology. In this case, the researchers studied the same type of rats that were utilized in the Monsanto study to demonstrate safety. (See appendix D7)

The study design is important, because this highlights a concern over GMOs. It is not necessarily the GMO *per se*, it is the *effects of the GMO* that may result in potentially significant and dangerous levels of pesticide ingestion. Given that the WHO classifies Roundup as a potential carcinogen, and given the distribution in terms of quantity and dispersion of such foodstuffs, this is no small matter.

It highlights the need to evaluate each GMO modification on its unique merits. The GMO, what it alters in terms of absence or addition, and what are the direct and/or indirect sequelae? A genetic modification that turns off the enzyme that causes exposed apple flesh to oxidize and turn brown, keeping cut apples fresher in appearance without adding acid, may be of little health import. Genetic modifications that cause rice to produce healthful carotenes may be a positive alteration.

Despite that preamble, the concern over the specific GMO modification that involves the use of Roundup *is* concerning. The liver and kidney problems noted at ninety days in the original Monsanto study developed into severe pathologies over the course of two years. The detrimental effects were seen in every treatment group; those that were fed genetically modified maize, those that were fed genetically modified maize treated with Roundup, and those that received Roundup in their drinking water.

The rats in the treatment group had two to three times the incidence of tumors. The female rats were given to the development of mammary tumors. There was a high level of pituitary tumors. These and other findings suggest a threshold effect causing significant disruption to the endocrine system. There was major disease and dysfunction of the hepatorenal system as well. The treatment groups, unsurprisingly, experienced increased mortality.

Such products like corn are ubiquitous in the MWD. Considering the amount of fried food Americans consume, and the use of oils containing GMO plants like corn and canola in their production, as well as the distribution of such oils in baked goods, condiments, and dressings, GMO alteration of these products is of grave concern. A 2018 U.S. Congressional report revealed that blood levels of glyphosate are detectable in over 90 percent of Americans.[631] Increased consumption of vegetable oils is not the equivalent of eating more fresh fruit and veg.

Vegetable oils are a category of oil that may vary by the type of oil and its predominant fatty acid (*i.e.*, saturated, polyunsaturated, and monounsaturated). Extra virgin olive oil (EVOO) contains oleocanthal, a phenylethanoid that binds cyclooxygenase (COX) 1 and 2 receptor. This is a contributor to the characteristic burning throat sensation, similar to that induced by chewing uncoated aspirin, experienced with real EVOO. Like aspirin, it exhibits anti-inflammatory properties with 50g of EVOO exhibiting about 10 percent of ibuprofen's anti-inflammatory activity.[632, 633, 634] There are differences in outcomes between regular olive oil and EVOO, suggesting that more than simply fatty acid content may be involved. [635] (See appendix D8)

As fruit and veg are a primary source of nutrients like potassium and magnesium, it is not surprising that they are deficient in the SAD. In randomized trials, potassium lowers BP and the risk of CVD, with stronger effects among individuals who have hypertension and when dietary sodium intake is high.[636]

Often, there is rationalization for eating less fruit and veg, and more processed and fried foods if a "heart healthy" oil like canola oil is used. Canola oil is touted for its health benefits and endorsed by the American Heart Association (AHA). The AHA healthy cooking oils guide said the following with respect to canola oil: "This was first introduced in the 1970s for home cooking and is made from seeds of the canola plant." This is the first, and rather egregious, error among many.

A good place to start is the beginning. Firstly, there is no such thing as a canola plant. What is referred to as the canola plant is really a cultivar of the rapeseed plant. That has been around and utilized by humans for at least four thousand years. It is a member of the *Brassica* family and is related to Brussels sprouts, mustard, rutabaga, turnips, and cabbage. In fact, the plant likely arose from natural crossbreeding between the turnip and the cabbage.

The oil has long been used for non-culinary applications, including use as a lamp oil. The natural compound is high in glucosinolates. These are compounds which add a bitter flavor to the liquid making it somewhat less than palatable. They are found in all members of this family and may actually be responsible for some of the health benefits associated with the consumption of cruciferous vegetables.

More importantly, naturally occurring rapeseed oil is extremely rich (30 to 60 percent) in erucic acid. Erucic acid, known as *cis*-13-docosenoic acid, is a monounsaturated omega-9 fatty acid. The name *"erucic"* is Latin for colewort, which is better known as kale. There have not been any significant morbidities in humans associated with the ingestion of plants containing this compound at naturally occurring levels. However, during the 1970s a series of animal experiments exposing them to high levels of ingestion suggested an association with the development of abnormalities involving the heart muscle.

In the 1970s, a variety of rapeseed was developed in Canada which was naturally low in erucic acid. This was accomplished through traditional seed crossbreeding and does not represent the creation of a genetically modified organism. The erucic acid was replaced by monounsaturated oleic acid, a prominent component of olive oil. By the end of the decade rapeseed oil produced by this cultivar contained less than 2 percent erucic acid. To consume levels of erucic acid which could potentially cause health concerns from canola oil derived from this variety, consumption would have to exceed 2 percent of total fatty acid intake.

It was during this time that the term canola was coined. Depending upon the source, it appears it was derived from a combination of Canadian ("can") and oil ("ola") or Canadian ("can"), oil ("o"), low acidity ("la"). The product was introduced into the United States in 1986 and touted as a healthful alternative due to its high smoke point (400°F/205°C), low saturated fat content (~6-7 percent), high monounsaturated fatty acid content (~63 percent) and favorable omega 6 to omega-3 polyunsaturated fatty acid ratio at 2:1.

However, in 1995 Monsanto introduced an herbicide resistant GMO version. Within a decade, almost 90 percent of the commercial rapeseed grown for canola oil in the United States was GMO. By 2009, 90 percent of Canadian rapeseed was GMO. The oil is currently commercially produced utilizing the hexane extraction method. In addition to the chemical exposure, the oil undergoes a steam distillation, bleaching, and deodorizing process.

Although currently marketed, likely based on serving size amounts, as trans-fatty acid (TFAs) free, some studies suggest that the oils contain anywhere from 0.56 to 4.2 percent TFAs. Recently, some canola oil has been labeled as organic. This refers only to the way the product was grown and processed; it may not address its GMO origin. Given the rat study suggesting pathology may develop due to the transgenic alterations alone, this is one reason specific GMO labeling is such a contentious topic.

The discussion, however, could be moot. The GMO is out of the can, literally. The GMO rapeseed has escaped the confines of commercial fields and has been found growing wild. Depending on your concern or comfort with such industrially produced products and GMOs, you can decide if, when it comes to culinary applications, canola is "oil" you want to use.

This is not a topic of discussion agribusiness wants us to have. The differences in the quality of food produced by different methods thus far have been constrained to those areas where the effects are potentially most concentrated. Farming fish can change both the amount and type of fat composition; grass fed, pasture raised organic beef is a superior meat; organic eggs are higher in critical nutrients; and most recently, studies demonstrated the healthier profile of organic milk and dairy products versus their conventional counterparts. And all of that tastes better from a culinary perspective.

But critics continually pointed to the fact that previous studies looking at fruits and vegetables, our base foundation, demonstrated no difference in terms of nutrition and only a slight reduction in pesticide levels. However, recent investigation has plowed that old agribusiness tale six feet under. A meta-analysis published in *The British Journal of Nutrition* contained almost three hundred and fifty different scientific papers.[637] It has over one hundred studies more than the previous most complete meta-analyses.[638] More than half of the studies in the most recent analysis have been published within the last decade. Here is the takeaway:

Organic fruits and vegetables are nutritionally superior. Organic fruits and vegetables are significantly higher in levels of critically important compounds like antioxidants. Organic products are 19 percent higher in phenolic acids, 69 percent higher in the flavanones, 28 percent higher in stilbenes, 26 percent higher in flavones, 50 percent higher in flavonols, and 51 percent higher in anthocyanins. Simply consuming organic produce could increase antioxidant levels in the diet from 20 to 70 percent.

Organic fruits and vegetables contain fewer toxic heavy metals. Organic fruits and vegetables were shown to be 48 percent lower in the toxic heavy metal cadmium. Cadmium is an extremely toxic heavy metal and its levels and exposure to it are heavily regulated. It can cause painful and significant bone, joint, respiratory (when inhaled), and kidney diseases. Cadmium toxicity from ingesting rice grown with contaminated water was the source in the early to mid-twentieth century Japanese epidemic called the *Itai-itai* (it hurts-it hurts) disease.

Organic fruits and vegetables contain less nitrogen. Concern is often raised over the nitrite content of processed foods like hot dogs and bacon. This is because of a perceived potential increased risk of certain carcinomas like gastric cancer. Because of the growing methods, organic crops contain significantly less nitrogen compounds. Organic crops are 10 percent lower in total nitrogen, 30 percent lower in nitrates, and 87 percent lower in nitrites compared to mass-produced, conventionally grown crops.

Organically grown fruits and vegetables contain significantly less pesticides. Lower pesticide levels with organically grown crops compared to conventionally grown crops have been a consistent finding. However, this study highlighted a significant difference:

- The highest pesticide levels were found in conventionally mass-produced fruit at a frequency of 75 percent.
- Crop-based products were the next highest at 45 percent, followed by mass-produced conventionally grown vegetables at 32 percent.
- There was a 10 percent frequency found in the organic produce, but this may have been from wind-borne contamination originating from conventionally grown fields.
- Overall, the detectable pesticide residue is four times higher in conventionally grown, mass-produced crops compared to those that are organically raised.

It is estimated that by switching to organic produce, the positive nutritional benefit is the equivalent of eating one to two additional servings of fruit and vegetables per day. This is critical because the PURE study found a significant health benefit to consuming fruits and veg. Hardly earth-shattering news, but they found that after consuming just three to four traditional servings, the benefits reached a plateau.

Current guidelines call for a minimum of five to six servings per day. With real world concerns, access to such amounts of fresh fruits and veg can be difficult, and expensive. Yet it is certainly attainable if we look at consuming just two servings of organic fruit and veg each day.[639] With organics, it is just as important to be wary of the compounds you are not ingesting.[640]

The vegetable and fruit checklist is as follows:

How was it bred? Is it from heirloom breeds? Is it from conventional breeds? Is it GMO? Is it organic? What is the country of origin? Is it in season?

What was it fed? Is it organically produced? Was it subjected to additional industrial fertilizer and/or pesticides? Is it raised locally or imported from a distance?

Where was it led? When was it harvested? Any post-harvest modifications besides simple packaging?

Herbs and Spices

Herbs and spices have shared the story of vegetables and fruits. In ancient times up to the Industrial Revolution, they occupied a much more prominent place upon our plates. Their use and utility has been global. Herbs and spices have been used in China and Southeast Asia for hundreds of years before the Christian era. For millennia, they have been part of true, authentic Mediterranean cuisine.

Thyme has been used as an herbal ingredient in food for centuries and in traditional medicine in connection with chest problems. Its value as an herb and its antimicrobial activity are due to several compounds, with thymol being the main component. Another well-known spice component with antiseptic properties is eugenol, a significant component of cloves and nutmeg. Up to the eighteenth century, cloves and nutmeg were only produced in the Moluccas, or Spice Islands. The value of herbs and spices has been appreciated throughout history; from the pepper paid as a ransom at the gates of Rome to the rise of the East India Trading Company (or as it was officially known, The Honourable East India Company).[641]

With the ascension of the MWD, the fate of herbs and spices followed the displacement pattern seen with fruits and veg as a group. Subtle tastes, textures, and flavor profiles were replaced by layers of sugar, salt, and fat plying the weakness of our genetic Achilles' heel, our individual bliss points.

The difference in taste, texture, flavor, and experience between a Japanese katsu, German schnitzel, Greek souvlaki, Chinese stir-fry, Italian parmesan, French paillard, or Mexican taco is not necessarily the meat or even the cut of meat. Strip away the supporting cast and the difference is in the herbs and spices. Herbs and spices form the basis for flavor profiles.

Utilizing chicken breast in the aforementioned dishes yields a week of tantalizingly different and savory meals. Yet because we cook with limited imagination, limited herbs and spices, it is inevitably, "Not chicken *again*, Mom!" Herbs and spices accentuate the variety inherent in global cuisines. Herbs and spices are the variety of life.

The herb and spice checklist is as follows:

How was it bred? Is it from heirloom breeds? Is it from conventional breeds? Is it GMO? Is it organic? What is the country of origin? Is it in season? Are the spices whole or ground?

What was it fed? Is it organically produced? Was it subjected to additional industrial fertilizer and/or pesticides? Is it raised locally or imported from a distance?

Where was it led? When was it harvested? Any post-harvest modifications besides simple packaging? Pure herb or spice or added filler?

The true chef is a culinary wizard only because they have mastered the Art of Source-ry. This craft is the key to toothsome textures and rarefied repasts. It is the antidote the Food Shaman administers to combat the dangers of the SAD.

CHEW THE FAT
(FOOD AS THERAPY™)

Long ago, our ancestors became masters of their domain, no longer at the mercy of what they could hunt and forage, but took charge of their food production, and in doing so brought choice to the table of their comestibles.

However, over the last seventy-five years or so, many consumers have traded choice for convenience. While a lap around a megamarket seems to offer unbridled choices that span the gamut of every conceivable foodstuff, it is a great illusion. It is estimated that approximately 70 percent of all processed foods contain GMOs in one form or another. Corn, a majority of which is GMO, is found in 25 percent of all supermarket products.[642]

Supposedly unbiased professional organizations dispense "eat this, not that" edicts with all the bluster of a tinpot dictator, and with an "evidence base" that has undergone more contortions than a hot yoga class. Worse yet, natural dietary constituents are replaced by industrial foods without any clear understanding of short or long-term complications or consequences. Gary Taubes expanded upon the ideas of Doctor

Geoffrey Rose, a leader in preventive medicine, when analyzing the American Heart Association's (AHA) condemnation of coconut oil in favor of polyunsaturated vegetable oils (PUFAs):

> *Geoffrey Rose...wrote an article in the BMJ on the strategy of preventive medicine, and he pointed out the same problem about vegetable oils that confronts us today. Again history keeps repeating itself in this world, in part because these researchers and authorities don't think we have to do the experiments necessary to resolve this controversy and find out if the AHA's hypothesis is indeed true. They're too hard....As Rose observed, it's one thing to tell people not to eat something because we evolved to eat very little of it and there's good evidence that eating less of it will reduce chronic disease risk. This is what Rose called removing an "unnatural factor and the restoration of 'biological normality'—that is, of the conditions to which presumably we are genetically adapted." As Rose put it, "Such normalizing measures [for instance, telling people not to smoke] may be presumed to be safe, and therefore we should be prepared to advocate them on the basis of a reasonable presumption of benefit."*
>
> *But telling people to eat something new to the environment—an unnatural factor, à la virtually any vegetable oil (other than olive oil if your ancestor happens to come from the Mediterranean or mid-East), which was what concerned Rose and*

concerns us today—is an entirely different proposition. Now you're assuming that this unnatural factor is protective, just like we assume a drug can be protective by lowering our blood pressure or cholesterol. So the situation is little different than it would be if these AHA authorities were concluding that we should all take statins or beta blockers. The point is that no one would ever accept such a proposal for a drug without large-scale clinical trials demonstrating that the benefits far outweigh the risks. So even if the AHA hypothesis is as reasonable and compelling as the AHA authors clearly believe it is, it has to be tested. They are literally saying (not figuratively, literally) that vegetable oils—soy, canola, etc.—are as beneficial as statins and so we should all consume them. Maybe so, but before we do (or at least before I do), they have a moral and ethical obligation to rigorously test that hypothesis, just as they would if they were advising us all to take a drug. Then, well, they should probably do it twice, since a fundamental tenet of good science is also independent replication. And what we need here is good science.[643]

When we see the French eat cheese, butter, and drink wine, living not only a more joyful culinary existence but a healthier one, when we see the Inuit people existing as practically carnivores only to have a cardiovascular event rate half that of the average America, we should start looking at what they are doing and re-examine our theories. Instead, the so-called experts of label all of these occurrences a "paradox."

This practice becomes a form of science faith that applies a unique "nutrilogic." It is a logical fallacy which utilizes a special form of reasoning, employing a built-in double standard: if evidence supports the preferred or established theory then it is accepted; if evidence does not, it is rejected, ignored or labeled a "paradox."

It is not the knowing that should drive science, but the doubt.[644] To seek out the natural foods that have sustained the human species requires discipline and diligence on the part of the consumer and a commitment, not to mention increased cost and paperwork, on the part of producers. A great place for the government and the so-called experts to introduce transparency would be the grocery store.

The previous chapters have outlined a rationale and a strategy regarding the proper acquisition of edibles. Sourcing like a chef for quality ingredients and proper preparation form the foundation of the food experience. It is important, critical even, yet there is so much more. The food experience is exactly that: an experience. As such, it is relational. The impact of our meals upon our health, well-being, and psyche extends far beyond isolated enzymatic reactions in laboratory test tubes and clinical trials. Consumption purely for nutrition's sake is no more the endgame than a lovers' stroll on the beach at sunset is strictly about physical exercise.

The Food Shaman understands this relational reality. It is reflected in the execution of mindfulness, sustainability, and implementation. These are the tools in your shamanistic toolbox. Mindfulness reflects how we approach the situation. Sustainability defines how our approach affects the larger whole, of which we are a part. Implementation is the course of action we pursue with respect to the former, given the circumstances that confront us at the time.

Quiet your mind, open your heart, and partake with abandon. Our dependence on food for survival, and particularly that we depend on a healthy gut microbiome as a living symbiotic organism, dismisses the idea that we exist separately from other life forms. As much as our technology, the modern food industry, and modern agribusiness might create the illusion of an isolated penthouse at the top of the food pyramid, we are every bit a link in the circle of life. As Ken Wilber observed, even what we regard as our own thoughts, they "arise in a cultural background that gives texture and meaning and context to my individual thoughts."[645]

Within this social and environmental fabric, as the Harvard Happiness Study affirmed, it is not the number of relationships, but the quality of those relationships that counts. Likewise, it is not the quantity of food that determines our well-being, but the quality of those food experiences. Utilizing shamanic tools allows us to develop that relationship with Nature every day through the Food Experience, through understanding Food as Therapy, through chewing the FAT™.

It is learning how to be still, and how to taste the silence. It is following the natural courses and rhythms of the seasons. We need to stop trying to push the river. The Food Shaman understands Nature and Nature's cycles, and works with them all. At first, it may be inconvenient; in our modern world, many of us have become addicted to being comfortable. It is always awkward when the chains come off. But engagement yields a powerfully positive synchronicity. This is The FAT Approach of The Food Shaman.

Mindfulness: Food is a Gift, Eat the Present

*"The mind is its own place, and in itself can
make a Heaven of Hell, a Hell of Heaven."*
—*John Milton, Paradise Lost*

The Bard summed it up another way in *Hamlet:* "There is nothing either good or bad, but thinking makes it so...nothing is really good or bad in itself—it's all what a person thinks about it."[646] Perhaps nothing demonstrates this concept better than the placebo effect.

The placebo effect is repeatedly dismissed because it is poorly understood. It is recurrently equated with a null effect, yet it is anything but that. The positive placebo effect or placebo response is a well-recognized phenomenon whereby an inactive treatment improves a patient's condition simply because the person has the expectation that it will. Research suggests that the more a person believes they are going to benefit from a treatment, the more likely it is that they will experience said benefit.

The power of such positive thinking is not new. It is a form of what the ancients referred to as "dreaming into being." The Talmud, a venerable Jewish text dating back thousands of years, records that: "Where there is hope, there is life." The modern term of the placebo effect dates to the work of anesthesiologist Henry K. Beecher in the 1950s. Beecher concluded in his paper, "The Powerful Placebo" published in 1955, that across the twenty-six studies he analyzed, an average of 32 percent of patients responded to placebo.[647]

In the 1950s a man dying of advanced cancer was given a highly publicized experimental drug called krebiozen. After a single dose, his huge cancers "melted like snowballs on a hot stove" and he was able to resume normal activities. Shortly thereafter, studies of krebiozen showed it to be ineffective. When the patient learned this, his cancer began spreading again. At this juncture, his doctor announced that there was now a new "improved" krebiozen and proceeded to give it to the patient. Once again, the man's tumors shrank, however, the doctor had given him only water.[648]

Subsequent research has confirmed that such placebo effects are widespread, and consistently approximately one-third of people treated with completely inactive placebos improve.[649] This effect, notes physician Lewis Thomas, points to "a kind of superintelligence that exists in each of us, infinitely smarter and possessed of technical know-how far beyond our present understanding."[650]

A review of fifty-three trials that compared elective surgical procedures to placebos found that sham surgeries provided some benefit in 74 percent of the trials and worked as well as the real surgical procedure in roughly half the cases.[651] Think about that for a moment. In half of the elective surgeries, patients essentially cured themselves simply because they believed it was possible. Attitude, like personality, goes a long way, and a positive attitude starts with gratitude.

Gratitude, Tasting, and Blessing. These are the actions of the mindful Food Shaman. Gratitude is "the quality of being thankful; readiness to show appreciation for and to return kindness."[652] Importantly, gratitude is an emotion expressing appreciation for what one *has*, as opposed to a consumer-driven emphasis on what one *wants*. Studies show that cultivating gratitude can increase well-being and happiness. Such an action is associated with increased energy, optimism, and empathy.[653]

Gratitude is an attitude and an orientation designed to open the heart. The heart, in the emotional and figurative sense, is a portal. When you are grateful, you connect to something outside of yourself. You establish a relation with some other thing and that creation becomes a node of its own, like a wave on the ocean. Shamans teach that gratitude is key to living a life filled with joy and harmony. The placebo effect is but one example of how it is our perception that creates our reality. The same dish enjoyed by one person is reviled by another; the pleasant or unpleasant all resides in your perception.[654] Approaching our meals with gratitude reframes our food experience.

Gratitude is an important aspect of mindfulness. It is currently an area of active investigation, as many of the mechanisms by which it clearly improves physical health remain unclear. Despite the lack of a clear biochemical pathway, incorporation of gratitude has been associated with improved kidney function, reduction of blood pressure, improved cardiovascular parameters, and significantly reduced stress hormone levels. According to Professor Christine Carter from the University of California, Berkeley, it appears that gratitude can rewire our brains as a counter to the fight or flight stress response. You simply can't be grateful *and* stressed or resentful at the same time.

Much like mindful meditation, gratitude increases the brain's production and release of dopamine and oxytocin, the "love" hormone.[655, 656, 657] Unlike simple reward gratification, which can habituate and attenuate over time, love reinforces itself with repeated exposure. The more we love, the more we love and are loved.

Tasting means that we are perceiving the truth and essence, and therefore there is no room on the palate for preconceptions, including negative feelings of hostility, blame, fear, or set decrees. It requires attention to the moment. The ordinary moments unfolding right in front of us, are anything but ordinary. In tasting the food and the moment, we extract the extraordinary from what we so often discount as mundane.

Our 24/7/365 techno-on-the-go society puts such a premium on successful multitasking that we forget there is beauty in monotasking as well. Paying attention in a particular way: on purpose, in the present moment, and nonjudgmentally has been cited by The American Psychological Association as a helpful tactic for alleviating depression, anxiety, and pain.

Such strategies for success include sitting down to eat. A study published in the *Journal of Health Psychology* performed at the University of Surrey in England revealed that eating on the go makes us prone to overeat later, according to lead researcher, Jane Ogden:

> *When you eat, eat: don't multitask. When you sit at your desk and continue to try to work while you eat, your brain is only able to completely pay attention to one thing at a time. Such inattention to what you are eating does not only lead to poor food choices, but a propensity to overeat as well.*[658]

Tasting involves the sensory experience of your food. When we slow down to pay attention to the flavors, tastes, and textures, we engage the moment and immerse ourselves in the experience. We help relieve ourselves of the dangers of eating on autopilot. While many fast food, junk food, processed, and ultra-processed foods of the modern Western diet are constructed so that minimal chewing is necessary, it is important that we do chew.

Both chewing and the textural "crunch effect" suggest that the *sound* of food is a key sensory cue that helps us regulate how much we consume. Likewise, varying consistency as well as taste helps to engage all our senses and keep us attentive and immersed in the food experience. The better the food experience, the more satisfied you are with the meal. The more satisfied you are with the meal, the less likely you are to overeat.

Many people have been taught to bless their food; they consider a blessing to be a few words mumbled over the meal that lack heart and meaning. This is hardly what shamans mean by blessing.[659] True blessing requires intent.

Intention is another powerful aspect of the Food Shaman's mindful approach to the food experience. Intent is one of the driving forces of creation. Intention in Sanskrit is *samkalpa* which, roughly translated, is an idea formed in the mind or heart. Such "right intention" is the second element of the Buddha's noble eightfold path. The eightfold path is a series of teachings that prescribe a way to avoid personal suffering and achieve enlightenment. This intention, in essence, says to treat yourself and others with kindness and compassion and try to live in alignment with your deepest values. In other words, don't eat hangry.

Blessing is the act of recognizing that Spirit is coming through what we are witnessing or experiencing. It is recognizing and acknowledging the grand flow of Beingness that is present as what we choose to eat.[660] This is the demiurgic force a chef feels in the creation and preparation of the meal. It is the pleasure and joy in the giving and sharing of a meal. To bless means that you become conscious that you are alive and so is your food, the company (whether there in person or in spirit), and the experience. The act of blessing is an act of awakening; it is positive energy in motion. These three movements, gratitude, tasting, and blessing, are a *sanshin*: a three-part spirit deed. It is a symphony of Love, Truth, and Energy.

"One of my favorite teachings is about the true meaning of abracadabra, which many of us used as children," recounts Sandra Ingerman. She goes on to note that this word comes from the Aramaic, *abraq ad habra*, which literally translates to "I will create as I speak."[661] It is important to be part of this creation by fully engaging the world you are dreaming into being, rather than passively watching as if it were movie. It is the awareness that consciousness, not matter, is the primary determinant of our individual reality. Eating—even a simple everyday meal—when approached with authenticity in the actions of gratitude, tasting, and blessing, can create ceremony.

True ceremony must be done with purpose. Without it, there is no meaning and passion. A chef without purpose or passion is merely a technician, assembling ingredients without any personal investment of energy. Keep things fresh beyond ingredients by using different approaches. Vary the flavor profiles, preparatory techniques, the plating, whatever calls to you to change your practice. Be committed to the endeavor, for energy follows attention. True cooking is energy, intention, and creation. True cooking sets the ceremony.

Ceremonies have always played an important role in shamanic communities. Ceremonies are a way for people living in community to support each individual and the collective. It is a way for us as humans to connect with the spiritual world and create a relationship. It is no coincidence that food plays a major role in the observance of many a ceremony.

Ceremonies have been used in shamanic cultures since the beginning of time. They have been a powerful agent of change and a way for communities to gather together, regardless of belief systems. The sharing of a meal is one of humanity's oldest formalities. True ceremony inaugurates thought and intention into action. Interlacing ceremony through mindful eating enriches your spirit by incorporating true ceremony into your life every day. In this way, you weave the sacred into your ordinary reality.[662]

The feast begins by enacting mindfulness. When we are not mindful, we are sleepwalking. Mindfulness starts with imperative action; a dialogue or internal monologue. Words, even spoken internally, are powerful. There is a congruence between who you say you are, to yourself and others, and who you really are.[663]

Every athlete knows you play the way you practice. People tend to die in the same way that they have lived, which is why it is important to bring mindfulness into our daily lives. We need to remember to enjoy the journey before we surrender the gifts that life has brought to us. That is why it is paramount to be fully present and savor the flavor, enjoy the moment in a positive, ultimately healthful way. Being focused in the moment releases an enormous store of energy otherwise held hostage to distraction. This is the power of living fully.

Ceremony creates change. Our forebears understood the power of food as ceremony, that a process of positive change begins with a wassail with Spirit on the path of Authenticity. There is a Haitian proverb, "The gods won't appear, the magic won't happen if you are not living your real life."[664]

The magic of mindfulness has real world consequences. Stress can affect the area of the brain known as the amygdala, specifically, the amygdala-subgenual anterior cingulate cortex (sgACC). Research from the University of Pittsburgh and Carnegie Mellon University revealed that mindfulness meditation could reverse these effects in stressed, unemployed adults. It is functional anatomic and physiologic correlation of what shamans have known for millennia. (See appendix E1)

Part of the problem in our modern society is that with constant multitasking there is no recovery time, exemplified by eating on the go. Wakeful mindfulness, such as a mindful approach to eating, benefits other areas such as improving sleep and thus allowing appropriate mental recovery. In all areas of your life you are going to be less prone to being hyperreactive. Research shows that a relaxed, alert state is optimum for any performance in any field.[665]

Distraction prevents deep thought and mental agility. Stress and ruminations tax our ability to be creative as well as to really immerse ourselves in experiences. Our brain normally switches between exploratory and exploitatory modes. Mindfulness, along with meditation, yoga, and aerobic exercise, have been shown to help people achieve a calmness of mind. In addition to decreasing stress and improving sleep, these practices can help avoid illness.[666]

Left untreated, stress can contribute to the development of serious illness such as heart disease, depression, anxiety, and diabetes. Research suggests it can accelerate the spread of breast and ovarian cancers. The mind perceives the threat of emergency and your body reacts. It is the fight or flight effect. The body responds with the release of hormones like adrenaline, norepinephrine, and cortisol, among others.

Over time, the chronicity of the condition wears the body down like a river carving a canyon. In 2012, researchers from Carnegie Mellon University revealed that chronic psychological stress is associated with the body losing its ability to regulate the inflammatory response. Their research showed that the effects of psychological stress on the body's ability to regulate inflammation can promote the development and progression of disease.

Specifically, it appears that chronic stress alters the effectiveness of cortisol to regulate the inflammatory response because it decreases tissue sensitivity to the hormone. When under stress, cells of the immune system are unable to respond to hormonal control, and consequently, produce levels of inflammation that promote disease.[667] These disabilities and diseases, such as cardiovascular, asthma, and autoimmune disorders, are associated with the lifestyle inherent to the modern Western diet. High cortisol levels have been associated with the breakdown of collagen and elastin in the skin, which is associated with accelerated aging.

Under chronic stress, cortisol can damage short-term memory and reduce gray matter in the brain. Constant stress can alter signals to the hypothalamus that results in a disruption of the hormones that trigger fertility such as gonadotropin releasing hormone (GnRH). Constant tension may cause pain and muscle spasms in the neck and back, particularly to those susceptible because of prior injury or illness. Others may be prone to releasing excess stress through bruxism (grinding of the teeth) which can result in jaw pain and headaches. Such physiological states are associated with a higher risk of migraines, seasonal allergies, irritable bowel syndrome, and arthritis.

Stress can act to reduce gastrointestinal transit time and increase inflammation. Research has shown that stress can change the balance of gut bacteria, altering the entire gut microbiome. Such changes can affect the metabolism and result in the accumulation of visceral adipose tissue, or belly fat. A 2014 study revealed that people under significant pressure at work have a 45 percent higher risk of type II diabetes, independent of other traditional risk factors.[668] Stress can affect cellular telomeres, in effect directly impacting our rate of physiologic aging.[669]

Positive social supports and practices such as mindfulness and meditation can dramatically reduce stress and strengthen our resilience. However, like many physiological responses, our stress response may be to some degree genetically pre-determined. A study from the National Institutes of Health found that stressor release, and anxiety reducing compounds are partly affected by genetic mechanisms.[670] But no matter the genes you were born with, it appears that exercise is a stress reducer for everybody. Yet it need not require hours in the gym or a personal trainer to achieve the desired result. A simple walk in nature can suffice.

In fact, as shamans have practiced for eons, immersion in nature may be superior in some ways to hitting the weights or cycling to Hell and back. The Japanese practice of forest bathing, *shinrin-yoku*, translates as "taking in the forest atmosphere through all of our senses."[671] It has been demonstrated to lower heart rate, blood pressure, reduce stress hormone production, boost the immune system, and improve overall feelings of wellbeing. All this without a Fitbit or even breaking a sweat. Based on such profound health benefits, as well as being immersed in the cultural legacy, *shinrin-yoku* has been part of a national public health program in Japan since 1982.[672]

A Japanese study has found that chemicals produced by trees, called phytoncides, lowered levels of stress hormones in humans.[673] Other research has found that such nature immersion for a few hours a week promotes lower concentrations of cortisol, lowers pulse rate, lowers blood pressure, increases parasympathetic nerve activity, and lowers sympathetic nerve activity. Similar results can be achieved in city environments by spending time in parks.[674] Research published in 2012 by Atchley and Strayer showed that spending time in nature, like engaging in mindfulness, may counteract the negative effects of too much tech time.[675]

In addition to exercise like nature walks, diet and adequate sleep are essential to effectively combat daily stressors. Humans deplete magnesium more quickly under duress, which is one reason among many that diet is an important factor in the equation. Good dietary sources of magnesium include leafy greens, bananas, nuts like almonds, and cocoa.

Sleep is the best meditation according to the Dalai Lama. Insufficient sleep has been linked to chronic diseases ranging from diabetes to depression. "Sleep is an experience, and it's important to start with that notion. Even though we try to measure it, is like trying to measure love. It's more like a feeling than it is a fact," according to Rubin Naiman, a clinical psychologist specializing in integrative sleep and dream medicine. Herbal tea, lavender, and chamomile are particularly soothing and helpful and relaxing prior to going to bed. Too much life throws off the body's circadian biological clock.[676] The Food Shaman, like the Buddha, understands that enlightenment, epicurean or otherwise, lies in the Middle Path.

Balance includes emotion as well as food and activity. Even a good cry can be therapeutic. In some types of shamanistic practice, the act of keening takes the participants through sorrow, to joy, to quiet contemplation. It is not only emotionally cathartic; stress hormones can be released through tears. The deep, slow, rhythmic breathing of introspection has been shown to improve exercise capacity in patients suffering from chronic heart failure.[677]

Concentrate on feeling each breath fully, then concentrate on the next breath. Such mindful meditation has been shown to increase the brain's production and release of serotonin, dopamine, oxytocin, and endorphins. In other words, it puts you in a good mood. And it may save your life. A study of African Americans with known CAD who meditated twice a day for twenty minutes showed that this activity lowered their measurable stress levels and their blood pressure by 5 mmHg. This is as effective an antihypertensive treatment as single pharmaceutical agent therapy. More importantly, it significantly reduced their risk for early mortality, myocardial infarction, and stroke.[678]

Meditation can lower blood pressure, slow Alzheimer's disease progression, and curb tobacco cravings. A review paper from Johns Hopkins University showed that mindfulness meditation may be as effective as antidepressants for treating anxiety symptoms. Such mindful pursuits are now recommended for conditions like insomnia and irritable bowel syndrome.

Other studies have shown that regular meditation can reduce subjective pain intensity by about 40 percent. It can reduce inflammation associated with stress and other conditions like arthritis and asthma. Meditation also seems to reboot the parasympathetic nervous system, which aids in proper digestion and functioning of the gastrointestinal tract. Meditation essentially acts to turn down the volume on the stress response.[679]

The purely physical realm of illness, where doctors diagnose with laboratory tests, is only part of the equation. The proof is in the tasting of the pudding, or perhaps the fresh squeezed veggie smoothie, as the case may be. Doctor Lissa Rankin expounds on this as she explored why so many of her "healthy" patients were so sick. These patients voiced physical complaints or exhibited physical ailments despite what by all measures would be considered a healthful lifestyle. She found that these patients were most often ill not because of bad genes, unhealthy habits, or even bad luck, but because they were lonely or unhappy in their relationships, stressed about work, worried about finances, or were deeply depressed.

Conversely, her patients who ate junk, took no supplements, and rarely exercised were often models of perfect physical health. Their lives were "filled with love, fun, meaningful work, creative expression, spiritual connection, and other traits that differentiated them from sick health enthusiasts."[680] Her findings are in complete agreement with the recent seventy-five-year results from the Harvard happiness study. Her conclusion, which recent research supports, is that lifestyle choices you make act to optimize your body's relaxation response, counteract the stress response, and result in physiologic changes that lead to better health. The body is a mirror of how we live our lives.[681]

A key component of mindfulness is to pay attention to the inner and outer experience in the present moment, without judgment. In clinical studies, it has been shown to decrease stress significantly in as little as eight weeks with regular repetition. In the practice of incorporating mindfulness, whatever puts you most at ease is more important than a particular regimen, such as standing, sitting, lying, eyes open, or eyes closed. It is important to settle your attention on the feeling of the normal, natural breath wherever and whenever it is most clear. In mindful eating, incorporation and execution of gratitude, tasting, and blessing is approached in parallel fashion.

Such an approach to mindful eating has its roots in the ancient shamanic practices, but extends into Hinduism with the sacred Vedic texts, Buddhism, and many, if not all faiths. Prince Siddhartha became the enlightened Buddha and introduced such mindfulness to the masses. But these basic components can be found in the world's three major religions: Judaism, Christianity, and Islam.[682]

The similar concept in Judaism is described by the word *kavanah*, which details total awareness and attention that you should strive to bring to every moment of your life. All of these are methods to notice and appreciate our surroundings and give meaning to our actions. When we give meaning to our actions we can get powerful results. The tale of the great Rabbi Zusya illustrates this:

> *Rabbi Zusya was lying on his deathbed, tears streaming down his face. When his followers asked him why he was crying, he said "If God asks me why I wasn't like Moses, I'll say I wasn't blessed with that kind of leadership ability or wisdom. But if God asks me, 'Zusya, why weren't you Zusya? Why didn't you fulfill your own highest potential? Why didn't you find your inner self? What will I say then?"*[683]

We engage in approximately two hundred distinct decisions per day regarding food and drink. When we apply mindfulness, we eat with intention and attention instead of inattention. With such engagement, we can train ourselves to become more conscious of every bite—mindful eating by simply being mindful. The research suggests that such a practice can significantly reduce stress and prevent overeating. Yet one of the real keys to extracting the health benefits associated with mindful eating is that it encourages and promotes people to enjoy a relaxed relationship with food; they participate in a pleasurable *food experience*.

So many modern diet approaches equate weight loss with health. These programs emphasize weight reduction through a series of external rules; eat this, don't eat that. When we eat mindfully, we are focusing on our own internal cues. Instead of counting calories (useless, as exposed in *The Fallacy of the*

Calorie), we determine whether we are hungry or whether we are full. Study after study has shown the healthiest people are not those with an "ideal" body weight, but those in the overweight and even mildly obese category, a phenomenon known as The Obesity Paradox.[684, 685]

Studies have shown that mindful eating reduces binge eating, emotional eating, and leads to a healthier body composition and weight. This approach eschews calorie counting or restriction of food choices. Yet the physiological benefits are not only real, but long-lasting.[686] Two hundred obese adults all had the same diet and exercise regimen. Half the group was given additional information on nutrition and exercise. The other half engaged in mindful eating, yoga, meditation, and breathing exercises. While weight was comparable between the two groups at the end of the study, the mindfulness group had significantly higher levels of HDL ("good") cholesterol and lower levels of triglycerides. They also had lower blood sugar levels.[687]

Engaging in the food experience is letting go and reveling in a very primal flow. As defined by Mihaly Csikszentmihalyi, a Hungarian psychologist, back in the 1970s, flow is a state of being totally and blissfully immersed in a task, to the exclusion of almost everything else, including the self. Such a state slows activation in the dorsolateral prefrontal cortex, according to research performed at Johns Hopkins University.

This is the area of the brain responsible for planning and self-monitoring. While activity slows there, the medial prefrontal cortex increases activity. This is the area of the brain responsible for expression. The result is that by entering a flow state, inhibitions fall, creativity rises, and we cruise into an almost subconscious mode. We enter the realm of the Food Shaman.

Stimulation here encourages the release of dopamine, serotonin, oxytocin, and endorphins. It makes us feel good. The bad news is that flow is a lot like love, you just can't intellectually will yourself to that place. The good news is that you can get there by immersing yourself in the experience, like falling in love. [688] Eat the foods of love, not the foods of addiction, and the flow will find you.

Sustainability: A Year and a Day

"Turning and turning in the widening gyre
The falcon cannot hear the falconer;
Things fall apart; the centre cannot hold;
Mere anarchy is loosed upon the world,
The blood-dimmed tide is loosed, and everywhere
The ceremony of innocence is drowned;
The best lack all conviction, while the worst
Are full of passionate intensity."
—W.B. Yeats, The Second Coming

Our modern world is one that is increasingly out of balance. The majority of us survive in a state of ongoing and pervasive disharmony, bobbing cacophonously on the tide of the moment. Yet at this moment there appears a shift in the realm of food and health within Western zeitgeist. Richard Sellin, in his book *The Spiritual Gyre*, observed that this revitalization movement is happening right on schedule. He suggests that our Western preoccupation with the linear development of our civilization is, in fact, a misconception, and that the zeitgeist—the spirit of the times embodied within the intellectual trends and moral values characteristic of any age—tends to express itself in cycles that repeat themselves on a regular basis.[689]

The cycles do not simply repeat like spokes on a turning wheel. They evolve with new faces, incorporating the past and forging it with the present to progress. We are our ancestors, yet we are our own individual selves as well. We view things with glasses colored by our personal experience, but against a wider backdrop. An individual's interpretation of phenomena in general, and of spirits in particular, are determined by their "world hypothesis": their fundamental assumptions about the nature of the world and reality.[690] This is influenced by and influences the underlying cultural milieu.

The purlieu in which we dwell can have huge consequences. The United States in the 1960s underwent a turbulent and at times violent rebirth from a monophasic into a polyphasic culture. Both the country and the people were deeply affected in a way that continues to resonate.

However meteoric or profound at the time, a single spiritual experience does not guarantee a spiritual life or an ethical lifestyle, either for individuals or societies. Yet long-term practice and multiple experiences, like a persistent wind upon the rock, can yield an impressive cumulative impact. It is a simple fact of existence that major enduring change often requires long-term effort.[691] Thus, these tumultuous times call to the visionary in each of us to restore equilibrium and harmony.[692] These times call to the shaman in each of us.

Like the shaman of old, we must look for inspiration and guidance in the natural world around us, the reality to which we are inextricably bound. Nature will provide much healing and insight in educating us on how to live a healthy, balanced life. Nature is a helping spirit.[693] As Andrew Steed has imparted to the masses, "Shamanism is a healing path."[694] As Albert Einstein advised, "Look deep into Nature, and then you will understand everything better."[695]

Whereas the mindful approach to eating concentrated on our individual needs, sustainability expands our focal point. In the manner of their ancient forebears, modern shamans always treat the individual within the context of community. Likewise, the Food Shaman must pursue an individual course that operates within the framework of delivering the greatest good for all beings. Sustainability is an approach that facilitates living in harmony with others within the larger community and with nature. As we create our reality, our outer world becomes but a reflection of our inner state of consciousness.[696]

As a society, the current health of our populace is one that is ill at epidemic proportions. We are sick at a pandemic level. The explosive increase across all sectors of the population in the incidence and prevalence of Type 2 diabetes mellitus (T2DM) is the case in point.

T2DM is an economically and physically costly chronic inflammatory illness that is linked to poor dietary choices—specifically, consumption of the modern Western diet. Diabetes related care accounts for more than one dollar of every five spent on healthcare in the United States, equating to two hundred and forty-five billion dollars in total costs in 2012. On a personal level, the average medical expenses for those with T2DM are more than double what they are for a person without diabetes.[697]

It is increasing in incidence and prevalence. One of the terrible tragedies of T2DM is that while the disease itself is debilitating enough, it is associated with many of the other chronic inflammatory disabilities and diseases associated with the modern Western diet. These diseases and disabilities which include cardiovascular disease (CVD), the number one cause of death in the United States and many other Western nations, are often heralded by the onset of

T2DM.[698] CVD is the cause of death in almost 65 percent of individuals with diabetes.[699]

For an individual without known CVD, but who suffers from T2DM, the risk for suffering a heart attack or myocardial infarction (MI) is the same in terms of a seven-year risk as someone who has already had a heart attack but has no T2DM.[700] However, successful treatment strategies for addressing the pathologies associated with T2DM utilizing lifestyle interventions date as far back as the 1940s.[701] Lifestyle modification, with a particular concentration on diet, is a preeminent and economical way to treat this rampant ailment.[702]

T2DM and CVD share many modifiable lifestyle risk factors: morbid obesity, physical inactivity, and diet, among others. These are additive to any genetic predisposition and other risk factors.[703, 704, 705] In the United States, diabetes affects at least 29.1 million individuals, the equivalent of almost 10 percent of the entire population and reflects 12.3 percent of the adult population. Depending on the study and the definition used, there may be as many as another 5.4 million people with undiagnosed diabetes.[706] Although pharmacological therapy is a cornerstone of treatment, lifestyle modifications and dietary approaches in particular still represent a core goal for primary and secondary prevention of CVD, diabetes, and related conditions.[707] Research demonstrates not only benefit, but achievable end points. Studies confirm that individual behavior can be shaped and behavioral interventions can help patients make better choices for their own diabetes self-management, even in the context of difficult circumstances.[708] Successful treatment of diabetes, like many chronic disabilities and diseases, is ultimately a case of self-management.

Among the central pillars upon which individuals can exert significant control and initiate meaningful behavior change, dietary patterns and physical activity emerge as two of the most obvious. Many studies and recommendations underscore the importance of diet, exercise, and education in the pursuit of successful treatment of diabetes.[709, 710] (See appendix E2)

Dietary and other practices which help the individual and the community need to be sustainable. Sustainable in the sense that the individual can maintain pursuing it. Sustainable in the sense that it behooves both the immediate and larger community from public health and economic considerations. And finally, sustainable from a planetary perspective. When we sacrifice Nature on the Altar of Convenience, we sacrifice a large part of ourselves in both body and spirit.

According to the Food and Agriculture Organization of the United Nations (2010):

> *Sustainable diets are those diets with low environmental impacts which contribute to food and nutrition security and to healthy life for present and future generations. Sustainable diets are protective and respectful of biodiversity and ecosystems, culturally acceptable, accessible, economically fair and affordable; nutritionally adequate, safe and healthy, while optimizing natural and human resources.*[711]

Contrary to these recommendations, many of our current industrial, agribusiness production programs in the West tend to pursue The Path of the Least Resistome. What is quickly becoming apparent is that *how we raise food mat-*

ters. It matters for the individual, for the immediate community, and for the society at large. Perhaps most importantly, it matters on a planetary scale.

Over 20 percent of the meat consumed in the United States is classified as processed.[712]Among these different protein options, chicken is currently the most commonly consumed.[713, 714] Most chicken produced for public consumption is done utilizing an industrial or CAFO (Concentrated Animal Feeding Operation) method. Studies looking at the production of animals in these types of settings is yielding results that have potentially far reaching consequences.

Upwards of 80 to 90 percent of all antibiotics employed in the United States may be administered to animals in the pursuit of food production.[715] Chicken gut microbiomes were examined after feeding chickens either control feed, feed with monensin (an antibiotic), or feed with virginiamycin (another antibiotic). Not surprisingly, subsequent analysis detected significant differences in the gut microbiome between the groups.

Antibiotic administration transiently alters the human gut microbiome. It is therefore no surprise that chronic administration of antibiotic enhanced feed permanently alters the gut microbiome of other animals. In another study, chickens fed GMO feed with enriched levels of glyphosate (the active ingredient in Roundup) experienced an altered gut microbiome with increased presence of *Salmonella* sp. It is not just the flora that is changing; there is an increased prevalence of antibiotic-resistant phenotypes in animals fed antibiotic-containing diets.[716, 717]

These antibiotic resistant microbes may not only affect an individual, but pose a risk to society at large.[718, 719, 720] Current practices of land disposal of animal wastes do not require pre-treatment. Chickens fed with antibiotic or GMO feed exhibited alterations in the normal poultry gut flora. With antibiotic resistant microbes, the bacteria escaped into the environment through waste.

Poultry waste moved resistance genes from poultry litter into the soil environment where poultry waste was deposited. Bacteria can confer antibiotic resistance to another bacterial species the way millenials retweet. These resistance "tweets" are known collectively as the resistome. Through such a mechanism, resistance genes first appearing in the gut bacteria of treated poultry have appeared in soil bacteria of the Chesapeake Bay, the dumping ground for much agricultural run-off and waste.

Because of the rapid and efficient transfer of resistance genes from one bacterium to another, even non-pathogenic, so-called commensal bacteria can carry and express resistance genes. This facilitates the spread of antibacterial resistance around the globe in short order. This reservoir of antibacterial resistance can thus include bacteria outside as well as inside our bodies, the collection of which is the resistome.[721, 722]

Alterations to our food pathways now include consideration of the impact of genetically modified organisms, or GMOs, like the aforementioned poultry feed. Unfortunately, at present there is no requirement for labeling foods if they contain GMO or animals are fed utilizing GMO feedstuffs. In point of fact, there are powerful forces working in the other direction. In the summer of 2015, with little fanfare, the U.S. Congress voted to pass HR 1599. This was a bill introduced into committee on March 25, 2015, in bipartisan fashion 275–150 with eight abstentions.

The proposed law, officially known as The Safe and Accurate Food Labeling Act, sought to amend the FDA

Federal Food Drug and Cosmetic Act to require developers of genetically modified organisms (GMOs), in this case plants, to submit premarket biotechnology notification. This notification includes the *developer's* determination that the "food from, containing, consisting of the GMO (GMO food) is as safe as a comparable non-GMO food."

In other words, if the maker of a GMO product deemed it safe, that's all that would be required. Only in the event that the FDA determined there was a material difference between a GMO food and a comparable non-GMO food may the FDA then specify labeling that informs the consumers of the difference.

The bill's main sponsor, then Rep. Mike Pompeo, R-Kansas, former Director of the CIA, and present Secretary of State, stated that there is "overwhelming" scientific evidence regarding the safety of GMO foods. He added that there is no credible evidence that "foods produced with biotechnology pose any risk to our health and safety." With respect to the purpose of the bill, he noted that "it is not the place of government—government at any level—to arbitrarily step in and mandate that one plant product should be labeled based solely on how it is bred, while another, identical product is free of government warning labels."[723]

The proposed bill was called the "Deny Americans the Right to Know," or DARK Act, by its opponents. With good reason. From the text of the original proposal the reason for the existence of such a bill was because:

> *an ever more vocal minority of citizens are creating doubt in the minds of many consumers and policymakers through misinformation regarding the safety and wise use of genetically engineered inputs.... This*

misinformation is influencing policymakers at the local, state, and federal levels and could threaten our farmers' ability to feed an ever growing population and increase the cost of food for consumers.... And so biotechnology activists continue to advocate for these proposals [GMO labeling laws] despite the clear scientific consensus on the issue. State labeling initiatives will produce a state-by-state patchwork of laws that lead to misinformation and confusion for consumers as well as costly disruptions to the food supply chain.[724]

Despite the fact that reliable polls show approximately 90 percent of Americans favor the labeling of GMOs foods, Congress felt it incumbent upon themselves to enact legislation which proposed precisely the opposite.[725] All because the simple-minded public and a few unenlightened policymakers were at risk, according to the Federal government, of being bamboozled by the balderdash and taradiddles of a few radical hippies.

Support for the governmental position was voiced by such food and health experts as a radiologist who likely never saw an actual patient and knows diddly squat about food. These self-proclaimed experts countered that the proposed law would not deny people the right to know what's in their food. The reason was because there was no impediment to "stop food manufacturers who avoid "genetically modified" ingredients from labeling and marketing their products accordingly."[726]

Except this solution is a non-sequitur. There are two key reasons why this is so. Rep. Pompeo argues that it is wrong to require the labeling of one plant because of how it is bred versus another plant that is "identical."

These plants are anything but identical.

These plants are modified at the level of their DNA. Corn that has the DNA of some bacteria inserted into it so it is resistant to the herbicide glyphosate is not *identical* to corn that does not. While it is true that people have been cross breeding plants that are naturally compatible for thousands of years, there is no scenario in this quadrant of the galaxy where a tomato will breed with a flounder. When the company DNA Plant Technology developed an experimental, genetically engineered tomato that included a modified gene from a breed of arctic flounder, it was hoped this would allow the tomatoes to be more resistant to frost and cold storage. This was unsuccessful and the product was never marketed.

The point of such examples is that these plants *are* distinctly different from their naturally occurring brethren at the level of their DNA, even though at face value they may look the same. This is not only the opposite of identical, but is actually an argument *for* the labeling of GMO products. A reason to label them is precisely because there is no easy way to differentiate them by casual inspection.

This proposed legislation was not a law that enforces or protects the consumer's right to know what is in their food. The clever pitch in this switch and bait was an onerous, complicated, and no doubt expensive certifying process if someone wished to tell you what was *not* in your food. The bill "amends the Agricultural Marketing Act of 1946 to require the Agricultural Marketing Service to establish a program to certify non-GMO food." Listing what your food is made from and declaring what is *not* in your food are not equivalent propositions. The proposed regulation, in practice, would have effectively barred the average consumer from knowing what was in their food.

The proposed certification process was legally empowered to encumber anyone attempting to officially label (like the current governmentally approved organic food label) their product non-GMO. It would have required an overbearing amount of recordkeeping, which of course was subject to any government investigation and enforcement at any time. All this to produce food naturally the way we have consumed it for millennia.

Any occurrence of set governmental standards which was deemed a violation was subject to a ten thousand dollar fine, however, "each day during which a violation described in subparagraph (A) occurs shall be considered to be a separate violation." Any violation carries an automatic five-year ban from producing and labeling any product non-GMO. The government had appropriated two million dollars in anticipation of the creation of such an oversight organization.

The law expressly stated that "labeling or advertising material on, or in conjunction with, such covered product shall not suggest either expressly or by implication that covered products developed without the use of genetic engineering are safer or of higher quality than covered products produced from, containing, or consisting of a genetically engineered plant."[727] In other words, even if you have a non-GMO certification you could neither claim nor imply that the food was safer or better than its GMO counterpart. Science be damned.

Speaking of science, despite the assurances of government, the data is far from complete and determined. The vast majority of studies done to demonstrate the safety of GMO products are performed by the corporations that make them. These are, invariably, short-term experiments. Independent evidence to the contrary of the company position, according to a congressional investigation, has been subject to a campaign of misinformation and bullying reminiscent of the Big Tobacco effort to hide the smoking-cancer connection.[728]

Even with this skewed perspective the universal laws hold: absence of evidence is not evidence of absence. Shortly after the bill was introduced in March of 2015, the International Agency for Research on Cancer (IARC), part of the World Health Organization (WHO), classified glyphosate a "probable carcinogen." Since that time, supporting data has led California to classify glyphosate as a carcinogen; "known to the state to cause cancer."[729] Roundup on your glyphosate resistant cash crop makes it particularly more profitable and easier to grow when you can kill every living plant within fifty parsecs of it. The new generation of GMO plants are not only resistant to glyphosate, but multiple potent pesticides like dicamba and others. Unfortunately, levels of the herbicides are increased in such plants and in us when we eat them. Inevitably, they find their way into our food supply in increasing levels.

As remarkable as it may seem, no regulatory agency currently requires any mandatory chronic animal feeding studies to be performed for GMOs destined for human consumption.[730] This proposed legislation, which was fortunately defeated, exposes only one of the many reasons to question former Rep. Pompeo's claim that "[p]recisely zero pieces of credible evidence have been presented that foods produced with biotechnology pose any risk to our health and safety."[731]

The government's track record in making such definitive statements would bankrupt a betting man. When refined white bread was first produced, May (Mary Anne) Yates

founded the Bread Reform League in 1880 because of a correlation between people consuming the refined product and
the development of disability and disease. She was dismissed
because the powers that be assured the public that the science
was sound and there was no issue. Decades later, it was found
that the refined white bread was extraordinarily deficient in
compounds that we call vitamins today. It is the reason white
bread is now a fortified food product.

Although trans-fats (TFAs) have been known since the
end of the nineteenth century, it was not until the 1990s
that evidence began to accumulate as to their harmful effects.
It took over a decade more for the FDA to then limit the
amount in the diet and only recently began to phase out
TFAs because of their incredibly detrimental health effects.
Even today, the labeling on packages is based on serving sizes,
determined by the manufacturer, so that foods with "zero
TFAs" can supply a lot of TFAs, depending on how much
you consume. And the list goes on. Suffice to say such governmental assurances should be taken with a grain of salt,
precisely because of the questions that surround the governmental recommendations concerning sodium intake.

And it seems that if you have the dollars to pursue labeling efforts, well it seems the government allows you to buy
an indulgence. The proposed bill required that a "food label
can only claim that a food is non-GMO if the ingredients are
subject to certain supply chain process controls. A food can
be labeled as non-GMO even if it is produced with a GMO
processing aid or enzyme or derived from animals fed GMO
feed or given GMO drugs."[732] So even if a small independent
producer went through the rigmarole and expense to obtain a
governmentally approved non-GMO label, they may have to

compete with industrially produced GMO containing foods legally labeled non-GMO.

Yes, you read that correctly. The proposed law allowed GMO products to be labeled non-GMO, which makes pursuing a non-GMO designation as worthwhile as seeking that mysterious inheritance you got in that email from Nigeria.

Resistance seems futile. The law "preempts state and local restrictions on GMOs or GMO food and labeling requirements for GMOs, GMO food, non-GMO food, or "natural" food."[733] The law was to be swiftly enacted once passed. The legislation required that this law be enacted within one year of passage.

The proposed law contained a section addressing the labeling of natural foods. This was an amendment to Section 403 of the Federal Food, Drug, and Cosmetic Act (21 U. S. C. 343). It was to include "the terms 'natural,' '100% natural,' 'naturally grown,' 'all-natural,' and 'made with natural ingredients' and any other terms specified by the Secretary." Because if you're not going to use the regulatory non-GMO certifying process, you sure as hell aren't going to be able to differentiate your non-GMO product by any other defining adjective.

The pathetic irony of the proposed law is that it was sold as a way to "ensure national uniformity regarding labeling of foods derived from genetically engineered plants by preventing a patchwork of conflicting state or local labeling laws which inherently interfere with interstate and foreign commerce."[734] If this was indeed the purpose, the United States Congress need only enact a national law which required the full disclosure of foods that are genetically modified.

Instead, there was an assemblage of a bureaucratic maelstrom that seemed more designed to camouflage and ubiquitously disseminate GMOs. Manufacturers needed only provide their own declaration that their product is safe and dismiss any troubling inconsistencies as "not biologically meaningful." Such regulations shift the burden of proof to proving that something is not a GMO. It is like being presumed guilty and having to prove you're not—exactly the opposite of the founding principles of the country. Are we learning nothing from the folly of the GRAS legislation?

Despite the continuing cries from modern US agribusiness and food industry that an approach that simply labels something genetically modified when it is genetically modified, is untenable and fiscally prohibitive, the other sixty-four civilized countries around the world seem to have implemented just such a strategy and the sky has not fallen. Even Russia, hardly a model of individual liberties and green environmental practices, has enacted legislation regulating GMOs. Vladimir Putin has signed legislation requiring the mandatory labeling of foods that contain GMOs in order to "protect its citizens from the overconsumption of genetically modified organisms and minimize risks to humans and the environment."[735]

The barbarians are not at our gates; they are in our fields. The invaders will enter not in a monument built for the gods, but hide in the small parcels we collect each day for sustenance. If we are not vigilant and wary, we will be bullied and beset by a corporate Agamemnon. We will unknowingly grant them entrance into our most personal temples, one bite at a time. Through poor choices, apathy, expediency, and a lack of caution, will we be fated like King Priam at the burning of Troy to realize, far too late: "I've suffered what no other mortal has, I've kissed the hand of one who killed my children."[736]

At the other extreme from malevolence, we must guard ourselves against frivolity, no matter how well-meaning. Recently, the state of New Jersey passed a well-intentioned law with unintended consequences. In an effort to protect consumers from foodborne salmonella poisoning, the state outlawed the serving of "sunny side up" eggs.[737] The increased risk of salmonella from "sunny side up" eggs is minuscule at best and seems to be based more on projecting an appearance of concern and action than on any actual data. In fact, the data suggests that there is a higher theoretical risk from poached and soft-boiled eggs.[738] In a rebuttal to such food fascism, it was the *vox populi* that overturned such governmental absurdity. When the people speak at the societal level, great transformation *can* occur.

All such shifts in the cultural zeitgeist must start with the individual. When we choose a wholesome, natural, and authentic diet the data supports a positive correlation to health and wellness and a decreased risk of the disabilities and diseases associated with the consumption of the modern Western diet. The lowest reported levels of coronary artery disease of any population recorded to date have been, as recounted, documented in the Tsimane.[739] These individuals exist as a tribal population in the Bolivian Amazon that subsists on hunting, gathering, fishing, and farming.

An approach based on such food and food pathways provides for a pleasurable palate experience. Innumerable combinations and variations of tastes, textures, and flavor profiles are available in an equally varied range of preparations. Such food of love makes us happy.

Reducing the incidence and prevalence of such disabilities and diseases associated with the modern Western diet yields positive benefits at the societal and cultural levels in both economic and non-financial measures. Production of such foodstuffs in a sustainable manner ultimately helps restore and continue a natural, planetary balance.

Enacting such a program begs an understanding of the foundation upon which any natural, wholesome, authentic, and sustainable diet is based. The bedrock for any such diet, regardless of whether individual or global, starts with plants. While we run to save cuddly pandas and protest the sale of whale meat, the diversity of which the crux of not just humanity, but the entire animal kingdom is based upon, is being decimated in an unprecedented fashion.

When the industrial agribusiness algorithms are introduced worldwide, they tend to favor particular plants over others. Often, those plants are the ones—increasingly of the GMO variety—for sale by the large suppliers. The loss of heirloom varietals, often preserved for flavor or unique growing characteristics, is a loss of plant diversity. The consequence is that certain genes are eliminated from the available gene pool. Once gone, they are lost.

Seeds should be viewed with the same urgency as endangered animals. Seeds are betwixt and between: between life and death; between the old plant and the new plant. Seeds are a form of reincarnation. Animals consume these plants. We consume these plants. These seeds are a magical life-force that "propagates the communal table."[740]

Hopi corn is a particular type of corn adapted to drought. According to Hopi, when it comes to their corn, "Every corn seed contains life." It can be grown without irrigation. Replacing it with higher yielding GMO corn requiring incessant irrigation is not necessarily the wiser choice. More is not always better.

There is a dance between plants and humans that many indigenous peoples still remember. Corn developed about ten thousand years ago in Central America. It founded empires we still regard with awe. About four thousand and seven hundred years ago it reached what is today the U.S. As recently as one thousand years ago corn was found throughout what is now the lower forty-eight states. The Blue Corn Maiden is revered by Native Americans everywhere. One Native American relates the words he was told by his elders that reflects this reverence with practical aplomb: "Seeds in the hand, in your pocket; this is life. When you are hungry a seed can feed you. You cannot eat money."[741]

The first lobbyist in the United States represented the American Seed Association. In the 1890s the US government gave away almost one billion seeds for free. Then the American Seed Association started lobbying against free seeds. By 1924, free seeds were no longer available. Seeds now had to be bought. The practice of farming was changed forever.[742]

Farming was changed again following World War II. Prior to that most everything had been grown by what today would be considered organic methods. Surplus nitrogen compounds and other relics of the war were found to make good fertilizers. Today we are finding that excessive fertilizers and pesticides disrupt the soil ecosystem. In a parallel fashion to the disruption of our own gut microbiome with the modern Western diet, we are destroying the complex microbial relationship plants have with the Earth, the soil, water, and air, through our additives.

Hybrid corn changed farming again. But this "green" revolution was not necessarily about sustainability. It was an effort to counter the Red revolution of communism. The premise was that if people got cheap food they would not riot. Happy and full, there would be less of an urge to heed the call of communism. It was a bit of the twentieth century version of "Let them eat cake."

Modern agricultural techniques were introduced to replace so called "peasant farming." Such techniques still hold valuable lessons. It is estimated that the farming techniques of the ancient Hawaiians could sustain three times the current population of the islands. Our modern industrial farming practices require lots of chemicals and terraforming. Much like the modern domestic turkey, as early as the mid-1800s the Broadbalk experiment had shown modern versions of wheat could not survive in the wild.[743]

Atrazine, an herbicide, use exceeded eighty million pounds in the recent past. There are over 1.4 billion pounds of Roundup sprayed each year. Seed plots are now continuously exposed to pesticides and chemicals without regulation.

There are currently roughly three hundred thousand plant species. Of these, there are approximately thirty thousand edible plants. Only about one hundred and twenty species are regularly consumed. In industrialized countries, the majority of people subsist on about ten plants: corn, rice, wheat, barley, and oats predominant among them. One only need to walk about the produce section of most grocery stores to see the same monotonous offerings that never seem to vary regardless of season or clime.

It is thus no surprise that over 90 percent of all seeds used worldwide to grow our food are owned by chemical or pesticide companies. Corporations own patents on seeds and all the offspring of those seeds. Native plants are being contaminated with GMO variants, like the wheat in US contaminated by a Monsanto experiment gone wrong. To this day there is no explanation of how this occurred.

In the recent past, Monsanto bought up all the seed companies in India. Now Indian farmers can only buy Monsanto seeds from the sixteen Indian seed companies that remain. Monsanto also bought up all the native seeds. In essence and in action, Monsanto formed a modern version of the Honourable East India Company, plying seeds instead of spices, with practices no less nefarious and results no less grim. There have been two hundred and seventy thousand suicides of Indian farmers correlating to the rise of the Monsanto monopoly.

There is only about 4 percent of seed diversity remaining. We have lost 96 percent of all vegetable seed diversity in the twentieth century. The last seed diversity count was 1983. It is currently estimated that:

- Among the five hundred and forty-four cabbage varietals, there are twenty-eight left;
- Among the one hundred and fifty-eight cauliflower varietals, there are nine left;
- Among the fifty-five kohlrabi varietals, there are three left;
- Among the thirty-four artichoke varietals, there are two left;
- Among the two hundred and eighty-eight beet varietals, there are seventeen left.

We have lost 98 percent of asparagus, 90 percent of pepper, 96 percent of corn, 98 percent of celery, 94 percent of onion, 94 percent of radish, 91 percent of watermelon, 91 percent of eggplant, and 94 percent of cucumber varieties.[744]

In the tale of "Jack and The Beanstalk", Jack is ridiculed for trading his valuable cow for a handful of worthless beans.

But Jack and the first peoples knew something we have yet to comprehend. A seed has secrets; a seed holds hope. Every bean is indeed magic.

Implementation: Text to Tapas

> *"It is the mind that maketh good or ill, that*
> *maketh wretch or happy, rich or poor."*
> —*Edmund Spencer*

What differentiates the shaman from other healers is the journey.[745] At the heart of shamanism lies the journey of body, mind, and spirit. All journeys first begin in the mind, no matter the ultimate physical destination. Thus as Food Shamans, we begin our food journey here as well. The words we tell ourselves, what we speak to ourselves in our minds are the first actions we take. Words are powerful seeds.[746] This makes words powerful magic, for good or ill.

The emerging field of psychosocial genomics explores how "psychotherapy and related cultural processes and rituals (such as meditation, prayer, and the deeply meaningful humanistic experiences of art, drama, dance, music, poetry and the like) can modulate alternative gene expression to facilitate health, rehabilitation, and healing." Depression and stress are known to alter the amount and even type of neurotransmitter produced by the body and affect the immune system. Presumably, we can bring ourselves back into healthy homeostasis by stress-relieving rituals.[747]

Potent examples can again be found in the exploration of placebo and nocebo effects. A nocebo effect is "harmful side effects or worsening of symptoms due to negative expectations or the psychological condition of the patient."[748] The placebo and nocebo effects have historically been viewed within the medical community as a "nuisance;" a viewpoint still prevalent today within basic and clinical research arenas. This, despite the fact that measurable beneficial effects have been documented in up to 50 percent of people being treated for Parkinson's disease, depression, and chronic pain syndromes.[749]

Recent experience with the process of renal denervation provides a sobering example of the underestimation of the placebo effect. Millions of people in the United States and around the world suffer from hypertension. Untreated hypertension is the most common cardiovascular disorder and a risk factor for a number of serious health sequelae including stroke and heart attack.

The prevalence and incidence of hypertension continues to increase worldwide. Approximately 10 percent of patients with diagnosed hypertension have resistant hypertension, defined as "a systolic blood pressure of 140 mm Hg or higher despite adherence to at least three maximally tolerated doses of antihypertensive medications from complementary classes, including a diuretic at an appropriate dose."[750] Such patients are at high risk for future cardiovascular complications.

Previous attempts to treat this condition focused on the sympathetic nervous system's role in the cross-talk between the kidneys and the brain. A surgical sympathectomy, cutting the nerve and thus the connection, was seen as an effective treatment for some patients with uncontrolled hypertension. Unsurprisingly, patients who underwent this procedure did suffer from serious side effects, and it fell into obsolescence.

Recent advances utilizing a catheter-based radiofrequency technique to cause denervation of the renal arteries renewed interest in the procedure. Initial studies in more than eighty countries, including parts of Europe, South America, Australia, the United States, and Canada were promising.

These trials demonstrated large reductions in blood pressure after renal denervation.[751]

Fortunately for the millions who might have been subjected to such a "cure," the SYMPLICITY HTN-3 trial was performed. It clearly showed that renal ablation was no better than a sham procedure—by comparing it to a sham procedure. Before the properly controlled trial, most of the experts predicted a new era in hypertension treatment utilizing this technique. Think about the ramifications of that very near almost-catastrophe.[752]

Now some researchers are questioning commonly performed but invasive procedures. Catheter ablation of atrial fibrillation (AF), an abnormal heart rhythm, consists of using a radiofrequency catheter to create a burn which forms a scar that in theory restores the normal sinus rhythm. In the DISCERN-AF study, the results revealed that the ratio of asymptomatic to symptomatic AF episodes increased more than threefold *after* ablation.[753] After almost twenty years of performing this procedure, academic papers tout the results as "promising."[754] The success rate in that promising study was 56 percent, which puts it squarely in the possibility of placebo range. (See appendix E3)

Recent medical history is rife with procedures that appeared revolutionary, only to prove that the effects were no better than placebo. Which is to acknowledge that the success of the early open label trials was due to the power of the mind. Pacemakers for prevention of fainting[755, 756] or to treat hypertrophic cardiomyopathy,[757] intracranial transplants of embryonic dopamine neurons for the treatment of Parkinson's disease,[758] the injection of cement into a fractured vertebra for the treatment of compression fractures,[759] the drilling of holes into the heart[760] or the ligation of coronary arteries[761] to relieve angina were all modern medical practices that have gone the way of recommending smoking a few Camel cigarettes for "good digestion."

The recently completed OBITA trial highlights the dangers of assumed benefit in the most profound and, to many interventional cardiologists, most unsettling way. For a lot of patients who currently receive intra-coronary stents (percutaneous coronary intervention or PCI), the goal of such a procedure is symptomatic relief of their chest pain or stable angina. However, there is no evidence from blinded, placebo-controlled, randomized trials to show if there is benefit in a procedure that is performed in over five hundred thousand individuals annually worldwide.

ORBITA was such a trial of PCI versus a placebo procedure for angina relief that was done at five study sites in the UK. The researchers enrolled two hundred and thirty patients with ischemic symptoms consistent with stable angina. The patients underwent cardiac catheterization, a common practice to evaluate angina in the United States, and they were included in the study if they had a single coronary artery with a severe (≥70 percent) stenosis. This degree of blockage was also measured physiologically with a device that calculates the fractional flow reserve (FFR). The mean value in the study was a FFR of 0.69. All of these findings would provide an incontrovertible rationale for the implantation of an intra-coronary stent in the US, according to current guidelines.

Patients either received such a device or underwent a sham procedure. All participants then underwent six weeks of medication optimization. Subsequently, they were questioned regarding their symptoms, and they underwent stress testing. There was no significant difference in the degree of chest pain or exercise (treadmill test) time between groups, and no one in either group died.

The researchers concluded that:

> *ORBITA has implications for our clinical understanding of stable angina. The concept of a simple linear link between a tight stenosis and angina is attractive to patients, easily explained by physicians, and biologically plausible. Moreover, since relieving the anatomical and haemodynamic features of stenosis by unblinded PCI is followed by the patient reporting angina relief, it is understandable that this link becomes generally accepted.*
>
> *However, forgetting the potential magnitude of placebo effects prevents exploration of the inevitably complex relationship between anatomy, physiology, and symptoms. Clinicians have hoped there might be a simple entity named ischaemia, which manifests as positive tests and clinical symptoms, and that treatment by PCI would eliminate all these manifestations concordantly. Perhaps this notion is too optimistic.*[762]

And, perhaps, too simplistic. We are complicated.

Modern healers, while utilizing the techniques and technologies of the age to propel medicine forward, practice an art that remains grounded in its ancient shamanic roots. A contemporary review of such elective surgical procedures, compared to sham or placebo procedures found that "in thirty-nine out of fifty-three (74 percent) trials there was improvement in the placebo arm and in twenty-seven (51 percent) trials the effect of placebo did not differ from that of surgery."[763] As Professor Olshansky surmised:

> *The beneficial effects of placebo, generally undervalued, hard to identify, often unrecognized, but frequently used, help define our profession. The role of the doctor in healing, above the therapy delivered, is immeasurable but powerful. An effective placebo response will lead to happy and healthy patients. Imagine instead the future of healthcare relegated to a series of guidelines, tests, algorithms, procedures, and drugs without the human touch. Healthcare, rendered by a faceless, uncaring army of protocol aficionados, will miss an opportunity to deliver an effective placebo response. Wise placebo use can benefit patients and strengthen the medical profession.[764]*

Likewise, the nocebo effect is real and actively impacts our health. The power of the voodoo curse to kill is often attributed to the strength of the victim's belief. Within the annals of recent medical history, data shows that women with similar risk factors were four times more likely to die if they believed they were prone to heart disease.[765] There is a strong correlation between emotions such as fear or depression, the development of cardiomyopathy and even death. Broken heart syndrome, or *Tako-tsubo* cardiomyopathy, especially prevalent in women, appears related to an adverse intense emotional stressor.[766, 767, 768] As Henry Ford supposedly said,

"Those who believe they can do something and those who believe they can't are both right."

How we journey is as important as the destination. The attitude of implementation of the action is as important as the action itself. The renowned psychologist, Abraham Maslow, cautioned: "If you deliberately plan to be less than you are capable of being, then I warn you that you will be deeply unhappy for the rest of your life."[769]

What is most important is not the crisis itself, but what comes out of it. For the shaman "is a sick man who has been cured, who has succeeded in curing himself." In the objective world of society, rituals can repair relationships, solidify and stabilize social structures, and affirm or challenge authority.[770] For the Food Shaman, the food experience is just such a ritual.

Each individual food experience has four aspects. There is the intending and the subsequent action or behavior. These two aspects are subject to cultural and social norms and are interrelated in a way that makes arbitrary divisions difficult. Each is a part of the circle like directions on a compass. Social systems influence the cultural worldview, which in turn sets limits to individual thoughts. These thoughts give birth to behavior and action.

Ken Wilber gives further insight:

You can traverse that circle in any direction you want. These quadrants are all interwoven. They are all mutually determining. They all cause, and are caused by, the other quadrants. Partial approach will never work. It seems instead that we need an integral approach which are not staring at exteriors but sharing of interiors. Not objective but intersubjective. Not surfaces but depths.

> *In medicine, for example, you can see that*
> *any effective care would have to take into*
> *account, not just the objective medicine or*
> *physical treatment that you give the person*
> *[Behavior], but also the person's subjective*
> *beliefs and expectations [Intention], the cul-*
> *tural attitudes, hopes, and fears about sick-*
> *ness [Cultural], and the social institutions,*
> *economic factors, and access to health care*
> *[Societal], all of which have a causal effect*
> *on the course of a person's illness (because all*
> *four quadrants cause, and are caused by, the*
> *others). This is an "all-level, all-quadrant"*
> *approach to consciousness, therapy, spiritu-*
> *ality, and transformative practice.*[771]

Such an attitude is in contradistinction to contemporary practices that are based on dualism; one *or* the other. The gluttonous tempts us with a buffet of pleasure comprised of misperception. The ascetic lures us with false promises of contradiction. The true middle path is a tree that branches into the various disciplines, each branch a unique aspect nourished from the same rootstock; a *Yggdrasil* connecting worlds of inquiry and encounter.

We need the proper food experience, not servile subsistence nor epicurean excess. The twin lions that guard the gates of Eastern temples are said to represent confusion and paradox, and anyone who seeks wisdom must be willing to pass through both.[772] We must, as Plotinus admonished, "Close our eyes and invoke a new manner of seeing...a wakefulness that is the birthright of us all, though few put it to use."[773]

One possible ill destination of such skewed *modi operandi* are exclusionary fad approaches. While a gluten free diet is a necessity for the 1 percent of the population with true Celiac disease, the practice has gotten completely of hand. The gluten free fad has expanded far beyond those with true gluten enteropathy and even beyond those who may have some form of gluten intolerance into the population at large.

Thanks in a large part to successful commercial marketing, roughly 30 percent of people pursue a gluten free diet. It continues to grow among people without these conditions, fueled by commercial opportunity, even though there is lack of evidence that reducing gluten consumption provides long-term health benefits. Such segregation is not without potential cost. Data presented at The American Heart Association meeting in 2017 suggested that low gluten diets may be associated with a *higher* risk of type 2 diabetes.

"We wanted to determine if gluten consumption will affect health in people with no apparent medical reasons to avoid gluten," said Geng Zong, Ph.D., a research fellow in the Department of Nutrition at Harvard University's T.H. Chan School of Public Health in Boston, Massachusetts and a contributor to the research. He further elaborated, "Gluten-free foods often have less dietary fiber and other micronutrients, making them less nutritious and they also tend to cost more. People without Celiac disease may reconsider limiting their gluten intake for chronic disease prevention, especially for diabetes." (See appendix E4)

The results revealed those with the highest gluten intake reduced their risk of T2DM by 13 percent.[774] But it is even more complex than simply analyzing the quantitative content of gluten in the diet. We don't eat gluten; we eat foods that contain gluten. Individual foods represent a complex matrix of fatty acids, proteins, carbohydrate quality, micronutrients, phytochemicals, and preparation and processing methods.[775, 776]

Because of this diversity, the cardiometabolic effects of total carbohydrates are modified by the *quality* of the carbohydrate. For people who consume mostly low-fiber, rapidly digested, refined grains, starches, and added sugars, a lowering of total carbohydrate will produce substantial metabolic benefits. Yet recommending a low-carbohydrate diet *per se* is not ideal: the focus should be on reducing less healthful carbohydrates, not *all* carbohydrates, which includes fruits and vegetables, and which there is consensus that most everyone should consume more of these.

Simply pursuing a plant-based diet, even a vegan diet, that is rich in sweets and refined grains may actually *increase* the risk of CVD, in contrast to the conventional assumption to the contrary. Plant-based diets are routinely recommended by many health care professionals to reduce the risk of obesity, diabetes, heart disease, and many other of the modern disabilities and diseases that afflict our contemporary culture. Yet a study published in the *Journal of the American College of Cardiology* suggested that, surprise, not all plant-based diets are created equal.

Broad recommendations so often dispensed to the public from high towers commonly treat all plant foods equally, even though certain plant foods like refined grains and sugar sweetened beverages are associated with a higher risk of cardio-metabolic disease. Likewise, they often lump comestibles together in a category like "meat," even though they are as distinct by well defining characteristics as Ozzy Osbourne and Pat Boone, though both versions of *Crazy Train* are fab.

When the researchers examined a plant-based diet that emphasized less healthy plant foods like sweets, including sweetened beverages and refined grains, the risk of CVD increased. Ambika Satija, ScD, a postdoctoral fellow at the Harvard T.H. Chan School of Public Health in Boston and the study's lead author concluded, "It's apparent that there is a wide variation in the nutritional quality of plant foods, making it crucial to take into consideration the *quality* [emphasis added] of foods in a plant-based diet."[777]

This may appear to be an obvious exercise in common sense, until you look at the discrepancies, contradictions, and pure poppycock that make up so much of the current dietary guidelines and expert consensus recommendations. There are many confounders in teasing out the data, in trying to sort out bane from benefit.

As different as we are as individuals, our gut microbiomes may be as unique as our fingerprints. Bread has been a staple of humankind for millennia and has evolved along with us. Even with the gluten-free craze, it is consumed daily by billions worldwide. People are told that whole grain breads are superior from a nutritional standpoint, and their preferred consumption is standard across different guidelines.

Yet the response of an individual may be more determined by gut microbiome composition than bread composition or human digestion and physiology. This may explain the observed contradictory effects of its consumption, depending on the population studied. Researchers performed a randomized crossover trial of two one-week-long dietary interventions comprising consumption of either traditionally made sourdough leavened, whole-grain bread, or industrially made white bread. They found *no* significant differential effects of bread type on multiple clinical parameters. *Videre licet*, there was no benefit or adverse effect to the group as a whole.

What they did find was that at the individual level there was a huge difference in the response to the different types of bread. In essence, the response at the individual level portended a beneficial or adverse outcome with continued consumption. However, the individual effects were washed out in the average result. But what predicted the individual response was fascinating.

The researchers demonstrated that:

> *The glycemic response to different bread types, suggest[s] that the lack of phenotypic difference between the bread types stems from a person-specific effect...[and] that the type of bread that induces the lower glycemic response in each person can be predicted based solely on microbiome data prior to the intervention...suggesting that understanding dietary effects requires integration of person-specific factors.*[778]

In other words, the individual's response to the bread type, their health or illness, could be predicted *entirely* on their individual gut microbiome. In fact, it could *only* be predicted by the gut microbiome. This huge piece of the puzzle is missing from every current dietary recommendation or guideline issued to date.

Discrepancies between observational studies and supplement trials may relate to residual bias in observational studies, e.g. from other lifestyle behaviors (i.e., observed benefits are not attributable to diet) or from other nutritional factors in vitamin-rich foods (i.e., observed benefits are caused by diet but not by the specific measured vitamins or nutrients). Diets higher in antioxidant vitamins tend to be rich in fruits, vegetables, nuts, and whole grains, and foods that contain multiple other beneficial factors including other vitamins, minerals, phytochemicals, and fiber. Because consumption is a zero-sum game, simply eating foods that can provide benefit means you don't eat unhealthful foods.

Sometimes the obstructions come in the form of pride, politics, or economics. Since the 1970s the government has been advocating fat reduction as the key to a healthful diet. As reported in *The British Medical Journal:*

> *Dietary recommendations were introduced in the US (1977) and in the UK (1983) to (1) reduce overall fat consumption to 30 percent of total energy intake and (2) reduce saturated fat consumption to 10 percent of total energy intake. No randomised controlled trial (RCT) had tested government dietary fat recommendations before their introduction. Recommendations were made for 276 million people following secondary studies of 2,467 males, which reported identical all-cause mortality. RCT evidence did not support the introduction of dietary fat guidelines. Dietary recommendations were introduced for 220 million US and 56 million UK citizens by 1983, in the absence of supporting evidence from RCTs.[779]*

It took almost half a century for the governmental recommendations to acknowledge the insurmountable weight of evidence contrary to their original recommendations. The 2015 Dietary Guidelines Advisory Committee stated, for the first time, that dietary guidelines should *not* focus on lowering total fat.

The experts remain non-committal when it comes to saturated fat. Saturated fat represents a highly heterogeneous category of fatty acids, with chain lengths ranging from six to twenty-four carbons, deriving from diverse foods, and possessing dissimilar biology. This biological and metabolic diversity does not support the grouping together of all saturated fatty acids based on only one chemical characteristic: the absence of double bonds.[780] (See appendix E5)

Dietary saturated fats are obtained from very different foods—e.g., cheese, grain-based desserts, dairy desserts, chicken, processed meats, unprocessed red meat, milk, yogurt, butter, vegetable oils, and nuts. Each of these possesses, in addition to saturated fat, numerous other ingredients and characteristics that modify their health effects. These complexities help clarify why total saturated fat consumption has little relation to health.

Judging a food or a person's diet as harmful because it contains more saturated fat, or as beneficial because it contains less, is unsound. In sum, these lines of evidence—complex lipid effects including little influence on ApoB, no relation of overall intake with CHD, and no observed cardiovascular harm for most major food sources—provide powerful and consistent evidence for absence of appreciable harms of total saturated fat. Continued prioritization of saturated fat reduction appears to rely on selected evidence: e.g., effects on LDL-cholesterol alone (discounting the other, complex lipid and lipoprotein effects); historical ecological trends in certain countries (Finland) but not in others (France); and expedient comparisons with polyunsaturated fatty acids (PUFAs).[781] In the end, we eat foods, not isolated molecules. (See appendix E6)

Thus, focusing on specific types of foods and oils, rather than monounsaturated fat content per se, may be most prudent. For example, extra virgin olive oil and mixed nuts appear to be good dietary choices to improve cardiometabolic health and as real, natural foods offer specific tastes, textures, and flavors.[782, 783, 784, 785, 786, 787] When we implement our selection of comestibles, it is more prudent to examine the food *quality* and its characteristics than generalized percentages of this or that.

Some foods, like some people, are to be avoided in their entirety. Trans-fatty acids (TFAs) are mono- or polyunsaturated fats with one or more double bonds in a *trans* position, rather than the mammalian synthesized *cis* position. Although as previously mentioned, small amounts of natural TFA are found in meats and milk of ruminants (e.g., cow, sheep, goat; formed by gut microorganisms), these contribute minimally to diet (<0.5 percent) and do not associate with CVD risk. Indeed, trans-palmitoleic acid (trans-16:1n-7), a trace TFA biomarker of dairy fat, is linked to a lower risk of diabetes mellitus and sudden cardiac death.[788, 789] Overall, naturally occurring TFAs form a very small part of a diet based on wholesome, authentic, and real foods, and they appear to be a healthful constituent.

Conversely, high levels of industrially produced TFAs can be consumed from partially hydrogenated vegetable oils, which typically contain thirty to 60 percent TFA. These fats have industrial advantages for commercial deep frying, baked goods, packaged snacks, and shortening. Higher TFA intake from partially hydrogenated oils is consistently associated with the risk of CHD and sudden death.[790, 791] It simply took the government decades to get around to telling us. (See appendix E7)

While attention to TFAs languished on the sidelines like three-day old fish, misdirected focus on isolated ingredients kept all eyes off the fact that it is the woefully adulterated foods that have ill health and ill taste in common. They served us red herrings. Believed to be the origin of the diversionary term, a "red herring" was a smoked kipper (usually herring) that was heavily treated with salt through brining and as a result would have its flesh turn a deep red.

There is continued belief, without adequate data, that salt consumption, or more precisely the sodium portion of the salt [sodium chloride] molecule, must be lowered and that it is the salt that is solely responsible for the untoward effects of the modern Western diet. Salt has become a modern day red herring.

For many years now, the consumption of salt, or more specifically, sodium, has been targeted as the major contributor to disability and disease associated with diet, specifically by contributing directly to the development or worsening of hypertension and cardiovascular disease. As cardiovascular disease remains the number one cause of mortality for both men and women in the United States, and many industrialized nations, this is a significant health issue.

Indeed, there are major governmental sponsored health programs like the American Heart Association's Million Hearts Initiative, of which part of their algorithm includes achieving their health objectives through reducing sodium consumption by 20 percent. This program consists of hundreds of millions of dollars in taxpayer funds as well as private corporate partnerships with similar allotments.[792] All in pursuit of a goal that has never yielded a single concrete health benefit. For full background description see The Fallacy of The Calorie.

In short, the purported benefit of a low sodium approach is based on the sodium hypothesis. The thought process goes like this: increasing your intake of sodium increases your intravascular volume. This is true, which is why when people are dehydrated they are treated with an intravenous solution of normal saline (salt water). More vascular volume increases blood pressure (albeit temporarily)—also true. Increased blood pressure, or hypertension, is a risk factor for stroke and cardiovascular disease and thus bad—also true. Therefore, by reducing intake of sodium, we lower blood pressure and save lives; this is not only *not* true but disturbingly reminiscent of the failed dietary cholesterol/fat hypothesis.

The foundation of this philosophy is mirrored in the statement by the U.S. governmental health agencies that utter because there is no harm in reducing sodium intake, it should be driven as low as possible. Current U.S. sodium consumption is roughly 3.5g per day; with many urging a decrease to 2.5g or even as low as 1.5g per day.

Reflecting the "you can't go too, too low" approach, anticipated benefit is modeled on a linear relationship in which there is increasing risk and adverse outcome with increasing sodium intake and conversely decreasing risk with decreasing intake, all in a linear fashion. This potential modeling is where many of the predictions of low sodium benefit are derived from: benefits that are remarkably lacking in prospective, real world trials and observations. In other words, when you get off the computer, do the experiment and look at the results from actual real people. The benefits don't appear.

A meta-analysis of four large, prospective trials helps solidify the reasons why, as well as the relationships that guide that them. This analysis compromised over one hundred and thirty thousand people from forty-nine countries who were examined for over four years. The population studied, importantly, compromised both those with hypertension as well as those without (normotensive). The researchers utilized urinary excretion of sodium, which is an accurate measure of dietary sodium intake from *all* sources.[793]

The results were striking and in agreement with recent, smaller studies. The relationship between sodium intake and cardiovascular morbidity and mortality is not linear. Regardless of whether one has hypertension or is normotensive, consumption of less than 3 g per day is associated with *increased* risk. The minimum amount of risk appears to be related to daily consumption of between 4g and 5g of sodium per day.

However, there does appear to be an increasing risk in cardiovascular disease in those persons *with hypertension* consuming more than 6g of sodium per day. In terms of actual numbers, this represents only about 24 percent of those people with hypertension. When the population includes all persons, those with and without underlying hypertensive disease, then the group at risk represents only about 10 percent of the entire population. For those without hypertension, significant potential harm did *not* exist until there was significant sodium consumption in excess of these levels. While approximately 95 percent of the world's population consumes more than 3g per day, only approximately 22 percent consume more than 6g per day (the level at which there is an association with increasing risk of cardiovascular disease). Also recall that far and away most dietary sodium is the result of consuming prepared and highly processed foodstuffs. (See appendix E8)

The failure of public policy due to incompetence, agendas, and politics does more than simply squander valuable resources. It erodes public confidence in the ability of the science at hand to successfully deliver on its promise of honesty, integrity, and improved health. Worse yet, misguided missions can set us off course for decades to come, leaving us marooned with disability and disease. We need only look back to the half century of admonitions to shun healthy, natural foods rich in fat for industrially produced, refined carbohydrates. Nobody told us the snack crackers came with a side of insulin.

The continued misguided push for so called "healthy" low salt or no-salt approaches is a straw man. Since over 70 percent of the daily sodium ingested comes from highly processed, refined, industrially manufactured foods, perhaps the correlation to disability and disease has to do more with the quality of the comestibles than quantities, sodium, calories or otherwise. The continued push with governmental labeling laws focuses on attempting to achieve healthful outcomes through caloric restriction. Just remember: cyanide is calorie-free.

Implementing dietary choices based on artificially broad food groups is another red herring served up by policy makers. High-protein diets are another fad pursuit. In meta-analysis of randomized trials, increased protein consumption has little effect on cardiometabolic risk factors including adiposity, lipids, blood pressure, inflammation, or glucose.[794]

This is not surprising. Like total fat or total carbohydrate, total protein represents the sum of very different foods (red meats, processed meats, milk, cheese, yogurt, fish, nuts, legumes) with widely divergent health effects. Thus, a focus on dietary protein *per se* appears much less relevant for health than a focus on specific types of foods. Judging the long-term health impact of foods or diets based on isolated macronutrient composition is simply unsound practice.[795, 796]

Yet there is a persistent pursuit to categorize and condition what we eat in terms of quantities, calories, and constituents in isolation. This approach is reiterated and reinforced at the highest levels until it becomes the conventional wisdom.

Throughout the history of humankind, there have been those among us that assert that *theirs* is the conventional wisdom. Some go further and proclaim that they themselves set or define the very convention itself. This conceited notion of superiority causes both caste and castigation among the different groups which necessarily comprise any society. The geometry of such an approach is inevitably a pyramid that has a single clique that sits upon its pinnacle.

The past has exposed the folly of such an approach time after time. The horrors and atrocities committed in the fanatical, single, and simple-minded approach to perfecting a master race still reside within generational telling. If the dangers and logic against such a pursuit are as unassailable as we declare them to be, why do we allow it to craft our menus and dictate our diets?

All the while, these elite experts ignore the fact that how the animal is bred, what it is fed, and where it is led, makes a world of difference. These concerns focus on the underlying *quality* of the product and speak to its true value. It's about the character of the comestible, about the personality more than the price. Great chefs are adamant in sourcing of authentic, wholesome, and natural ingredients. It is why they seek out organic or organically equivalent heirloom vegetables and heritage breeds.

As we set about and engage in implementing our food choices, the three questions we must ask of all our potential comestibles bears repeating here:

- *How is it bred?* (What are its genetics?)
- *What was it fed?* (How was it raised and what did eat?)
- *Where was it led?* (If there was any post-processing, what and how was it done?)

Real flavor and real health quite simply demand real food. Take pause, breathe, and engage.

Imagine if you will a stroll into the garden in the deep of summer, or a meander about the farmers market; real food can be found here. It is as real as the heat that reaches profoundly into us. Carried quite literally on heavy water vapors, the humidity is palpable with each breath. With each long, slow lungful of the dog days that drag on, the oppressive moisture clings to us. It hangs on us, an unwanted, heavy cloak. It is a hothouse that seems fit for neither man nor beast.

But it is a produce paradise. This is the time of year it is easy to be green. And purple. And orange. And red. And every nuance and shade that covers the horticultural spectrum. So when we enter the air-conditioned corridors of the market, enjoying a brief respite, when we see that unblemished, perfectly round, intensely red tomato, we cannot but help but reach the conclusion that has been so insidiously and meticulously crafted for us to stumble upon.

It is an assumption planted for us to grasp. That this is a real, fresh garden tomato. That this has spent its entire life up until its most recent arrival to our market becoming the fruit of the vine. There it blossomed from bud to flower, lazing sunnily in God's own green acre; it captured the essence of sunlight. It drew deep of the Earth itself, swelled with the waters of life. It transformed all of these to a sweet succulence that is the taste and texture of a perfectly vine-ripened, fresh garden tomato picked at the perfect moment of peak flavor and brightness. So sweet on the palate, it is obvious why this is actually a fruit, not a vegetable. This, quite simply, is the real food that nature intended.

Yet not all that glitters is gold, nor is all that is red in the produce department a tomato. When we grasp the fruit, its flesh does not yield gently to our soft caress. It is hard and uncaring, like some plastic doppelgänger. When we bring it close, it does not greet us with the soft perfume of summer, but with a cold indifference that offers no hope of either taste or texture.

For this tomato never saw the sun. It knew only the harsh glow of the grow light. The soil was no loamy nest, but dirt enhanced for rapid growth. The species of tomato was not picked for flavor, but for function. It was produced for large size, water retention—especially useful when sold by weight—and uniformity of product, each tomato so exactly like the rest that mechanical harvesting is not only possible, but profitable.

It did not develop the distinctive deep vermillion solar blush that marks this summer berry being sun kissed. It was picked green. Under ripe, rock-hard, and green, it travels well with minimal damage during its long transport. Just before it makes its faux debut amongst the fruits and vegetables, it is gassed with ethylene oxide. And with the application of some horrible botanical spray tan, the fake food makeover is complete.

That is one of the dark sides of our modern food pathways. What looks truly at its penultimate and desirable, may not be. Real, freshly harvested foods can be on your grocer's shelf, on ice at the fishmonger, or in the craft butcher's display case quite literally overnight. The average fish travels five thousand, four hundred and seventy-five miles before making an appearance on your dinner plate.

That distance creates openings for nefarious tampering and tinkering. A decade ago, *Consumer Reports* tested twenty-three salmon fillets that were labeled as wild caught. Only ten were in fact wild salmon.[797] We can no longer simply rely on our sight to convey to us if the information about our food is accurate, not when we cannot tell if the vibrancy of the carrots is due to carotenes or orange dye.

We must engage all our senses. Most importantly, we must engage our brains. We must no longer be consumers blindly accepting what is proffered to us. We must become chefs, at least to the extent that we learn how to, and we properly engage in, sourcing our food. Authenticity has its own *terroir*.

Although there is no universally accepted literal translation of the word *terroir*, the concept is widely recognized. It speaks to the place from which our sustenance comes. It is most commonly associated with wine in the sense that certain geographic areas have a unique set of constituents. These combine in such a way that the wine from this vineyard or region cannot be duplicated anywhere else. A true French champagne can only be produced in the French region of Champagne, and nothing else on Earth will ever taste like it.

All real food has its own *terroir*. It is the simple realization that our food should be wholesome and authentic; it should reflect the pitch and yaw of seasonality and experience. It should, like our lives, reflect variety and vitality, give pleasure and purpose, and at all costs avoid homogeneity and sterility. This is the food we seek out with the action of implementation. This is the stuff of the food experience. This is what transforms subsistence into symbol and victual into ritual.

Because of their highly-charged meaning, the symbolic elements that are used in rituals penetrate the mind-body system and elicit powerful psychological responses, causing a cascade of corresponding biological responses throughout the body. These responses extend across organ systems such as the brain, endocrine, and autonomic nervous systems. It extends across biological levels from organs to physiology, to biochemistry, and even down to gene expression (the ways in which genes create new cellular building blocks). It affects our symbiotic partner in existence; the organisms of our microbiome. In the reduction and separation to acquire knowledge, we tear down and create borders. But these are artificial constructs that reflect the limits of our understanding. The body functions as a whole and knows none of the artificial divisions we create for our own understanding.

As we act to implement, we engage not only those personal intentions and their behaviors, but the cultural influences and societal norms that we are a part of and are a part of us. We engage them in concert as the wheel turns. Nobel Laureate Eric Kandel summarized a new way of understanding. Simply stated, the regulation of gene expression by social factors makes all bodily functions, including all functions of the brain, susceptible to social influences. Because its effects penetrate so widely, an effective food experience is simultaneously:

- Cultural Therapy: Healing and cohering culture and creating *communitas*
- Sociotherapy: Repairing relationships, harmonizing social structures, and stabilizing society
- Psychosomatic Therapy: Diminishing disease and its complications
- Gene Therapy: Modulation of gene expression
- Psychotherapy: Healing the subjective dis-ease of illness
- Spiritual Therapy: Relieving a sense of alienation and estrangement from the universe, creating a sense of connection and alignment with the sacred, and fostering a transpersonal/ transegoic sense of identity.[798]

The action of implementation is done with the same care and consideration as choosing a friend. Look past the labels and examine for yourself the character, the *quality*, of the comestible. Carefully prepare your food experience with a mindfulness of personal gratitude and a sustainability for the greatest benefit of all. It is the soft edges of the food experience, so often overlooked in contemporary Western medicine, which is central to the Food Shaman. It is this that implements the transmutation from meal to miracle.[799]

QUANTUM FOOD FOR A
CHANGING WORLD

*"A man searching for lost Paradise, can seem a fool
to those who never sought the other world."*
—*Jim Morrison,* The American Night

Food is life and life is a miracle.

The origin of Life, like that of the Universe, still escapes us. Sir Fred Hoyle (1915–2001), an English astronomer and former director of the Institute of Astronomy at Cambridge, co-authored the book *Evolution From Space* with mathematician Professor Chandra Wickramasinghe. Hoyle argued that the notion that not only the constructs, but that the operating program of a living cell were the result of chance combination in some primordial organic soup here on the Earth, was simply rubbish.

Hoyle and Wickramasinghe calculated that the chance of obtaining the required set of enzymes for even the simplest living cell without panspermia was one in $10^{40,000}$. Since that exceeds the number of atoms in the known universe by a factor of five hundred (10^{80} estimated for the number of known atoms), they argued life could not have originated on Earth. The spontaneous emergence of life on Earth, Hoyle would contend, was the equivalent to "a tornado sweeping through a junkyard and assembling a Boeing 747 from the materials therein."

The opportunity for obtaining even a single functioning protein by chance combination of amino acids was, according to his estimation, "equivalent to a solar system full of blind men solving Rubik's Cubes simultaneously."[800] This seems to be on the order of chance that a monkey types a Shakespearian play. The time needed for that is estimated at about a billion, billion years. The entire known universe is only fourteen billion years old. The invoking of such chance is a taboo of the traditional scientific doctrine that comforts us with certainty of prediction and reproducibility of outcome.

Hoyle and Wickramasinghe's support for the concept of panspermia, a hypothesis proposing the methods of life's distribution in the universe—not its origin—was echoed in 2009 by physicist Stephen Hawking. He acknowledged that, "Life could spread from planet to planet or from stellar system to stellar system, carried on meteors."[801]

Though Hoyle declared himself an atheist, the implied integration of a larger whole led him to conclude that "a super intellect has monkeyed with physics, as well as with chemistry and biology, and...there are no blind forces worth speaking about in nature."[802] Albert Einstein contributed to the discussion on this relational nature of reality:

> *A human being is a part of the whole, called*
> *by us "Universe," a part limited in time and*
> *space. He experiences himself, his thoughts*

and feelings, as something separated from the rest—a kind of optical delusion of his consciousness. This delusion is a kind of prison for us, restricting us to our personal desires and to affection for a few persons nearest to us. Our task must be to free ourselves from this prison by widening our circle of compassion to embrace all living creatures and the whole nature in its beauty. '803

We are a part of the Universe, and as such we are indivisible from Nature. This is something indigenous peoples, living closely with Nature, were able to intuit. In a rare occurrence of insight, the United States government in 1988 acknowledged:

Indigenous peoples have rich storehouses of information about nature, man, and the balanced relationship of the two. From their beliefs about the spiritual world to their traditional knowledge of rainforests, healing, and agriculture, these societies provide the opportunity for new interpretations about the world and ourselves. Many of these populations face severe discrimination, denial of human rights, loss of cultural and religious freedoms, or in the worst cases, cultural or physical destruction.... If current trends in many parts of the world continue the cultural, social and linguistic diversity of humankind will be radically and irrevocably diminished...immense undocumented repositories of ecological, biological and pharmacological knowledge will be lost, as well as an immeasurable wealth of cultural, social, religious, and artistic expression.[804]

What native cultures and the great scientific minds of our time both grasped as they probed the true nature of reality at the edges of observation, was the singularity of what we might term scientific and spiritual thought. As humankind has always perceived, ultimately the experience cannot be divorced from the experiencer. Reality is finite and granular. At some sub-atomic level of Planck-space, the Universe is constructed of particles that cannot be further subdivided.[805] At some level you can no longer remove the observer from the observed, or in the case of food, the diner from dinner.

Einstein, as was his wont, put the paradox succinctly: "Science without religion is lame, religion without science is blind."[806] He further probed the fundamental question:

What is the meaning of human life, or of organic life altogether? To answer this question at all implies a religion. Is there any sense then, you ask, in putting it? I answer, the man who regards his own life, and that of his fellow creatures as meaningless is not only unfortunate, but almost disqualified for life.

What an extraordinary situation is that of us mortals! Each of us is here for a brief sojourn; for what purpose he knows not, though he sometimes thinks he feels it....

By way of the understanding he achieves a far-reaching emancipation from the shackles of personal hopes and desires, and thereby

attains that humble attitude of mind
toward the grandeur of reason incarnate
in existence, and which, in its profoundest
depths, is inaccessible to man. This attitude,
however, appears to me to be religious, in the
highest sense of the word. And so it seems to
me that science not only purifies the religious
impulse of the dross of its anthropomorphism
but also contributes to a religious spiritual-
ization of our understanding of life....The
further the spiritual evolution of mankind
advances, the more certain it seems to me
that the path to genuine religiosity does not
lie through the fear of life, and the fear of
death, and blind faith, but through striving
after rational knowledge.[807]

It was in this pursuit of such knowledge that Einstein unwittingly and irreversibly propped open the door to the Atomic Age. Although the ideas that form the basis of quantum theory have been debated since at least the times of Democritus in ancient Greece, Einstein, like Newton before him, provided the science, the methodology, and the math to usher us across the threshold.[808]

With that door opened, others like Alan Turing described the concept of self-organization and quantitated this phenomenon in a mathematical construct. This led to a further understanding of Nature's rhythms: fractals. A fractal is a simple equation: $Z \leftrightarrows Z^2 + C$; the Mandelbrot equation. It describes a concept of self-similarity. The pattern continues to repeat itself in ever smaller iterations but with minute variation. To see it in action, observe the branching of a tree. Yet among humanity's greatest gifts is the potential to *self-transcend.* Self-transcendence is a novel emergence as opposed to self-organization or self-similarity seen in other aspects of Nature.

Such quests have brought us ever closer to understanding the reality of being, what fabric lines the heart of the Universe. This is the search of quantum mechanics. It deals with the ultimate reality of existence. Following this path toward its logical conclusion has led us to the end of logical science as we know it. We are at the inception of a new paragon.

Our current paradigm is a representation, a theory to explain the world. It is based on the scientific method. This process requires a model maker who cannot be part of the model. Scientific method by necessity must exclude the scientist from the equation. It must be free from bias; including effects brought about, consciously or un, by the observer; a form of error known as observer bias. Such a model represents the limits of logical thought in a quantum world. We need to expand into a quantum model that accounts for observer.

A contemporary way to think about this problem would be to realize the subtle implications of quantum entanglement. Imagine a mother gives birth to identical twins, Pat and Chris. The twins are separated at birth and raised without human contact and in isolation at different places halfway around the world. Even their biological mother does not know the sex of the twins.

Then one day you meet Pat and observe that she's biologically female. Instantaneously, because they are identical twins and the pair must be either both male or both female, you know the identity of her twin Chris, halfway across the world. You know that even though you have never met Chris. You have acquired information about a person (or a particle in quantum theory) faster than the speed of light. In terms of quantum mechanics, these twins are entangled. Knowing the sex of one immediately identifies the sex of the other.[809]

To move forward, it is important to understand that with respect to quantum mechanics, knowing whether the twin across the world was either male or female is more consequential than simply resolving a knowledge deficit. In the world of quantum mechanics, prior to defining whether the twins are male or female, they do not have a definite biological sex. In other words, until you have met one of the twins, they both have the *potential* to be male or female. There is a 50 percent probability Pat and Chris are male and a 50 percent probability that they are female. Until you meet them, their biological sex exists as a probability function. This ability to exist in a potentiality of all possible states, both male and female, is called superposition.

This idea of quantum indeterminacy is expressed through the famous thought experiment known as Schrödinger's cat. One of the key principles of this concept is that until an observation has taken place the physical reality is unknown. In other words, until there is an observation or measurement the physical reality remains undefined. This of course, by inference acknowledges the role of an observer. Without an observer, there is no physical reality. There is simply a state of potentiality. It is the observer that brings the physical reality into existence.[810] Without the observer there is no certainty, simply a range of probabilities.

This is a critical concept. Humankind first sought to understand the world around us through the creation of myth. Humankind's thought process evolved from archaic to magical to mythical to rational. Moving beyond myth, we proceeded into our present-day world of science and rationality. With the development of the scientific method we formalized logic, and propelled forward into our modern, technological age.

Yet the strength of the scientific method is based on reproducible experiment. The pursuit of this methodology yields predictability via the minimization of all biases, including observation bias. And therein lies the conundrum. From a certain perspective, pushing the boundaries of logic and rationality into the world of quantum mechanics yields uncertainty because this reintroduces the concept of an observer to validate any physical reality.

The architecture of the Universe thus becomes relational. It cannot exist independently outside of the observer. We find ourselves back at Immanuel Kant's Copernican Revolution: the mind forms the world more than the world forms the mind. Georg Wilhelm Friedrich Hegel, who through his writings furthered the concept of *aufheben,* or sublation, professed that thoughts are not merely a reflection on reality, but a movement on that reality itself.

When we taste and engage the Food Experience it affects our physiology and biology in profound ways. Brillat-Savarin in his *The Physiology of Taste: Or Meditations on Transcendental Gastronomy,* challenged his readers to reflect on what they ate. "Show me what you eat and I will show you who you are."[811] Now we are just beginning to comprehend the enormity of the venture. It is not just what you eat, but how. We are not just what we eat, we eat what we are.

We find ourselves on the verge between rational and existential. Clinging to outdated logic in the face of a contrary data set is the definition of the irrational; a crossroads where we risk substituting science faith for science fact.

There is danger if as a society we slip into replacing scientific fact with scientific faith. The famous physicist Richard

Feynman remarked that the true pursuit of science was to "bend over backward to prove ourselves wrong."[812] This must include acknowledgement of our methodologies as we strive to perceive the reality of creation. We evolved in thought and technology because evolution involves incorporation and understanding, not flat rejection or indifference. Ken Wilber examines our peril in ignoring the human relation to the Cosmos, the danger as we currently sit:

> *All smug and confident that nothing higher will sweep out of the heavens and completely explode our solid perceptions, undoing our very foundations. They transcend and include. Because they are more inclusive, they are more adequate. So, it's not that the earlier worldview is totally wrong and the new worldview is totally right. But of those emotions, of course, you will not find much description, because emotions pertain to the interior experience of the limbic system. These emotions and the awareness that goes with them are what the holon with a limbic system experiences from within, on the inside, in its interior. And objective scientific descriptions are not much interested in that interior consciousness, because that interior space cannot be accessed in an objective, empirical fashion. You can only feel these feelings from within. When you experience a sort of primal joy, for example, even if you are a brain physiologist, you do not say to yourself, Wow, what a limbic day. Rather, you describe these*

feelings in intimate, personal, emotional terms, subjective terms: I feel wonderful, it's great to be alive, or whatnot, so that we can see something of ourselves in each other, and treat each other with care and concern. The great and undeniable advances in the empirical sciences from the Renaissance to the Enlightenment made it appear that all of reality could be approached and described in it-language, in objective scientific terms. And conversely, if something couldn't be studied and described in an objective, empirical fashion, then it wasn't "really real." The Big Three were reduced to the "Big One" of scientific materialism, scientific exteriors and objects and systems.[813]

In conducting experimental analysis, a whole is reduced into parts, but then you have parts not the original whole. In figuring out how a car works, the parts can be removed. But the parts on the garage floor will not transport you anywhere, it only works once reassembled. In our Western approach, we sometimes mistake the parts for the whole; we suffer from too much reductionism. We mistake a holon for *the* whole.

The term holon was first described in 1967 by Arthur Koestler in his book *The Ghost in the Machine*, to describe something that was simultaneously a whole and a part. Although the origins of such a system of hierarchies can again be traced back at least to Democritus and his atomic theory. In his descriptions of holons, Koestler identified sub-wholes or parts of systems that were wholes and parts at the same time.

As a thing which could be identified, it was to that degree a whole. Yet as that same item was part of a larger system, it was also a part. Thus, he concluded that absolute wholes or parts do not exist anywhere; everything exists in relation to something else. Holons exist simultaneously as self-contained wholes in relation to their subordinate parts, and as dependent parts when considered from the inverse direction. Furthermore, these relations *must* be hierarchical in nature.

Each holon builds upon the previous. Sentences contain words, meals contain ingredients, not vice-versa. There is a directionality of progress that establishes hierarchies. These hierarchies are pyramidal in construction with both a horizontal span and a vertical axis, or depth. In this form by design as verticality increases, population decreases.[814]

People existing as holons can be viewed as comprised of four quadrants sitting within the cardinal directions or gateways. For descriptive purposes, they could be seen as the North-East quadrant: Behavior, the South-East quadrant: Social, the South-West: Cultural, and the North-West: Intention. These are the four facets of the human holon and transformation correlates to the successful integration of these four gateways.[815]

Intention is the internal driver of the individual. It is the internal thought process known only to that individual. The behavior is the observable action of the individual. These are influenced by and influence the cultural aspects of which the individual is part. These cultural attitudes are manifest in the observable society at large. We are not removed from the world in which we live, although we often act in an isolationist manner. Quite the converse, we are at every level inextricably twisted into every facet of existence, the hidden and the mundane.

The Northern gateway is one of behavior, integrity, and bringing our truth into the world through action. The Eastern gateway is one of societal action, hospitality, and community. The Southern gateway is cultural legacy, the story of art and attitude. The Western gateway is one of intention. Authenticity and sovereignty stand at the center and lie at the heart of the circle.[816] Such a description of reality incorporates both observable and hidden, subjective and objective, components.

The intention and cultural influences are the subjective "I" and "We." The behavior and observable society are the quantifiable "It." Our current approach is to ignore the "I" and "We" quadrants and evaluate only in terms of quantifiable "It." This is the remnant of the Enlightenment Paradigm. To evolve is to differentiate and integrate both the interior and exterior.

Koestler describes this relationship between subjective and objective knowledge as it reflects both the interior and exterior aspects of life:

> *Einstein's space is no closer to reality than Van Gogh's sky. The glory of science is not in a truth more absolute than the truth of Bach or Tolstoy, but in the act of creation itself. The scientist's discoveries impose his own order on chaos, as the composer or painter imposes his; an order that always refers to limited aspects of reality, and is based on the observer's frame of reference, which differs from period to period as a Rembrandt nude differs from a nude by Manet.*[817]

In focusing on only empirical observation we lose an understanding of the interior. It is like judging a book by its cover, a restaurant solely on its exterior façade, a meal by appearance only without tasting it. The value simply does not depend on location or an easily quantifiable quantity or measurement.[818] Objectively analyzing a play by William Shakespeare might include a word count, a page count. Subjectively analyzing a play by William Shakespeare requires reading it.

Subjective does not equate to arbitrary. The subjective is relational and must be understood in terms of context. Ultimately, the objective must be realized in context. What does it do versus what does it mean? Eating x increases glucose. That is what it does. But that must be understood in terms of what it means to the biological system consuming it. Those effects include the interior or effect on intention. Changes derived from interior actions like mindfulness are no less valid than pharmacological interventions. Is Truth not Truth?

Quantum mechanics, ushered in by Einstein's theories of special and general relativity, predicted phantasmagorical truths that were initially met with skepticism because they simply appeared to the casual intellect as if they could not possibly be "real," whatever that means. Yet the proofs accrued, verifying prediction and theory. Space is a gravitational field that encompasses time. There is neither space nor time as independent variables, only space-time. In 1919 the curvature of light around the sun, the curvature of space-time was proved. The prediction of the fluidity of time, which is it expands and shrinks according to the vicinity of masses, was verified. Sensitive clocks run faster at higher altitudes as the Earth's mass slows time at the surface.

The existence of black holes, originally dismissed as an abstract theoretical anomaly is accepted science fact today. The origin of the universe predicted to be fourteen billion years ago was confirmed by astronomers Penzias and Wilson in 1964. The proof of gravitational waves that ripple across space-time like the aftermath of a stone on a placid lake won Hulse and Taylor the Nobel Prize in 1993. The list goes on. The quantum world may seem an outlandish world of dreams, yet this strangeness may ultimately prove to be more substantial than our illusory interpretation of this reality.

When we see a child on the beach and wave to them, we are not seeing "them." The physicist Carlo Rovelli explains:

> *We only see vibrating Faraday lines. To "see" is to perceive light, and light is the movement of the Faraday lines. Nothing leaps from one location in space to another without something transporting it. If we see a child playing on the beach, it is only because between him and ourselves there is this lake of vibrating lines that transport his image to us.*

This lake of vibrating Faraday lines is a field, an electromagnetic field that we perceive. We interpret the quanta, or photons, of this field as color and image. It is the quanta in quantum fields that give quantum theory its granularity. It is a knowable dimension defined as the Plank-length; 1.6×10^{-33}cm or about one millionth of a billionth of a billionth of a billionth of a centimeter. But as small as it is, it is not infinitely small. Unlike classical physics, quantum mechanics sets limits. There is a finiteness to the Universe and everything in it, including information.

In loop quantum gravity theory, it is covariant quantum fields upon which the universe is built. It is gravitational fields that give us the universe of space-time and gravity in which we dwell. It also gives us uncertainty. This unpredictability, this quantum indeterminacy, is a feature of our reality. Niels Bohr first described in the atomic model every schoolchild recognizes as resembling the solar system, with electrons in discrete orbits about a nucleus like planets about the sun. But it was Werner Heisenberg, he of the Uncertainty Principle, who helped us understand that "the more we look at the world the less constant it is. The world is not made up of tiny pebbles. It is a world of vibrations, a continuous fluctuation, a microscope swarming of fleeting microevents."[819]

Electrons do not orbit, but only appear and disappear according to probabilities. These probabilities can be calculated utilizing Feynman's sum over paths, but they can never be *known*. Quantum indeterminacy means that randomness operates at the atomic level. There are no certainties. Chance is an innate characteristic of the Universe. It is only because we exist at the macroscopic level where the average effect of microscopic processes creates the illusion of determinism and inevitability that the Universe appears to act in a contrary manner.

Heisenberg's musings opened a Pandora's Box of quantum weirdness. For he, along with subsequent work from Paul Dirac, verified that electrons *literally* appear and disappear according to probabilities. Electrons only exist when they interact. This is the third tenet of quantum mechanics, existence is relational. For electrons:

> *They exist when they interact. They materialize in place when they collide with something else. The "quantum leaps" from*

one orbit to another constitute their way
of being real: an electron is a combination
of leaps from one interaction to another.
When nothing disturbs it, an electron does
not exist in any place...every object...has no
property in itself, apart from those that are
unchanging, such as mass. Its position and
velocity, it angular momentum and its elec-
trical potential only acquire reality when
it collides-interacts-with another object. It
is not just its position that is undefined, as
Heisenberg had recognized: no variable of
the object is defined between one interac-
tion and the next. The relational *aspect of*
the theory becomes universal.[820]

Knowledge is likewise relational. It depends upon both subject and object. States of systems, information, refer implicitly or explicitly in relation to some other system. Rovelli concludes:

Classical mechanics misled us into thinking
that we could do without taking account of
this simple truth, that we could access, at
least in theory, a vision of reality entirely
independent of the observer. But the devel-
opment of physics has shown that, at the
end of the day, this is impossible.[821]

Our interaction with food on all levels can likewise not be separated. Pursuit of health and wellness through nutrition and strictly medical avenues has been like seeking the fundamental constructs of the Universe with a strictly classical physics approach. It has been false. Food affects our human physiology but also our gut microbiome. The Food Experience works in the limbic system but also functions on a level of consciousness unto itself; it is both subjective and objective. We must understand the true nature of the Food Experience is relational in its entirety.

Meals can be better or worse, but currently we study them only in terms of quantities; bigger, smaller, more or less. Their value is defined only in terms of some quantity like calories. A quantum food approach seeks to peer into the ultimate reality of our relationship with food; the ultimate reality of the Food Experience.

Quantum food is natural food, the real and authentic food of our ancestors. It is what we and our symbiotic gut microbiome have co-evolved to co-metabolize. Like the honeybee and the flower, we are so bound to this good Earth. We are not bound as if in chains, but as a microcosm of a living eco-system. We are a holon of the planet we inhabit. It is an umbilical tie to the Universe we should rejoice in and celebrate. And what better way to do that, than with a good meal?

Quantum food is not molecular gastronomy, but beyond predictable, clinical approaches such as calories, RDAs, nutrients. We have dissembled food to understand the components, now we must reassemble the whole foods. We have artificially differentiated our food and created labels to better comprehend their functions and effects. But—much like Humpty Dumpty—once disassembled, real, authentic food cannot so easily be put back in place. Our attempts have been marred by a process of reduction, destruction, and concretion, not integration and evolution. Without a clear direction, the path of the quick fix becomes a narrow one, ultimately leading to a mine of despair and a cessation of progress.

A human being is essentially 99 percent air, water, coal, and chalk. You can add a bunch of trace minerals and elements like iron, zinc, phosphorus, sulfur, and a few others to the mix. The total sum value of the elements that comprise the human body is roughly ten dollars. But understanding this in no way allows us to answer the question of what human *life* is worth. We are transcendent in that we have novel or creative properties that are not merely the sum of our components. We have the ability, if we choose, to use the gifts to advance ourselves and others; to become unlike other species on this planet, self-transcendent and self-actualized.

In our clinical fashion, we may break down the core constituents of natural food into carbohydrates, proteins, fats, minerals, elements, vitamins, and the like. We may measure our food on graphs and charts, and assign values like calories. But none of this helps us unlock and understand the Food Experience. Is happiness really just so much serotonin?

In such an objective only approach we go from a value to valueless. Consciousness is intrinsic to the Food Experience. We cannot have dinner without the diner. The Food Experience, like us, is transcendent in all the ways that defy quantification.

Mainstream medicine is just beginning to comprehend the magnitude of the Food Experience. As a recent review observed:[822]

> *Many current approaches to improving nutrition—e.g., clinical counseling, food labels, menu labeling, dietary guidelines— arise from an implicit assumption that dietary habits are primarily a function*

of individual choice. In reality, multiple complex factors influence dietary choices. At the individual level, dietary habits are determined not simply by personal preference but also by familial norms, education, income, nutritional and cooking knowledge and skills, and health status. Additional relevant factors include attitudes toward food and health, incentives, motivation, and values. Other lifestyle behaviors such as television watching and sleep influence patterns of food consumption.

Outside the individual quadrant, the social and cultural quadrants contain drivers like cultural norms, social pressures, and social networks. Additional environmental or societal influences include neighborhood accessibility (*e.g.*, food availability, cost, and convenience). Each of these individual, environmental, and sociocultural determinants is shaped by, and in turn shapes, much broader drivers of food choice such as agricultural policy and production practices, food industry formulations and marketing, national and international trade agreements, other market forces, climate, and agricultural policies.[823, 824, 825, 826] (See appendix F1)

Integrated, multicomponent approaches that include upstream policy measures, midstream educational efforts, and downstream community and environmental approaches may be especially effective. Successful, sustainable improvements in population dietary behaviors will require close collaboration among multiple stakeholders, including academics, clinicians, health systems, insurers, community organizations, schools, workplaces, advocacy groups, policy makers, farmers, retailers, restaurants, and food manufacturers.[827, 828]

This is the unity that the quantum approach to the Food Experience seeks to bring. It is all of those seemingly random parts that sometimes appear at odds with logic. This is because logic is based on intellectualism. Taste is an experience beyond intellect. We are more than an animated carcass. Engaging our senses in the quantum food experience awakens our minds and spirit; it is truly a *Bodhicitta*, awakening mind, encounter. One proper solution births several new questions. (See appendix F2)

The predominant influence of environmental risk factors such as the quality of food choices in unmasking or mitigating genetic risks must be demonstrated to the public at large in a way that speaks to not only external physical, nutritional needs, but internal psychological and spiritual needs as well. It is an unfamiliar vision: "For now we see through a glass, darkly; but then face to face: now I know in part; but then shall I know even as also I am known."[829]

The human gut microbiome functions to reflect upon us, sometimes darkly, that phenomenon of what might be termed "human entanglement." In the world of quantum mechanics, entanglement is what Albert Einstein referred to as, "Spooky action from a distance."[830] Quantum entanglement can be described to mean "that multiple particles are linked together in a way such that the measurement of one particle's quantum state determines the possible quantum states of the other particles. This connection isn't depending on the location of the particles in space."[831]

The human gut microbiome is entangled with its human host. The character and composition of the individual gut microbiome correlates not just with our physical health and biological functioning, but with our very wellbeing. It mirrors our health and wellness or disability and disease through active participation. It can influence our emotional state, and cause us to action, like signaling to our brain we are full and thus to stop eating. The recent bread study shows that our idiosyncratic response to ingesting bread is completely predictable, not by any measure of *Homo sapiens*, but strictly by the characteristics of the individual gut microbiome.[832]

The gut microbiome is also a holon. If we destroy our gut microbiome, we destroy ourselves. Yet, destroy us and the bacteria survive. In the hierarchical nature of holons, we need to understand there are no *value* judgements. There are only holders of location in the hierarchical order. Therefore, the gut microbiota as holons are components of *our* being.

To destroy them is suicidal. You are no longer eating a meal, you *are* the meal. Is what we choose to consume poison or medicine? It is in the dose, and the character. You are the experience; you consume both. We must exhibit super-consciousness, for in reality we are not a single unique organism. We are a supra-organism.

What do you choose to eat?

The average person encounters over eighty thousand different manmade chemical compounds per day.[833] Many are not only added to our food, but enter food pathways through such innocuous doorways as the packing in which our food is delivered. [834, 835] (See appendix F3)

Food expresses a type of ultimate truth. The history of food is the history of us; our conscious and unconscious, individual and societal, development. The role of food is preponderant to our personal physiology and biology, but because unlike any other species the human celebration of food involves complex societal and psychological parameters as well, it has holistic implications. The celebration of food and the pursuit of the celebration of food is shared by cultures and civilizations throughout the world and throughout history. As something so treasured by humanity throughout antiquity into our modern age, we should take note of its profundity.

A meal can and should be Spirit-in-action, where every moment and movement unfolds into a tiny microcosm of who we are and who and where we want to be, or it can be a mindless walk to the gallows pole. A meal is a microcosm because each ingredient is a holon—a whole (spice, herb, vegetable) that becomes a part of the repast that in turn is but part of the Food Experience.

Quantum food is a holonic and holistic approach to food. It moves beyond solely the comestibles as an isolated afterthought but engages the totality of the Food Experience; taste and taster. It is a child of both logic and intuition. Within the Food Experience there is a directive to seek those natural, wholesome, and authentic foods to which we have evolved to positively relate.

There is a desire to honor the Earth and respond to the alienation from Nature that is so much a part of modern life and that is producing "nature-deficit disorder" in individuals and ecological disaster for our planet.[836, 837] What a quantum perspective shows us is that the reality is relational. The Food Experience is relational in the context and intersection between the dinner and the diner, the observer and the observed, the taste and the taster.

The magic of the Food Experience is in the doing. It is not an abandonment of modern progress, technology, or knowledge. Things may not necessarily be "wrong," but perhaps we have been looking at it the wrong way. Perhaps in some cases it is merely an adjustment of our own perspective.

Our journey will bring us new tastes and treasures, but these must exist within the purview of realities. Fire will not cool our food, and modern society, for all its ills, offers us tremendous benefits. We must seek to integrate, not denigrate, both the interior and exterior. Only this way can we move beyond the overly simplistic view of reality as a duality. Quantum mechanics demonstrated early on that light is neither a particle nor a wave, but exists as both. Certainly, it is time for us to move beyond the dualistic view that a meal must be either delicious or healthy, that there is food and there is us.

We must try. In this fashion the Food Shaman through the Food Experience, applying the Art of Quantum Food, seeks to engage Spirit. Without trying one has no reference of failure or success. As Einstein was so keen to observe, it is our point of reference that helps shape our reality. Our reference point places us in relation to others, Nature, Spirit, and the Universe not in an arbitrary location, but in a relative relation given our point of reference. As Satprem observed on the relativity of seeking:

> *This is why it is so difficult to explain the path to one who has not tried; he will see only his point of view of today or rather the loss of his point of view. And yet, if we only knew how each loss of one's viewpoint is a progress, and how life changes when one passes from the stage of closed truth to the stage of the open truth—a truth like life itself, too great to be trapped by points of view, because it embraces every point of view...a truth great enough to deny itself and pass endlessly into a higher truth.*[838]

Ken Wilber further stewed Truth and Spirit into seeking the Food Experience:

> We can describe Spirit subjectively as one's own Buddha-mind—the "I" of Spirit, the Beauty. And we can describe Spirit objectively as Dharma—the "It" of Spirit, the ultimate Truth. And we can describe Spirit culturally as Sangha—the "We" of Spirit, the ultimate Good. Individual "pathologies" as but the tip of an enormous iceberg that includes worldviews, social structures, and cultural access to depth. You are the Kosmos. The universe of One Taste announces itself, bright and obvious, radiant and clear, with nothing outside, nothing inside, an unending gesture of great perfection, spontaneously accomplished. So what is the sound of that one hand clapping? What is the taste of that One Taste? When there is nothing outside of you that can hit you, hurt you, push you, pull you—what is the sound of that one hand clapping? See the sunlight on the mountains? Feel the cool breeze? What is not utterly obvious? Who is not already enlightened? As a Zen Master put it, "When I heard the sound of the bell ringing, there was no I, and no bell, just the ringing." There is no twiceness, no twoness, in immediate experience! No inside and no outside, no subject and no object—just immediate awareness itself, the sound of one hand clapping. This nondual state, this

state of One Taste, is the very nature of every experience before you slice it up. This One Taste is not some experience you bring about through effort; rather, it is the actual condition of all experience before you do anything to it. This uncontrived state is prior to effort, prior to grasping, prior to avoiding. It is the real world before you do anything to it, including the effort to "see it non-dually." And precisely because this is the simplest thing in the world, it is the hardest. This effortless effort requires great perseverance, great practice, great sincerity, great truthfulness. It has to be pursued through the waking state, and the dream state, and the dreamless state. And this is where we pick up the practices of the Nondual schools. You and the universe are One Taste. Your Original Face is the purest Emptiness, and therefore every time you look in the mirror, you see only the entire Kosmos.[839]

Live like someone who matters. Have an authenticity of presence. Change your mind or change your consciousness. These things can only be done through experiences. Currently we sit upon the cusp and we can either collapse or evolve and transcend. For the Food Shaman the Food Experience, the food service, is Spirit-in-action. For the Food Shaman, the Food Experience becomes a shamanic journey; a chance to meld the internal realms of intention with the external realms of behavior and to bring that tasty nugget to the community at large through cultural and societal means.

By taking charge of your cuisine, you empower your-self to reclaim your creativity. Sandra Ingerman presents the opportunity:

> We create our lives with our thoughts and words. In our culture, few are encouraged to use their imaginations in a way that helps develop creative abilities. Most of us are taught early on that there are only a few creative geniuses in the world and that we are not among them. Throughout our lives, we were taught to give our power away to authority figures who then determined the shape of our world according to their wishes.
>
> These activities reaffirm the shaman as a person who can move out of the mental state and become a "hollow bone" or "hollow reed" through which the Navajos say the many colored winds may blow. Inherent in the practice of shamanism is the under-standing that the shaman opens himself or herself to allow the power of the universe to flow through them and bring healing to those in need. By serving as the bridge between the worlds, the visionary can liter-ally merge with and act as a conduit for the power of the universe. One way to do this is through making art.[840]

Or in the case of the culinary arts, the creation of the Food Experience. A chef, like a shaman, becomes:

> a facilitator who, through ceremony, can help others achieve a new mind state. A

*shaman is the harmonizer between human-
kind and the natural world. By engaging
all your senses, you may work with an inner
process that engages your body-soul—a process that can be expressed into the physical
world. It is important to see, hear, feel, smell,
and taste this world as it already is and as it
is coming into existence. Otherwise you are
always creating it in the future.*

*You can do this with anything you make,
including food. Through daily activities
such as cooking...we can focus our thoughts
on a healing intention, and love will fill our
lives with power, harmony, and beauty.* [841]

With the eyes and heart of child we can rejoice at the
simple enjoyment of a food experience. In some ways, the
way of the shaman is the way of the child. For too often in
our modern world we have forgotten the magic in our lives.
Rediscover the mysteries. Reignite the light and joy that are
the result of a rich inner life. As we relish the physical meal,
let it feed our souls as we partake of the rich layers of the
Food Experience. This restores equilibrium and homeostasis.
We reclaim our innate right to dream and discover.

The path of the Food Shaman allows a rediscovery, a
re-experiencing, and a reinvigoration of the foods that fed
our forebears. It is dinner with the ancestors. And yet it is
more, because we infuse that food experience with our own
unique technology, insight, and knowledge. Through the
shamanic process our modern food experience integrates and
evolves and transforms into something more than the sum
of its disparate parts. It is a quantum leap forward and every
experience is unique.

A meal is like the river that Heraclitus of Ephesus observed. Just as you could not step twice into the same river, in consuming a meal you can never have the same food experience. You may combine the identical ingredients in a similar manner, but they are never exactly the same. The service is never quite duplicated. The dining transpires from a new reference point. A proper food experience is always sacramental; "shamanic ritual is always different in that its outer form is suggested, not prescribed, by tradition."[842]

Our current modern Western diet is a mumpsimus. With the use of the previously described approaches, the Food Experience can be "reworked in our time to do something entirely new, something that reflects who we are today and what we are becoming. There's the need to achieve an upgrade that reflects who we are as modern people in our own time."[843]

At the same time, it must sing to the past and stay true to its roots. Hence, we find:

> *Things hidden, to which we may learn that everything that exists is alive and has a spirit (and a voice), and that there is a field of energy that connects us to all to of life.... Healers and shamans actually create changes in reality by singing their intent into the "now point," or what quantum physicists call the quantum field.... [Although] the quest of the seeker is intensely personal...this awareness, the inevitable realization that everything, everywhere, is interconnected is shared by tribal shamans at one end of the human continuum and by quantum physicists and Zen Buddhists at the other.*[844]

But you do not need to be a theoretical physicist, a Zen priest, Michelin-starred chef, or a tribal shaman to practice as a Food Shaman. Anyone can incorporate the shamanic approach of the Food Experience into the simple ceremonies of daily repasts. The Food Shaman does this through the Art of Quantum Food.

We speak of ethnic foods: Chinese, Mexican, Italian, and the like. By that we mean a use of certain ingredients and flavor profiles along with what may be preparation and cooking techniques indigenous to those areas or regions. We speak of fast foods and junk foods, by which we refer primarily to processing and production as the defining characteristics. We speak of vegetarian, vegan, and gluten-free foods that highlight the exclusion of certain dietary components. We speak of Paleo foods by which we reject the inclusion of certain items based on time and technology. Quantum food is none of these things and all of these things.

Quantum food is the foundation of the Food Experience. Infusing the spirit of the Food Shaman in the true reality of existence, quantum food is an evolution. In the fashion of *aufhebung* or sublation, it fuses apparently contradictory elements into a new whole. It is like an emulsion of oil and water, seemingly incongruous and intractable parts come together into something new.

The food itself is not new. In this sense, it is a return to the old ways. It is about sourcing like a chef and understanding the critical importance of the quality of the ingredients. It is understanding that more volume is not necessarily more value. But it goes beyond obtaining our food in a state of anoesis with nothing but pleasure on the palate.

We undertake the endeavor with an understanding of the symbiotic supraorganism we truly are. We understand the wee beasties that we harbor give us life, and in turn we must give them life. To do otherwise is to tip the scales toward disability and disease.

We undertake the endeavor with an understanding that the very nature of reality is finite and granular. It is also relational. Within the laws of the Universe, we create our reality. For the Food Shaman this is not new. But with bright knowledge we bring focus to the soft edges; we acknowledge the reality and importance of the interior effects. We do not deny ourselves, the "I/We" in favor of the overtly quantifiable "It." We integrate the subjective and the objective, seen and unseen, and claim our sovereignty in authenticity at the center. We bring a bit of Epicurean enchantment back into our food, meals, and lives.

Despite all we know about the production of food, nutrition, and the science of cookery, the Food Experience retains an air of personal mystery. The event remains slightly unpredictable, slightly unknowable, and indescribable until it is tasted and acquired. Thus, there is always an enigmatic character to it; a bit of magic within the meaning. The ordinary is the sublime in disguise. The Japanese phrase, *Shikin Haramitsu Daikomyo* can roughly be translated as "Every experience brings the potential for enlightenment." Or every meal. Become a Food Shaman and find the Divine in the pedestrian; it awaits in every bite.

It is up to all of us. And all of us starts with you.

> *"Believe nothing, no matter where you read it, or who said it, no matter if I have said it, unless it agrees with your own reason and your own common sense."*
>
> —*The Buddha*[845]

APPENDIX OF SCIENTIFIC STUDIES

A. Food and Sex: Can You Smell What's Cooking?

1. These are a class of seven transmembrane domain G protein-coupled receptors that function in the olfactory epithelium as chemo-sensors. The capacity of the olfactory system to distinguish among a staggeringly large universe of chemical compounds depends upon these ORs, which are encoded in the mammalian genome. The results of any sniff test are gathered up by the ORs and funneled through a single common signaling pathway. When an OR binds to its odorant, it activates a single species of G protein, the olfactory trimeric G protein (G_{olf}), which then activates the olfactory isoform of adenylate cyclase (AC3).[846]

2. Interestingly, there is no thalamic intermediary to odor-evoked signals to central brain areas. The thalamus receives sensory information from all the other senses and processes this prior to it being interpreted by the brain's higher functioning areas of consciousness. This is another unique characteristic of olfaction among all the sensory modalities.[847]

3. It may be worth noting that there is no such mention of the seven deadly sins within the text of the Torah, Bible, or Koran. Their identification originated with the writings of Evagrius Ponticus in the fourth century A.D. They are first listed in his *Practical Guidebook to an Ascetic Life*, a title which pretty much tells you everything you need to know.

4. The central olfactory brain regions that process the olfactory input, the areas that detect and process smell, taste, and flavor, are more extensive in humans than is usually realized. These dedicated olfactory regions include the aforementioned olfactory cortex, the olfactory tubercle, the entorhinal cortex, parts of the amygdala, parts of the hypothalamus, the mediodorsal thalamus, the medial and lateral orbitofrontal cortex, and parts of the insula.

There is no doubt that these regions are involved in immediate processing of odor, taste, and flavor input and probably subserve the specific tasks of smell detection and simple smell discrimination. But where it becomes uniquely human is in the performance of more complex tasks. Here memory becomes important in comparing smells. This then involves areas of higher function such as the temporal and frontal lobes; and the specifically human higher association areas. It may be hypothesized that these regions enable humans to bring far more cognitive power to bear on odor discrimination than is possible in the rodent and other mammals.

5. Bourgeonal is potent aromatic with a fragrance reminiscent of lily of the valley. It also turns out to be an incredibly a powerful agonist for the type of OR,

hOR17-4, found in human sperm cells. Such odorants and receptors may turn out to play crucial roles in human sperm chemotaxis and may be a critical component of the fertilization process. In other words, male sperm may sniff their way to the feminine objective of their desires. It is likely no small coincidence that such a compound is also a mainstay of perfumery.[848]

In contrast to bourgeonal and related compounds, undecanal is a potent OR antagonist. Undecanal, also known as undecyl aldehyde, is a colorless, oily liquid, that occurs naturally in citrus oils.[849]

6. There is a specific OR, human OR51E2, also named prostate-specific G-protein-coupled receptor (PSGR), that is vigorously expressed in prostate cancer cells. By activating these receptors with certain smell compounds, the cancer cells turn off. One of the compounds which turned off the cancer cells was the odorant β-ionone.

The ionones are a series of closely related chemical substances that are part of a group of compounds known as rose ketones. They are common ingredients in a variety of essential oils, including rose oil. The specific compound, β-ionone, is largely responsible for the aroma associated with roses. The combination of α-ionone and β-ionone is characteristic of the scent of violets and both are common components used in the manufacture of perfumes. It is intriguing to note that this class of compounds, the ionones, are derived from the degradation of carotenoids. Carotenoids are a class of phytochemicals fundamental to a healthy diet. They supply many of the various and distinctive colors found in fruits and vegetables throughout the world.

The carotenes α-carotene, β-carotene, γ-carotene, and the xanthophyll, β-cryptoxanthin; can all be metabolized to β-ionone. Because of this ability to undergo enzymatic modification, they all have vitamin A activity. All these compounds can be converted by plant-eating animals to retinol and retinal. Carotenoids that do not contain the β-ionone moiety cannot be converted to retinol, and thus have no vitamin A activity.

When the prostate cancer cells were exposed to β-ionone, it resulted in the activation of members of the mitogen-activated protein kinase (MAPK) family and inhibition of cell proliferation. Diets rich in such plant derived compounds could provide benefit to both sexes because the isoprenoids β-ionone and geraniol also have been shown to inhibit mammary carcinogenesis by a so far unknown mechanism.[850]

7. It was recently discovered that solitary pulmonary neuroendocrine cells (PNECs), which are morphologically distinct and physiologically undefined, serve as chemosensory cells in human airways. Upon further investigation, some human PNECs are actually members of the odorant receptor family.

These cells are anatomically positioned in the airway epithelium to respond to inhaled volatile chemicals. Upon exposure of primary-culture human airway epithelial cells to volatile chemicals, the cells decreased their levels of serotonin. This then led to the release of the neuropeptide calcitonin gene-related peptide (CGRP). CGRP can stimulate the lung epithelium, which may then cause constriction of the airways. This is a potential mechanism by which inhaled irritants cause difficulty breathing.

These smell receptors may also be involved in the development of diseases like chronic obstructive pulmonary disease (COPD). There are changes in the distribution of serotonin and neuropeptide receptors in patients suffering from COPD that suggest that these cells could contribute to acute exacerbations.[851]

8. Although being the body's most abundant endocrine cell type, EC cells are difficult to study because they constitute only a minor proportion of the total intestinal epithelium and have a diffuse distribution.

Together with other enteroendocrine cells such as cholecystokinin and secretin-producing cells in the small intestine, they sense the luminal content of the gut and control the function of the stomach, the gall bladder, the pancreas, and the intestine. Serotonin, secreted by EC cells, is an important regulator of peristalsis and epithelial transport. This is why many of the drugs that are used for the treatment of gastrointestinal motility disorders, such as irritable bowel syndrome, focus on serotonin and serotonin receptors.

In the oral cavity and the nose, sensor cells endowed with gustatory and olfactory receptors begin the processing of food before we even take a bite. Previous animal research has demonstrated that EC cells express similar olfactory receptors. Human research suggests OR ligands, present in the chyme or produced during digestion, are important stimuli of intestinal EC cells. These EC cells in turn regulate motility and other functions of the human gastrointestinal tract.

Specifically, human gastrointestinal enterochromaffin cells may yet be another form of smell receptor.

They contain odorant receptors. These cells, when stimulated, release serotonin. Once released, serotonin can stimulate the submucosal sensory branch of the enteric nervous system, and via inter-neurons and motor neurons, control gut motility and chloride secretion by enterocytes.

9. Smell plays a key role in regulating migration and adhesion of muscle cells. Both migration and adhesion are necessary for proper muscle tissue repair. Bathing the receptors in Lyral, a synthetic fragrance redolent of lily of the valley, promotes the regeneration of muscle tissue.

Conversely, blocking these receptors inhibits muscular regeneration. An inability for the cells to smell, a loss of MOR23, leads to increased myofiber branching, commonly associated with muscular dystrophy (MD). Although preliminary in nature, such research identifies "a functional role for an OR outside of the nose and suggest a larger role for ORs during tissue repair."[852]

10. As the outermost barrier of the body, the skin is exposed to multiple environmental factors, including temperature, humidity, mechanical stress, and chemical stimuli such as odorants that are often used in cosmetic articles. Keratinocytes, the major cell type of the epidermal layer, serve as a barrier, protecting the body against pathogens and excessive water loss.

They also sense the environmental information. Epidermal keratinocytes express a variety of different sensory receptors; transient receptor potential channels, ATP receptors, and endocrinology receptors that enable them to react to various environmental stimuli and process information. Keratinocytes form the forefront of skin surface perception and communicate this information to the nervous system. To accomplish this task, they express functional ORs. One particular OR, OR2AT4, appears to be significantly involved in wound healing. This particular OR responded to Sandalore, which is a synthetic sandalwood odorant. Once activated, there was initiation of a cAMP-dependent pathway with subsequent phosphorylation of extracellular signal regulated kinases (Erk1/2) and p38 mitogen-activated protein kinases (p38 MAPK). That is, there was a positive effect on cell proliferation, migration and regeneration. Wound healing was kickstarted and turbocharged to such a degree that in a series of human tests, skin abrasions healed 30 percent faster.[853]

OR2AT4 also responded positively to Brahmanol, another sandalwood analog. Phenirat, which is a synthetic food flavor ingredient with a sweet, fruity, rose-honey scent, and Oxyphenylon, which is a raspberry ketone and the primary aroma compound of red raspberries, inhibited the sandalwood enhanced healing. Apart from keratinocytes, OR2AT4 could also be detected in melanocytes and dendritic cells. Interestingly, melanocytes are proposed as key sensory cells in human skin.[854]

B. Hunger Games

1. There is some suggestion from scientific literature that people switching to low-fat dairy products compensate elsewhere in their diet by increasing consumption of carbohydrates, that children who habitually drink low-fat milk gain more weight, and

those who drink whole-fat milk gain less weight, over time.[855, 856]

2. The gut microbiome also appears increasingly important; e.g., probiotics in yogurt appear to interact with microbiota to reduce weight gain.[857, 858, 859, 860, 861]

3. For instance, independent of calories and body weight, one's dietary pattern strongly influences metabolic dysfunction including the risk of developing diabetes mellitus.[862, 863] This is analogous to the weight-independent metabolic benefits of physical activity; diet *quality* has similar robust metabolic benefits independent of *quantity*.

4. For long-term weight gain, foods rich in refined grains, starches, and sugar appear to be major culprits.[864, 865] Such rapidly digested, low fiber carbohydrates drive many obesogenic pathways.[866, 867, 868, 869, 870] Additionally, there is the phenomenon of displacement. Since food consumption at any time is to a degree finite, as relative portions of the plate are occupied by refined grains, sugar, and other nutrient poor, energy dense foodstuffs, more healthful choices are excluded.

5. Focusing on overall diet patterns, rather than individual nutrients or foods, can also facilitate individual behavioral counseling and population dietary recommendations, because such patterns permit greater flexibility and personal preferences in diet choices.[871] The quality and the quantity of the food, the processing of the food, and the method of food preparation all impact the final flavor and the ultimate health effects.[872, 873, 874, 875]

6. As a dietary approach, the pathways of benefit appear diverse including effects on BP, glucose-insulin homeostasis, blood lipids and lipoproteins, inflammation, endothelial function, arrhythmic risk, coagulation and thrombotic risk, paraoxonase-1 activity, and the gut microbiome.[876, 877]

7. The basic Okinawan diet is vegetable heavy but with a low glycemic index (GI). There is widespread consumption of green and *kohencha* (a semi-fermented) tea. Like the Mediterranean and other healthful diets, the use of fresh, wholesome ingredients makes the Okinawan diet very anti-inflammatory. Three main characteristics of Okinawan longevity cuisine include *shingi gusui*, which means using a concoction of foodstuffs as herbal medicine. A combination of multiple items is the second characteristic. For example, *chimu* and *shinji*, which is a combination of pig's liver and vegetables like island carrot and garlic in a broth, is used to treat various illnesses. The third characteristic is a combination of foods into a meal such as *choumigusu* (long-life grass) that is eaten with sashimi.

8. Mediterranean cuisine focuses on fresh, quality foods based upon a regimen that includes whole grains, vegetables, legumes, fruits, fish, and seafood. The Mediterranean diet also includes moderate alcohol consumption. This combination of vino and victuals has resulted in both the prevention and reversal, in certain groups, of obesity, diabetes, cardiovascular disease and a number of other untoward conditions.

9. This was a study that examined the effects of darapladib (a selective lipoprotein-associated phospholipase A2 (LpPLA2) inhibitor) therapy.

10. The objective of one particular study was to examine trends in the proportion of packaged food and beverage purchases with a nutrient claim, whether claims are associated with improved nutritional profile, and whether the proportion of purchases with claims differs by race/ethnicity or socioeconomic status. The study reported that approximately 13 percent of foods and 35 percent of beverages claimed that they had superior health benefits because they actually contained less of something; sodium, fat, cholesterol, sugar, calories, or the like. When critically investigated, "the association between particular claim types and specific nutrient densities varied substantially, and purchases featuring a given low-content claim did not necessarily offer better overall nutritional profiles or better profiles for the claimed nutrient, relative to products without claims." [878]

C. Fire in the Belly: The Gut Microbiome

1. In effect, this experiment reproduced the mouse to mouse experiment of transferrable obesity, but used the human gut microbiome. Subsequently, researchers have identified greater than three hundred microbial genes associated with obesity. Some of them also indicate a microbial contribution to host carbohydrate metabolism as well as carbohydrate transport, nitrate reduction, and xenobiotic metabolism. The gut microbiota contributes to the efficiency of energy storage, can disrupt metabolic homeostasis, and confer cardiometabolic risk independent of host genetics.[879, 880]

2. The microbiota from the lean twin had a high efficiency to ferment short-chain fatty acids (SCFA),

thus promoting good metabolic health. The effect of the gut microbiota on host metabolism is mediated in part by its capacity to process indigestible, complex dietary carbohydrates via numerous hydrolytic enzymes that facilitate the intestinal absorption of SCFA; such as acetate, propionate, and butyrate. Gut microbiota regulate enzyme activity in the digestive tract and produce metabolites that are important for host signaling.[881, 882]

3. *F. prausnitzii* is involved in proper function of the immune system. A reduction of *F. prausnitzii* has been reported in patients with Crohn's Disease, obesity, asthma and depression. A decrease has also been reported in patients with metabolic syndrome or overt T2DM compared to levels in healthy controls. Conversely abundance of *F. prausnitzii* has been associated with normal glycemic status in humans.[883]

4. Bacterial DNA has also been detected in the bloodstream of those patients with T2DM. The DESIR study aimed to identify characteristics that can predict the future development of T2DM using variables available in the clinic. The researchers followed three thousand patients without T2DM for nine years. Baseline circulating bacterial DNA for *Proteobacteria* was increased in the patients who developed T2DM during the follow-up period compared to those who did not develop T2DM. Adiposity development paralleled DM development. Although *Proteobacteria* is found in the oropharynx as well as the gut, the gut concentration is tenfold higher compared to the mouth, throat, and gums.[884]

Overweight patients with metabolic syndrome, a precursor to T2DM, were transferred microbiota from either their own feces (autologous transfer) or from lean healthy controls (allogeneic transfer). After six weeks of follow-up, the allogeneic fecal transfer had improved hepatic and peripheral insulin sensitivity by 119 percent and 176 percent, respectively.[885]

The allogeneic fecal transfer induced an increase in overall gut microbial richness, and more specifically, increased the abundance of butyrate-producing bacteria, such as *Roseburia*. This correlates with previous results that showed an association between *Roseburia* and glucose homeostasis. The decrease in *Roseburia* seen in patients with T2DM compared to healthy controls is also seen in patients with atherosclerotic disease.[886]

5. The use of this therapeutic approach is growing and is already well-established for the treatment of *Clostridium difficile* infection, where fecal transplantation induces an over 80 percent long term remission rate.

6. Some of the species identified were similar to those found in the microbiota of the oral cavity of those with T2DM; high levels of *Proteobacteria*, and low levels of *Firmicutes*. The amount of bacterial DNA recovered in the atherosclerotic plaque correlated with CVD risk factors.[887]

Patients with symptomatic atherosclerotic cardiovascular disease have been found to have increased intestinal concentrations of bacteria from the *Collinsella* species. Conversely, patients without disease were found to have higher levels of the bacteria from *Roseburia* and *Eubacterium* species.[888] While all three of these species are gram-positive types of bacteria, it is possible that certain species like *Collinsella* produce products that initiate or participate in the inflammatory process.

At variance with inflammation producing bacteria, other species of gut bacteria like *Roseburia* and *Eubacterium* may be cardioprotective through the production of compounds like beta-carotenes and lycopenes.[889, 890] The consumption of foods rich in these carotenoids is associated with a number of health benefits. However, trials with supplements of these compounds alone have been disappointing. Many of these compounds when they are consumed orally failed to reach the large intestine intact. It is possible that some of the health benefits associated with these compounds may actually depend on their bacterial production in the large intestine.

Other bacterial pathways that may produce beneficial, or anti-inflammatory, compounds are also possible. The bacterium of the *Roseburia spp.* have been proven to metabolize linoleic acid (LA); the omega-six polyunsaturated essential fatty acid. The bacteria metabolize LA into two precursors of the c9, t11-conjugated linoleic acid (CLA) isomer. This form of CLA, a bacterial metabolite, has shown potential in the attenuation of inflammatory disorders such as cardiovascular disease.[891, 892]

7. The FMO3 enzymatic activity is regulated by bile acids via the nuclear hormone farnesoid X receptor, which is also expressed in the liver.[893] Another by-product of TMAO can form a cancer producing nitrosamine under weekly acidic conditions.[894]

8. A study examined more than four thousand people over three years who underwent elective coronary

angiography and then were followed for the development of a major cardiovascular event like death, heart attack, or stroke. Those with the highest levels of TMAO had over two and a half times the likelihood of having one of those events over a three-year period when compared to those with the lowest levels.[895] Cardiovascular diseases represent among the most fatal maladies world-wide. CVD is currently responsible for an estimated 30 percent of mortalities globally, each year.[896]

The measurable, circulating TMAO level is a robust prognostic marker of adverse cardiac events during a five-year follow-up, even after adjustment for other known CVD risk factors like age, kidney function, and NT-pro-BNP hormone levels. TMAO was increased in patients who developed notable cardiac events during follow up compared to those who remained stable.[897]

9. *Prevotella* and *Peptostreptococcaceae incertae sedis* are increased and associated with increased TMAO levels. L-carnitine ingestion induced a reduction in reverse cholesterol transport.[898]

Reverse cholesterol transport is a multi-step process resulting in the net movement of cholesterol from peripheral tissues back to the liver via the plasma. Cholesterol from non-hepatic peripheral tissues is transferred to high density lipoproteins (HDL or "good" cholesterol) by the ABCA1 (ATP-binding cassette transporter).

Another type of lipoprotein, apolipoprotein A-1 (ApoA-1) then acts as an acceptor, and the phospholipid component of HDL acts as a sink for the mobilized cholesterol. Uptake of HDL2 is mediated by hepatic lipase, a special form of lipoprotein lipase found only in the liver. Hepatic lipase activity is increased by androgens and decreased by estrogens, which may account for higher concentrations of HDL2 in women.

The cholesterol is converted to cholesteryl esters by the enzyme lecithin-cholesterol acyltransferase (LCAT). The cholesteryl esters can then be transferred, with the help of cholesterylester transfer protein (CETP) in exchange for triglycerides, to other lipoproteins; such as low density lipoproteins (LDL or "bad" cholesterol) and very low density lipoproteins (VLDL). These lipoproteins can be taken up by secreting unesterified cholesterol into the bile or by converting cholesterol to bile acids.

10. L-carnitine is currently used to treat angina or chest pain, congestive heart failure (CHF), cardiac complications of diphtheria, acute heart attack, leg pain caused by intermittent claudication, and high cholesterol. It is also being investigated in the use of muscle disorders associated with certain AIDS medications, male infertility, Rett syndrome, anorexia, chronic fatigue syndrome, diabetes, overactive thyroid, attention deficit-hyperactivity disorder (ADHD), leg ulcers, Lyme disease, and in athletics to enhance performance and endurance.[899]

11. The control mice were fed normal chow (NC) and demonstrated zero plaque burden. The study mice were fed a diet that led them to develop aortic atherosclerotic plaques.

PSE also attenuated cholesterol accumulation, and nearly abolished atherogenesis. PSE significantly reduced the total aortic plaque percentage from 15.2 percent to 2.4 percent Paradoxically however, PSE supplementation produced the heaviest mice with the greatest degree of adiposity. It made healthy—but fat—mice.

12. OBG also significantly reduced the aortic plaque percentage to 7.4 percent.

However, in the mouse model neither Statin nor a bile salt hydrolase-active probiotic (BSH-*Lactobacillus reuteri APC 2587*) significantly reduced plaque formation. Possible confounders include identifying the right species of probiotic. For example, a different *Lactobacillus sp.*, *Lactobacillus reuteri NCIMB 30242* has demonstrated the potential to reduce LDL-C, non-LDL-C, and apo-B100, as well as several inflammatory markers associated with atherogenesis.[900, 901]

The highest mean fecal TMA levels were found in the OBG treated mice. Despite this, OBG mice appeared to be protected from atherogenesis. Both PSE and OBG provide potential substrate for microbial fermentation and the production of short chain fatty acids (SCFAs).

SCFAs are key microbial fermentation metabolites which, through activation of G protein-coupled receptors (GPCR)-41 and 43, can have important implications for host metabolic function. Commonly produced SCFAs include acetate, butyrate and propionate. In contrast to acetate; butyrate and propionate have previously been found to protect against diet-induced obesity in a murine model.[902] In the mouse model, PSE, OBG, and Statin all appeared to have considerable impact on the host serum metabolome, including alterations in several acylcarnitines previously associated with a state of metabolic dysfunction.[903]

13. *A. muciniphila* produces propionate, which affects intestinal L-cells and GLP-1 production via receptors expressed in the gut, such as GPR43 via direct luminal action. Some aspects of the gut microbiome appear to be hereditary in nature, namely the *Christensenellaceae* family. *Christensenellaceae* and associated bacteria are more abundant in individuals with a decreased BMI.[904, 905]

14. Studies performed in the French cohort found that low and high microbial gene counts are associated with differential gut microbiota signatures; there was a difference in both quality *and* quantity of the bacteria in the gut microbiome.[906]

Studies performed in the Danish cohort found that forty-six genera differed between the low and high gene count groups. At the phylum level, those with less microbial diversity had higher numbers of *Proteobacteria* and *Bacteroidetes*. Those with greater diversity of bacteria in their gut also had higher numbers of *Verrucomicrobia* (*A. muciniphila*), *Actinobacteria,* and *Euryarchaeota.*[907]

15. There is decreased passive carrier mediated transport across the intestinal wall. There are higher levels of IgA-anti-lipopolysaccharides (LPS) in CHF. There is an increase in the bacterial biofilm. All of these perturbations cause qualitative and quantitative changes in the gut microbiome. In CHF patients, this often involves *Bacteroides/Prevotella, Eubacterium rectale,* and *Fusobacterium prausnitzii.*[908] Inflammatory

mediators like TNF-α and interferon gamma disrupt epithelial barrier function.

16. The majority of risk factors for CVD are also risk factors for CKD. Therefore, certain changes in the gut microbiota that affect CVD might also be expected to be associated with CKD. A total of 190 bacterial operational taxonomic units (OTU) were increased in patients with ESRD; among the more prominent were *Firmicutes*, especially subphyla *Clostridia*; *Actinobacteria*; and *Proteobacteria*, primarily *Gammaproteobacteria*. These phyla are also associated with other chronic and common diseases.[909] Certain species are dramatically increased in patients with ESRD: *Klebsiella, Proteus, Escherichia, Pseudomonas,* and an entire *Enterobacter* species that is unique to those with ESRD.[910]

Critically, these patients with ESRD receive dietary interventions geared to reduce the risk of hyperkalemia, or high potassium in the blood. Unfortunately, this means patients consume less fruits, vegetables, and fiber. Accordingly, the gut microbiota becomes depleted in bacteria that can produce beneficial SCFA. There is also an increased concentration of systemic D-lactate in patients with ESRD. This is believed to be caused by increased gut permeability in these patients and is associated with increased markers of inflammation: CRP and Interleukin-6 (IL-6).[911]

17. DMB is degraded by liver alcohol dehydrogenase. There were no signs of toxicity in chronic murine models, or any effect on glucose metabolism. As expected, if the mechanism worked by favorably affecting the gut microbiome, DMB did alter gut

microbiome composition. The presence and levels of Clostridiaceae correlated with TMAO and atherosclerotic lesions for both male and female mice. For females, there was also a positive correlation with Ruminococcus. For both sexes, Bacteriodetes negatively correlated with plaque and TMAO. These findings suggest a meta-organismal pathway.[912] With the administration of DMB to the diet, there was a decrease in Clostridiaceae and a resurgence of Bacteriodetes in both male and female mice.[913]

18. Faecalibacterium prausnitzii is a butyrate-producing bacterium that exerts anti-inflammatory effects by blocking the activation of nuclear factor kappa-light-chain-enhancer of activated B cells (NF-κB), and induces a reduction in bacterial-produced proteins that can modulate the NF-κB pathway.[914]

NF-κB is a protein complex that controls transcription of DNA, cytokine production, and cell survival. It is found in almost all animal cell types and is involved in cellular responses to stimuli such as stress, cytokines, free radicals, ultraviolet irradiation, oxidized LDL, and bacterial or viral antigens. Incorrect regulation of NF-κB has been linked to cancer, inflammatory and autoimmune diseases, septic shock, viral infection, and improper immune development.

There are differences in bacterial gene composition indicative of alterations in microbiota metabolic function. An enrichment in butyrate-acetoacetate CoA-transferase genes negatively correlate with systemic inflammation. There is a negative association between butyrate and inflammation.[915] The more bacteria that produce the SCFA butyrate, the less systemic inflammation. Healthy control patients also have an enrichment of bacterial groups with phytoene dehydrogenase functions. These are involved in lipid-soluble antioxidant metabolism and serum β-carotene production.[916]

19. This gradient of species reflects correlated genera or co-abundance groups that are frequently found together. This probably reflects the co-colonization of the species and their nutritional cross-feeding as a result of a dependence on similar nutritional sources.[917]

20. Mice that underwent four weeks of a WD exhibited an increase in LPS levels. As their markers of gram negative endotoxin exposure increased they developed insulin resistance concomitant with modifications to the composition of the gut microbiota. This was reproduced when the mice underwent a LPS infusion, exposing their circulating blood to bacterial endotoxins and activating their immune systems.[918]

LPS forms part of the gut bacterial membrane and binds to the CD14 receptor that is expressed on human immune cells and adipocytes. Mice that lack this receptor and thus have an immune system that cannot respond normally are designated Cd14–/– mice. When these mice were exposed to a WD or LPS infusion, they were protected from weight gain and metabolic impairments, such as the insulin resistance and systemic and adipose tissue inflammation that was observed in similarly treated wild-type mice. These results indicate the importance of the LPS-CD14 pathway in mediating the metabolic consequences of a WD.[919]

21. Mice display a high systemic level of Escherichia coli just one week after initiation of a WD. The WD induces a continuous increase in E. coli over the course of four weeks. Mice fed a WD also exhibit a marked increase in the presence of bacterial DNA in various tissues, including mesenteric adipose tissue and mesenteric lymph nodes, from low baseline levels. This effect was blunted in Cd14–/– mice fed a WD. This systemic inflammation continues to rise until a diabetic status is established. These results suggest that dietary factors affect glucose homeostasis.[920]

22. A. muciniphila is a mucin-degrading gram-negative member of the Verrucomicrobia phylum that produces SCFAs and other metabolites. The mechanisms of action of A. muciniphila are not fully understood, but it is thought to induce changes in the production of lipids involved in the endocannabinoid system that trigger the secretion of gut peptides, such as Glucagon-like peptide-1 (GLP-1).[921, 922]

23. The pathways involved were microbial metabolic pathways related to antioxidant and bile biosynthesis, and fat and carbohydrate metabolism. The effects of probiotics could be measured in the hippocampus, and involved the expression of many genes related to neuroplasticity and serotonin.

D. Double, Double, Toil and Trouble: Understanding Food Choices

1. A prospective trial of three thousand seven hundred and thirty-six US adults showed that higher concentrations of plasma trans-palmitoleic acid (trans-

16:1n-7), a fatty acid mainly found in whole-fat dairy foods, was associated with significantly higher concentrations of high density lipoprotein (HDL), lower concentrations of triglycerides (TG) and C reactive protein (CRP), and reduced insulin resistance. This correlated with a clinically observable almost 60 percent reduction in the incidence of diabetes in adults.[923]

2. The mechanism of intestinal cholesterol and sterol uptake from the lumen of the small intestine is poorly defined. The Niemann-Pick C1Like1 (NPC1L1) protein plays a critical role in the absorption of intestinal cholesterol. NPC1L1 expression is enriched in the small intestine and is found in the brush border membrane of enterocytes.

Although otherwise phenotypically normal, NPC1L1-deficient mice exhibit a substantial reduction in absorbed cholesterol, which is unaffected by dietary supplementation of bile acids. Ezetimibe, a drug that inhibits cholesterol absorption, had no effect in NPC1L1 knockout mice, suggesting that NPC1L1 resides in an ezetimibe-sensitive pathway responsible for intestinal cholesterol absorption.

However, if dietary cholesterol absorption was critical to lipid levels then using such a drug as ezetimibe which affects such a critical pathway should yield a reduction in significant clinical events. Yet clinical trials of ezetimibe and other medications which only lower cholesterol through blocking dietary absorption fail to yield any significant clinical benefits. This is behind the recent change to guidelines which no longer recommend drugs other than statins for primary and secondary prevention of CAD because of the unimpressive results obtained with such gastrointestinal cholesterol blocking agents.

3. This rapid digestion and production of glucose may induce multiple adverse health effects, including; potentially stimulating reward and craving areas in the brain, activating hepatic de novo lipogenesis, increasing uric acid production, and promoting visceral adiposity.[924, 925, 926, 927, 928, 929] In other words, it initiates an addictive cycle of ever increasing fat, particularly "belly fat," and inflammation.

4. Wheat bran is the "gold standard" in use for fecal bulking and decreasing gastrointestinal transit time. Transit time can affect both health and satiety. Slower gastric emptying may decrease rate of glucose absorption in small intestine. Fiber also affects the production of hormones such as ghrelin (the hormone that makes you hungry), polypeptide YY (PYY), and glucagon-like peptide 1 (GLP-1). There are other mechanisms that affect satiety as well: increased chew time, gastric distension, increased distention due to water, vagal afferent signals of fullness, and butyrate production in the colon.

5. Andrastins are potent inhibitors of the enzyme farnesyltransferase. This enzyme plays a key role in cholesterol synthesis and its inhibition decreases cholesterol production. In fact, while the total cholesterol is overall minimally unchanged, some studies suggest that consuming these types of foods shift cholesterol toward the less inflammatory, less atherogenic type A LDL molecule.

An interesting observation arises from these studies. The decrease in oxidative stress and inflammation markers seen with diets rich in foodstuffs like cheese (and other fats) is independent of body weight. More evidence that eating fat does not make you fat. Nor are the benefits simply the result of losing weight or caloric considerations. The healthful effects also occur quite rapidly before weight loss is seen. This suggests not just a correlation, but a causation.

6. Spermidine appears to act via a different pathway than impacting TMAO production. Spermidine enables a process called autophagy. In essence, it allows cells to disable dysfunctional and unnecessary parts of themselves. This natural polyamine is found in greater quantities in younger men and women.

7. They examined the health effects of a Roundup-tolerant NK603 genetically modified (GM) maize (from 11 percent in the diet), cultivated with or without Roundup application and Roundup alone (from 0.1 ppb of the full pesticide containing glyphosate and adjuvants) in drinking water. There was also a control group. Of note, these amounts are significantly less than the MRL. The rats were studied at intervals over two years.

8. In the PREDIMED randomized trial, participants receiving extra virgin olive oil and dietary advice to consume a Mediterranean diet experienced approximately a 30 percent lower risk of stroke, MI, or death, in comparison with control. In the intervention group, approximately 60 percent of the extra virgin olive oil simply replaced regular olive oil, commonly used in Spain. This suggests that fatty acid profiles

may not be the only relevant determinant of health effects of oils.[930]

E. Chew the FAT

1. Studies such as this provide evidence that mindfulness promotes functional neuroplastic changes, suggesting an amygdala-sgACC pathway for stress reduction effects.[931]

2. A healthful attitude is a key in the prevention and management of conditions like diabetes and CVD. It must include an approach which is realistic in both implementation and sustainability for the individual. Contemporary programs like The Mediterranean diet and its offspring like the DASH (Dietary Approaches to Stop Hypertension) diet, as well as some low carbohydrate diets have proven effective in treating diabetes and lowering CVD risk factors. The Prevención con Dieta Mediterránea (PREDIMED) trial group has been extremely active in investigating the potential healthful benefits of a Mediterranean style approach. One of their randomized trials demonstrated a 30 percent reduced risk of CVD events in diabetic patients randomized to the Mediterranean diet.[932]

In the Adventist Health Studies, when compared to the modern Western diet, the prevalence of diabetes was reduced by 23 percent with a semi-vegetarian diet, 38 percent with a pesco-vegetarian diet, and 55 percent with a lacto-ovo-vegetarian diet.[933] There is no doubt that any dietary approach that increases the proportion of fresh fruits and vegetables on the American plate is an improvement over the current state of the SAD. Other regimens focusing on increasing consumption of foods with a lower glycemic index or decreasing consumption of processed food products, like some processed meats, have also been associated with a lower risk of developing diabetes.[934, 935]

Combining a proper diet with a practice like mindfulness only enhances the benefit. Researchers have examined the potential benefits of meditation, both mindfulness and transcendental, for diabetes management. A randomized trial published in JAMA found that meditation reduced blood pressure, decreased insulin resistance, and significantly reduced the rates of CVD events.[936]

Adding increased physical activity to a proper diet reduced the incidence of diabetes by nearly 60 percent over four years in the Diabetes Prevention Study and the Diabetes Prevention Program.[937] The Da Qing study compared diet, exercise, and diet plus exercise with a no-treatment control group and found that all three lifestyle approaches reduced the risk of developing diabetes by 31 to 46 percent.[938] The Finnish Diabetes Prevention Study obtained similar results in over five hundred overweight subjects with impaired glucose tolerance. They demonstrated that lifestyle intervention reduced the risk of diabetes by 58 percent.[939, 940]

3. So poor is the data for success that the Agency for Healthcare Research and Quality (AHRQ) after an analysis of almost three thousand and five hundred papers, failed to find enough evidence to support the procedure's efficacy or safety. The AHRQ concluded that there is:

- insufficient evidence to draw conclusions regarding its effectiveness and safety in the Medicare population,
- no impact on all-cause mortality,
- no firm conclusions regarding health-related quality of life due to heterogeneity across studies.[941]

4. The study estimated daily gluten intake for almost two hundred thousand participants in three long-term health studies—sixty-nine thousand, two hundred and seventy-six from the Nurses' Health Study (NHS), eighty-eight thousand, six hundred and ten from the Nurses' Health Study II (NHSII) and forty-one thousand, nine hundred and eight from the Health Professionals Follow-up Study (HPFS). Over the course of the study there was a total of 4.24 million person-years of follow-up. The major dietary sources of gluten were pastas, cereals, pizza, muffins, pretzels, and bread.

   The researchers found that most participants had gluten intake below 12g/day. Within this group, those who ate the most gluten had a significantly lower risk of developing Type 2 diabetes. Those in the highest 20 percent of gluten consumption had a 13 percent lower risk of developing T2D in comparison to those with the lowest daily gluten consumption, which was fewer than 4 grams per day.[942]

5. Even within the realm of evaluating single types of fats, the effects are pleiotropic. For instance, in comparison with carbohydrate, palmitic acid (16:0) raises blood LDL-cholesterol, yet simultaneously raises HDL-cholesterol, reduces triglyceride-rich lipoproteins and remnants, and has no appreciable effect on ApoB, the most salient LDL-related characteristic.[943]

Saturated fats also lower lipoprotein (a), an independent and causal cardiovascular risk factor; in comparison with monounsaturated fat or carbohydrate.[944, 945]

6. The most common PUFAs are n-6 linoleic acid (LA, 18:2n-6) and n-3 α-linolenic acid (ALA, 18:3n-3), derived principally from vegetables and their oils (e.g., soybean, canola, flaxseed, walnuts). Seafood is the major source of long-chain n-3 polyunsaturated fats, principally EPA and DHA. Humans cannot synthesize or interconvert LA or ALA, making them essential fatty acids that must be consumed in the diet. Humans also synthesize relatively little EPA and DHA, for which diet remains the major source.

    The recommendations for consuming other fats like monounsaturated fats (predominantly oleic acid, 18:1), is based on data looking at the fat in isolation. When all the information that has examined such fats in isolation is taken together, the evidence for cardiometabolic benefits is not strong.[946] Total saturated fat, carbohydrate, and protein each appear relatively neutral for CVD. The effects of total monounsaturated fat remain uncertain.[947] The relatively neutral effects of each of the former macronutrients reflects substantial heterogeneity in nutrient subtypes and food sources within each of these categories. When *diets* rich in oleic acid, like the Mediterranean diet, are analyzed, the benefit is much more robust and is linked to lower risk.[948] The food source may indeed modify these health effects.

7. These artificially introduced TFAs have unique adverse effects on blood lipids and lipoproteins, including raising LDL-cholesterol, ApoB, triglycerides, and lipoprotein(a), and lowering HDL-cholesterol and ApoA1.

These particular TFAs also appear to have non-lipid adverse effects, promoting inflammation, endothelial dysfunction, insulin resistance, visceral adiposity, and arrhythmia. Emerging evidence suggests that 18:2 TFA isomers may be the most adverse; these can be formed through not only partial hydrogenation, but also other industrial processes such as oil deodorization and high-temperature cooking.[949, 950]

8. As we are learning, it appears that almost all the natural relationships we have with food, nutrients, vitamins, and minerals take this form. The body mass index or BMI likewise exhibits a "J" shaped relationship. There is a weight/height relationship below which there is an increased risk, despite the pervasive mantra that thinner is better at all expense.

The EPIC trial revealed an interesting "J" shaped trend with relation to vegetarian/vegan consumptive patterns and animal protein. There seemed to be an increased risk of morbidity and mortality when animal protein (meat, poultry, fish, seafood and insects) consumption was below a certain threshold level.[951] In fact, the linear straight-line relationships that exist between what we consume and adverse outcomes seem to primarily identify toxins and poisons, not nutrients and necessities.

Sodium is an element, an essential cation, necessary for life itself. It is critical for the proper functioning of every single cell in the body and, not surprisingly, its control is tightly regulated. Einstein noted that God does not play dice with the Universe; he does not play dice with our salt either.

The benefits of blood pressure lowering, even in those with concomitant inflammatory disease like diabetes seem to apply to only those with a systolic (top number) blood pressure greater than 140mmHg. The recent HOPE-3 trial shows that for those with a blood pressure greater than 143mmHG a 25 percent reduction in cardiovascular disease can be achieved with a 6mmHg decrease.[952] An amount, by the way, shown to be achievable in another recent study by consuming just 30g per day of Grand Padano cheese, a Parmesan-like cheese from Italy with the sodium equivalent of a one ounce serving of potato chips.[953]

F. Quantum Food for a Changing World

1. These complex determinants each represent a potential barrier, but also a promising opportunity for encouraging healthful and delicious diets.[954, 955] For many healthcare providers, a variety of barriers within the current healthcare system can limit their ability to fully implement effective behavior change strategies. Such barriers include limited patient visit time to focus on behavior change, insufficient financial or other provider incentives for health promotion, suboptimal knowledge or experience on the most effective behavior change strategies and relevant behavioral targets, and inadequate tools for assessing and monitoring behaviors over time.[956]

A systematic review identified numerous randomized trials and quasi-experimental studies evaluating these approaches for dietary change and/or weight loss. Most were internet based or combined

Internet and mobile approaches. The great majority had durations between six weeks and six months; very few extended beyond one year. Approximately two-thirds of these studies identified improved dietary behaviors or greater weight loss with the use of these novel technologies, in comparison with usual care. Although promising, little is known on their long-term effectiveness and sustainability, and longer-term studies are required.[957] What is clear is that technological advances operating through cultural influence can change individual behaviors that impact physical joy and well-being. Every quadrant counts; every gateway is important.

2. While personalized nutrition; the ability to provide customized dietary advice specialized to each person's unique profile of genes and other underlying characteristics, is a tangible goal it remains elusive.[958] In broadening perspective to address interior and exterior variables, achievement has been hampered by a lack of replication and methodology to demonstrate relevance and efficacy.[959, 960, 961, 962, 963] Personalized cognitive-behavioral and culturally and socioeconomically sensitive strategies are needed to increase effectiveness of clinical approaches to behavior change.

3. Bisphenol A (BPA) is a chemical used in the manufacture of plastic bottles and the inner lining of beverage cans. It is almost ubiquitous in terms of its exposure to the population. BPA has been associated with the risk of developing hypertension. Consuming just two canned beverages compared with consuming two glass bottled beverages increases the level of BPA

exposure and subsequently significantly increases blood pressure.[964]

A recent study found that blood levels of phthalates correlated to risk of cardiovascular disease, T2DM, hypertension, and increased levels of chronic low-grade inflammatory biomarkers. Phthalates are a class of chemicals commonly used in plastic packaging of foods. Researchers from the University of Adelaide and the South Australian Health and Medical Research Institute (SAHMRI) demonstrated an independent association between chronic diseases among over two thousand men and concentrations of phthalates. The risk increased with time and intensity of exposure. Phthalates were detected in urine samples of 99.6 percent of those aged thirty-five and over.[965]

Age and western diets were directly associated with higher concentrations of phthalates. Previous studies have shown that men who ate less fresh fruit and vegetables and more processed and packaged foods, and drank carbonated soft drinks, have higher levels of phthalates in their urine. Even after adjusting for other known risk factors, the association remained robust.

Although the mechanism is unknown, phthalates are known to impact the human endocrine system. While that is disruptive enough, any disruption here can alter the gut microbiome above and beyond the direct effects. This is just one of many examples of how the addition of non-naturally occurring compounds into our food and food pathways can wreak havoc. This does not even begin to consider the potential for calamity when those eighty thousand different man-made compounds have the opportunity to interact.

REFERENCES

Global Burden of Disease Study Collaborators 2013. (2015). Global, regional, and national incidence, prevalence, and years lived with disability for 301 acute and chronic diseases and injuries in 188 countries: 1990-2013: A systematic analysis for the Global Burden of Disease Study 2013. *Lancet., 386,* 743-800

The World Health Organisation. (2014). *Global status report on noncommunicable diseases.* The World Health Organisation

Whole Grains Council. (2013). *Definition of whole grains.* Retrieved from Whole Grains: http://wholegrainscouncil.org/whole-grains-101/definition-of-whole-grains

Looft, T., Allen, H. K., Cantarel, B. L., Levine, U. Y., Bayles, D. O., Alt, D. P....Stanton, T. B. (2014). Bacteria, phages and pigs: the effects of in-feed antibiotics on the microbiome at different gut locations. *The ISME Journal, 8,* 1566–1576; doi:10.1038/ismej.2014.12

Abdullah, M., Jones, P., & Eck, P. (2015). Nutrigenetics of cholesterol metabolism observational and dietary intervention studies in the postgenomic era. *Nutr Rev., 73,* 523–543. doi: 10.1093/nutrit/nuv016

Abete, I., Romaguera, D., Vieira, A., Lopez de Munain, A., & Norat, T. (2014). Association between total, processed, red and white meat consumption and all-cause, CVD and IHD mortality: A meta-analysis of cohort studies. *Br J Nutr., 112,* 762-775. doi: 10.1017/S000711451400124X

Ablow, K. (2017, March 9). *Now, there's proof: Love keeps people alive longer.* Retrieved from Foxnews.com: http://www.foxnews.com/opinion/2017/03/09/now-theres-proof-love-keeps-people-alive-longer.html

Abumrad, N. A., & Davidson, N. O. (2012). ROLE OF THE GUT IN LIPID HOMEOSTASIS. *Physiol Rev, 92:* 1061-1085

Adams, J. (2017, March 27). *Regio III - Insula X - Terme dei Sette Sapienti (III,X,2).* Retrieved from Ostia-Antica.org: http://www.ostia-antica.org/regio3/10/10-2.htm

Ader, R., & Cohen, N. (1985). CNS-immune system interactions: Conditioning phenomena. *Behavioral and Brain Sciences, 8*(3), 379-395. doi: https://doi.org/10.1017/S0140525X00000765

Ader, R., Cohen, N., & Felten, D. (1995). Psychoneuroimmunology: Interaction between the nervous system and and immune system. *Lancet, 345*(8942)0, 99-103

Afshin, A., Micha, R., Khatibzadeh, S., & Mozaffarian, D. (2014). Consumption of nuts and legumes and risk of incident ischemic heart disease, stroke, and diabetes: A systematic review and meta-analysis. *Am J Clin Nutr, 100*(278)-288. doi: 10.3945/ajcn.113.076901

Afshin, A., Micha, R., Khatibzadeh, S., Schmidt, L., & Mozaffarian, D. (2014). Policies to reduce non-communicable diseases. In G. Brown, G. Yamey, & S. Wamala, *The Handbook of Global Health Policy, 1st ed.* West Sussex, UK: John Wiley & Sons, Ltd

Ahmadi-Abhari, S., Luben, R., Powell, N., Bhaniani, A., Chowdhury, R., Wareham, N., ... Khaw, K. (2013). Dietary intake of carbohydrates and risk of type 2 diabetes: The european prospective investigation into cancer—norfolk study. *Br J Nutr., 23*,1-11

Ailhaud, G., M. F., Alessandri, J.-M., & Guesnet, P. (2007). Fatty acid composition as an early determinant of childhood obesity. *Genes Nutr, 2,* 39–40. doi: 10.1007/s12263-007-0017-6

Alabas, O., Hall, M., Dondo, T., Rutherford, M., Timmis, A., B. P., & . Gale, C. (2016). Long-term excess mortality associated with diabetes following acute myocardial infarction: A population-based cohort study. *J Epidemiol Community Health*, doi:10.1136/jech-2016-207402

Alderman, M. (2010, May 10). *Einstein on salt: Is sess sodium always better?* Retrieved from Einstein School of Medicine, http://www.einstein.yu.edu/video/?VID=162#top

Alexander, C., & Rietschel, E. (2001). Bacterial lipopolysaccharides and innate immunity. *J Endotoxin Res., 7*(3), 167-202

Algoe, S. B., & Way, B. M. (2014). Evidence for a role of the oxytocin system, indexed by genetic variation in CD38, in the social bonding effects of expressed gratitude. *Soc Cogn Affect Neurosci., 9*(12), 1855-1861 doi: 10.1093/scan/nst182

Alhazmi, A., Stojanovski, E., McEvoy, M., & Garg, M. (2012). Macronutrient intakes and development of type 2 diabetes: A systematic review and meta-analysis of cohort studies. *J Am Coll Nutr., 31*,243-258

Al-Lamee, R., Thompson, D., Dehbi, H.-M., Sen, S., Tang, K., Davies, J., & Francis, D. P. (2017). Percutaneous coronary intervention in stable angina (ORBITA): A double-blind, randomised controlled trial, *The Lancet,* doi: 10.1016/S0140-67

Alpern, R., & Sakhaee, S. (1997). The clinical spectrum of chronic metabolic acidosis: Homeostatic mechanisms produce significant morbidity. *American Journal of Kidney Disease, 29,* 291-302

Amar, J., Chabo, C., Waget, A., Klopp, P., Vachoux, C., Bermúdez-Humarán, L. G., & Rautonen, N. (2011). Intestinal mucosal adherence and translocation of commensal bacteria at the early onset of type 2 diabetes: Molecular mechanisms and probiotic treatment. *EMBO Mol. Med. 3,* 559-572

Amar, J., Serino, M., Lange, C., C. C., Iacovoni, J., Mondot, S., & Burcelin, R. (2011). Involvement of tissue bacteria in the onset of diabetes in humans: Evidence for a concept. *Diabetologia, 54,* 3055-3061

America Heart Association. (2016, January 15). *America Heart Association and Stroke Encyclopedia: Eggs.* Retrieved from Heart.org: http://www.heart.org/HEARTORG/

American Diabetes Association. (2013). Economic costs of diabetes in the US in 2012. *Diabetes Care., 36*(4), 1033-1046. doi: 10.2337/dc12-2625

American Diabetes Association. (2015). Standards of medical care in diabetes—2015. *Diabetes Care, 38*(1), S1-S89. doi: https://doi.org/10.2337/dc15-S001

American Heart Association. (2016). *History of the American Heart Association.* Retrieved from American Heart Association: http://www.heart.org/HEARTORG/General/History-of-the-American-Heart-Association_UCM_308120_Article.jsp#.VxGON0mTU2w

American Heart Association. (2017, March 30). *Gluten may lower risk of Type 2 diabetes.* Retrieved from American Heart Association News: http://news.heart.org/gluten-may-lower-risk-of-type-2-diabetes/

American Heart Association. (2017, March 30). *Prevention & Treatment of High Cholesterol.* Retrieved from Heart.org: http://www.heart.org/HEARTORG/Conditions/Cholesterol/PreventionTreatmentofHighCholesterol/The-Skinny-on-Fats_UCM_305628_Article. jsp#.WbUf3LpFyo4

American Heart Association. (2013). *American Heart Association 2020 Impact Goal.* Retrieved from Heart.org, http://www.heart.org/idc/groups/heart-public/@wcm/@sop/@smd/documents/downloadable/ucm_319831.pdf

American Heart Association. (2014). *Healthy Cooking Oils 101.* Retrieved from Healthy Cooking Oils 101: American Heart Association. Retrieved fromhttp://www.heart.org/HEARTORG/GettingHealthy/NutritionCenter/SimpleCookingwithHeart/Healthy-Cooking-Oils-101_UCM_445179_Article.jsp

Anderson, J. J., Kruszka, B., Delaney, J. A., He, K., Burke, G. L., Alonso, A.,...Budoff, M. M. (2016). Calcium intake from diet and supplements and the risk of coronary artery calcification and its progression among older adults: 10-year follow-up of the multi-ethnic study of atherosclerosis (MESA). *J Am Heart Assoc. 5*(e003815) doi: 10.1161/JAHA.116.003815)

Anderson, J., & Gilliland, S. (1999). Effect of fermented milk (yogurt) containing lactobacillus acidophilus 11 on serum cholesterol in hypercholesterolemic humans. *J Am Coll Nutr., 18*(1), 43-50

Anderson, J., Smith, B., & Gustafson, M. (1994). Health benefits and practical aspects of high fiber diets. *Am J Clin Nutr, 59*(supplement), 1442S-1247S

Andrade, J., Mohamed, A., Frohlich, J., & Ignaszewski, A. (2009). Ancel keys and the lipid hypothesis: From early breakthroughs to current management of dyslipidemia. *BCMJ, 51*(2), 66-72.

APA. (2015, May 20). *Stress a major health problem in the U.S., warns APA.* Retrieved from American Psychological Association Web Site: http://www.apa.org/news/press/releases/2007/10/stress.aspx

Appel, L., Sacks, F., Carey, V., Obarzanek, E., Swain, J., Miller, E. 3.,...Bishop, T. (2005). OmniHeart Collaborative Research Group. Effects of protein, monounsaturated fat, and carbohydrate intake on blood pressure and serum lipids: results of the omniheart randomized trial. *JAMA. 294,* 2455-2464. doi: 10.1001/jama.294.19.2455

Arena, R., G. M., Lianov, L., Whitsel, L., Berra, K., Lavie, C. J., & Pinto, F. J. (2015). Healthy lifestyle interventions to combat noncommunicable disease—a novel nonhierarchical connectivity model for key stakeholders: a policy statement from the American Heart Association, European Society of Cardiology. *Eur. Heart J. 36,* 2097-2109

Aron-Wisnewsky, J., & Clément, K. (2015). The gut microbiome, diet, and links to cardiometabolic and chronic disorders. *Nature Reviews Nephrology,* doi:10.1038/nrneph.2015.191

Astrup, A., Dyerberg, J., Elwood, P., Hermansen, K., Hu, F., Jakobsen, M.,...LeGrand, P. (2011). The role of reducing intakes of saturated fat in the prevention of cardiovascular disease: Where does the evidence stand in 2010? *Am J Clin Nutr, 93,* 684-8

Atchley, R. A., Strayer, D. L., & Atchley, P. (2012). Creativity in the wild: Improving creative reasoning through immersion in natural settings. *PLOs One, 7*(12)=, doi:10.1371/journal.pone.0051474

Aune, D., Norat, T., Romundstad, P., & Vatten, L. (2013). Whole grain and refined grain consumption and the risk of type 2 diabetes: A systematic review and dose-response meta-analysis of cohort studies.. *Eur J Epidemiol, 28*(845)-858. doi: 10.1007/s10654-013-9852-5

Aung, T., Halsey, J., Kromhout, D., Gerstein, H. C., Marchioli, R., Tavazzi, L.,...Clarke, R. (2018). Associations of omega-3 fatty acid supplement use with cardiovascular disease risks: Meta-analysis of 10 trials involving 77,917 individuals. *JAMA Cardiology*, doi:10.1001/jamacardio.2017.5205

Azad, M. B., Abou-Setta, A. M., Chauhan, B. F., Rabbani, R., Lys, J., Copstein, L.,... Zarychanski, R. (2017). Nonnutritive sweeteners and cardiometabolic health: A systematic review and meta-analysis of randomized controlled trials and prospective cohort studies;. *CMAJ 189*(28) E929-939, doi: 10.1503/cmaj.161390

Backhed, F., Ley, R., Sonnenberg, J., Peterson, D., & Gordon, J. (2005). Host-Bacterial Mutualism in the Human Intestine. *Science 307*, 1915-1920

Badkar, M., & Lubin, G. (2012, April 20). *18 facts about mcDonald's that will blow your mind.*Retrieved from *Business Insider*: http://www.businessinsider.com/19-facts-about-mcdonalds-that-will-blow-your-mind-2012-4/#mcdonalds-daily-customer-traffic-62-million-is-more-than-the-population-of-great-britain-1

Bae, S., & Hong, Y.-C. (2014). Exposure to bisphenol a from drinking canned beverage increases blood pressure: Randomized crossover trial. *Hypertension*, doi: 10.1161/HYPERTENSIONAHA.114.04261

Bai, P., Wittert, G., Taylor, A., Martin, S., Milne, R., Jenkins, A.,...Zumin, S. (2017). The association between total phthalate concentration and non-communicable diseases and chronic inflammation in South Australian urban dwelling men. *Environmental Research 158*, 366-372

Ballesteros, M., Valenzuela, F., Robles, A., Artalejo, E., Aguilar, D., Andersen, C.,... Fernandez, M. (2015). One egg per day improves inflammation when compared to an oatmeal-based breakfast without increasing other cardiometabolic risk factors in diabetic patients. *Nutrients 7*(5), 3449-63. doi: 10.3390/nu7053449

Baranski, M. S.-T. (2014). Higher antioxidant and lower cadmium concentrations and lower incidence of pesticide residues in organically grown crops: A systematic literature review and meta-analyses. *British Journal of Nutrition*, doi:10.1017/S0007114514001366

Barclay, A., Petocz, P., & McMillan-Price, J. (2008). Glycemic index, glycemic load, and chronic disease: A meta-analysis of observational studies. *Am J Clin Nutr, 87*(3), 627-637

Barclay, E. (2012, June 27). *A nation of meat eaters: See how it all adds up.* Retrieved from NPR.org: http://www.npr.org/sections/thesalt/2012/06/27/155527365/visualizing-a-nation-of-meat-eaters

Barnsley, M., Devaney, R., Mandelbrot, B., Peitgen, H.-O., & Saupe, D. (1988). *The science of fractal images.* New York: Springer-Verlag

Barrett, H., Dekker, N. M., Conwell, L., & Callaway, L. (2014). Probiotics for preventing gestational diabetes. *Cochrane Database Syst Rev. 2*, CD009951. doi: 10.1002/14651858.CD009951.pub2

Basaranoglu, M., Basaranoglu, G., Sabuncu, T., & Sentürk, H. (2013). Fructose as a key player in the development of fatty liver disease. *World J Gastroenterol 19*, 1166-1172. doi: 10.3748/wjg.v19.i8.1166

Basu, A., & Lyons, T. (2012). Strawberries, blueberries, and cranberries in the metabolic syndrome: clinical perspectives. *J Agric Food Chem. 60* 5687-5692. doi: 10.1021/jf203488k

Bea, F., Blessing, E., Bennett, B., Levitz, M., Wallace, E., & Rosenfeld, M. (2002). Simvastatin promotes atherosclerotic plaque stability in apoE-deficient mice independently of lipid lowering.. *Arterioscler Thromb Vasc Biol, 22*(11), 1832-7

Beauchamp, G., Keast, R., Morel, D., Lin, J., Pika, J., Han, Q.,...Breslin, P. (2005). Phytochemistry: ibuprofen-like activity in extra virgin olive oil. *Nature 437*, 45-46. doi: 10.1038/437045a

Beck, D. L. (2015, April 15). *Changing diets, saving lives: Mediterranean, vegetarian, vegan, and More | CardioSource World News*. Retrieved from American College of Cardiology: http://www.acc.org/latest-in-cardiology/articles/2015/04/29/14/34/changing-diets-saving-lives-mediterranean-vegetarian-vegan-and-more?wt.mc_id=cvnewsdig

Beckie, H. J., Harker, K. N., Legare, A., Morrison, M. J., Seguin-Swartz, G., & Falk, K. C. (2011). GM canola: The canadian experience. *Farm Policy Journal*, 43-49

Beilharz, J., Kaakoush, N., Maniam, J., & Morris, M. (2017). Cafeteria diet and probiotic therapy: Cross talk among memory, neuroplasticity, serotonin receptors and gut microbiota in the rat. *Molecular Psychiatry*, doi:10.1038/mp.2017.38

Benatar, J., Sidhu, K., & Stewart, R. (2013). Effects of high and low fat dairy food on cardio-metabolic risk factors: A meta-analysis of randomized studies. *PLoS One, 8*, e76480

Benbrook, C. M., B. G., Latif, M. A., Leifert, C., & Davis, D. R. (2013). Organic production enhances milk nutritional quality by shifting fatty acid composition: A united states-wide, 18-month study. *PLOS One*, doi: 10.1371/journal.pone.0082429

Bennett, B., de Aguiar, V. T., Wang, Z., Shih, D., Meng, Y., Gregory, J....Crooke, R. (2013). Trimethylamine-N-oxide, a metabolite associated with atherosclerosis, exhibits complex genetic and dietary regulation, *Cell Metab, 17*(1), 49-60

Bentley, J. (2017). *U.S. trends in food availability and a dietary assessment of loss-adjusted food availability, 1970-2014, EIB-166*. Washington, DC: U.S. Department of Agriculture, Economic Research Service

Berglund, L., Lefevre, M., Ginsberg, H., Kris-Etherton, P., Elmer, P., Stewart, P.,... Investigators, D. (2007). Comparison of monounsaturated fat with carbohydrates as a replacement for saturated fat in subjects with a high metabolic risk profile: studies in the fasting and postprandial states, *Am J Clin Nutr., 86*, 1611-1620

Bertoia, M., Mukamal, K., Cahill, L., Hou, T., Ludwig, D., Mozaffarian, D.,...Rimm, E. (2015). Changes in intake of fruits and vegetables and weight change in United States men and women followed for up to 24 years: Analysis from three prospective cohort studies, *PLoS Med, 12*, e1001878, doi: 10.1371/journal.pmed.1001878

Bhatt, D. L., Kandzari, D. E., O'Neill, W. W., D'Agostino, R., Flack, J. M., Katzen, B. T.,... Bakris, G. (2014). A controlled trial of renal denervation for resistant hypertension. *N Engl J Med, 370*, 1393-1401, doi: 10.1056/NEJMoa1402670

Bhupathiraju, S., Tobias, D., Malik, V., Pan, A., Hruby, A., Manson, J.,...Hu, F. (2014). Glycemic index, glycemic load, and risk of type 2 diabetes: results from 3 large US cohorts and an updated meta-analysis. *Am J Clin Nutr., 100*, 218-232, doi: 10.3945/ajcn.113.079533

Billings, T. (1999). *Comparative anatomy and physiology brought up to date: Are humans natural frugivores/vegetarians, or omnivores/faunivores?* Retrieved from Beyond Vegitarianism: http://www.beyondveg.com/billings-t/comp-anat/comp-anat-1a.shtml

Binia, A., Jaeger, J., Hu, Y., Singh, A., & Zimmermann, D. (2015). Daily potassium intake and sodium-to-potassium ratio in the reduction of blood pressure a meta-analysis of randomized controlled trials. *J Hypertens., 33*, 1509-1520. doi: 10.1097/HJH.0000000000000611

Bittman, M. (2008, November 15). A seafood snob ponders the future of fish Retrieved from *The New York Times*: http://www.nytimes.com/2008/11/16/weekinreview/16bittman.html?scp=1&sq=bittman%20farm-raised&st=cse

Bittman, M. (2009, April 10). *The bottom line on salmon.* Retrieved from *The New York Times*: https://dinersjournal.blogs.nytimes.com/2009/04/10/the-bottom-line-on-salmon/?_r=0

Bittman, M. (2014, March 25). *Butter is Back..* Retrieved from *The New York Times*: http://www.nytimes.com/2014/03/26/opinion/bittman-butter-is-back.html?_r=0

Bittman, M. (2015, June 24). Trust me. Butter is better. Retrieved from *The New York Times*: http://www.nytimes.com/2015/06/24/opinion/the-trans-fats-that-wontleave.html

Bloom, D., Cafiero, E., Jané-Llopis, E., Abrahams-Gessel, S., Bloom, L., Fathima, S.,... Weinstein, C. (2011). The global economic burden of noncommunicable diseases. Geneva, Switzerland: World Economic Forum.

Bloom, P. (2015, November 24). Scientific faith is different from religious faith. Retrieved from *The Atlantic*: https://www.theatlantic.com/science/archive/2015/11/why-scientific-faith-isnt-the-same-as-religious-faith/417357/

Bloomfield, H., Koeller, E., Greer, N., MacDonald, R., Kane, R., & Wilt, T. J. (2016). Effects on health outcomes of the mediterranean diet with no restriction on fat intake: A systematic review and meta-analysis. *Annals of Internal Medicine*, doi: 10.7326/M16-0361

Bolland, M., Barber, P., Doughty, R., Mason, B., Horne, A., Ames, R. G.,...Reid, I. (2008). Vascular events in healthy older women receiving calcium supplementation: Randomised controlled trial, *BMJ.*, *336*, 262-266

Bolland, M., Grey, A., Avenell, A., Gamble, G., & Reid, I. (2011). Calcium supplements with or without vitamin D and risk of cardiovascular events: Reanalysis of the women's health initiative limited access dataset and meta-analysis. *BMJ.*, *342*, d2040.

Bonthuis, M., H. M., Ibiebele, T., Green, A., & van der Pols, J. (2010). Dairy consumption and patterns of mortality of Australian adults. *Eur J Clin Nutr,64*, 569-577. doi: 10.1038/ejcn.2010.45

Boulton, T. (2013, April 2). *The origin of "say cheese" and when people started smiling in photographs.* Retrieved from todayifoundout.com: http://www.todayifoundout.com/index.php/2013/04/the-origin-of-say-cheese-and-when-people-started-smiling-in-photographs/

Braam, J. (2013, June 21). NPR science friday: vegetables respond to a daily clock, even after harvest. (I. Flatow, Interviewer)

Brand-Miller, J., McMillan-Price, J., Steinbeck, K., & Caterson, I. (2009). Dietary glycemic index: Health implications. *J Am Coll Nutr.*, *28*(suppl), 446S-449S

Braun, T., Voland, P., Kunz, L., Prinz, C., & Gratzl, M. (2007). Enterochromaffin cells of the human gut: Sensors for spices and odorants. *Gastroenterology, 132*, 1890-1901

Brillat-Savarin, J. A., & Robinson, F. (2014). *The physiology of taste or transcendental gastronomy.* South Adelaide, Australia: The University of Adelaide Library

Brown, I., Tzoulaki, I., Candeias, V., & Elliott, P. (2009). Salt intakes around the world: Implications for public health. *Int J Epidemiol.*, *38*, 791-813

Browning, J., Baker, J., Rogers, T., Davis, J., Satapati, S., & Burgess, S. (2011). Short-term weight loss and hepatic triglyceride reduction: Evidence of a metabolic advantage with dietary carbohydrate restriction. *Am J Clin Nutr.*, *93*, 1048-1052. doi: 10.3945/ajcn.110.007674

Brug, J. (2008). Determinants of healthy eating: Motivation, abilities and environmental opportunities. *Fam Pract.*, *25*(suppl 1), i50-i55. doi:10.1093/fampra/cmn063

Brug, J., Kremers, S., Lenthe, F., Ball, K., & Crawford, D. (2008). Environmental determinants of healthy eating: In need of theory and evidence. *Proc Nutr Soc.*, *67*, 307-316. doi: 10.1017/S0029665108008616

Buchbinder, R., Osborne, R. H., Ebeling, P. R., Wark, J. D., Mitchell, P., Wriedt, C.,... Murphy, B. (2009). A randomized trial of vertebroplasty for painful osteoporotic vertebral fractures. *N Engl J Med*, *361*, 557-568 doi: 10.1056/NEJMoa0900429

Buckley, D., Fu, R., Freeman, M., Rogers, K., & Helfand, M. (2009). C-reactive protein as a risk factor for coronary heart disease: A systematic review and meta-analyses for the u.s. preventive services task force. *Ann Intern Med*, *151*, 483-95

Buettner, D. (2012). *The blue zones : Lessons for living longer from the people who've lived the longest.* Washington, D.C.: National Geographic Society

Buijsse, B., Boeing, H., Drogan, D., Schulze, M., Feskens, E., Amiano, P.,...Wareham, N. (2015). InterAct Consortium. Consumption of fatty foods and incident type 2 diabetes in populations from eight European countries. *Eur J Clin Nutr.*, *69*, 455-461. doi: 10.1038/ejcn.2014.249

Bunner, A., Wells, C., Gonzales, J., Agarwal, U., Bayat, E., & Barnard, N. (2015). A dietary intervention for chronic diabetic neuropathy pain: A randomized controlled pilot study. *Nutr Diabetes.*, *5*, e158. doi: 10.1038/nutd.2015.8

Burdge, G., & Wootton., S. (2002). Conversion of alpha-linolenic acid to eicosapentaenoic, docosapentaenoic and docosahexaenoic acids in young women. *British Journal of Nutrition*, *88*, 411-420.

Burdge, G., J. A., & Wootton, S. (2002). Eicosapentaenoic and docosapentaenoic acids are the principal products of alpha-linolenic acid metabolism in young men. *Br J Nutr.*, *88*(4), 355-63

Burke, M., & Small, D. (2015). Physiological mechanisms by which non-nutritive sweeteners may impact body weight and metabolism. *Physiol Behav.*, *152*(pt B):381-388. doi: 10.1016/j.physbeh.2015.05.036

Bushinsky, D. (1996). Metabolic alkalosis decreases bone calcium influx by suppressing osteoclast and stimulating osteoblasts. *American Journal of Physiology, 271*, F216-222

Busse, D., Kudella, P., Gruning, N.-M., Gisselmann, G., Stander, S., Luger, T., ... Benecke, H. (2014). A synthetic sandalwood odorant induces wound-healing processes in human keratinocytes via the olfactory receptor OR2AT4. *Journal of Investigative Dermatology*, *134*, 2823-2832, doi:10.1038/jid.2014.273

Byelashov, O. A., Sinclair, A. J., & Kaur, G. (2015). Dietary sources, current intakes, and nutritional role of omega-3 docosapentaenoic acid. *Lipid Technology, 27*(4), 79-82 doi: 10.1002/lite.201500013

Cai, X., Wang, C., Wang, S., Cao, G., Jin, C., Yu, J.,...Ding, F. (2015). Carbohydrate intake, glycemic index, glycemic load, and stroke a meta-analysis of prospective cohort studies. *Asia Pac J Public Health, 27*, 486-496. doi: 10.1177/1010539514566742

Cancer, I. A. (2015). Carcinogenicity of consumption of red and processed meat. *The Lancet*, doi: 10.1016/S1470-2045(15)00444-1

Cani, P. D., Bibiloni, R., Knauf, C., Waget, A., Neyrinck, A. M., Delzenne, N. M., & Burcelin, R. (2008). Changes in gut microbiota control metabolic endotoxemia-induced inflammation in high-fat diet-induced obesity and diabetes in mice. *Diabetes*, *57*, 1470-1481

Cani, P., Geurts, L., Matamoros, S., Plovier, H., & Duparc, T. (2014). Glucose metabolism focus on gut microbiota, the endocannabinoid system and beyond. *Diabetes Metab.*, *40*(4), 246-57

MICHAEL S. FENSTER, MD

Carlin, G. (2012, April 1). *George carlin: we've added years to life not life to years.* Retrieved from Venugopal: https://venugopalmn.wordpress.com/2012/04/01/george-carlin-weve-added-years-to-life-not-life-to-years/

Carmody, R. N., Weintraub, G. S., & Wrangham, R. W. (2011). Energetic consequences of thermal and nonthermal food processing. *Proceedings of the National Academy of Sciences, 108*(48), 19199-19203

Catry, E., Pachikian, B., Salazar, N., Neyrinck, A., Cani, P., & Delzenne, N. (2015). Ezetimibe and simvastatin modulate gut microbiota and expression of genes related to cholesterol metabolism. *Life Sci., 132,* 77-84

CBS News. (1977, July 26). Exchange between dr robert olson and senator george mcgovern from the united states senate select committee on nutrition and human needs. Washington, DC, USA.

CDC. (2009). *Health, united states 2008.* Retrieved from CDC.gov: http://www.cdc.gov/nchs/data/hus/hus08.pdf

CDC. (2011, August 17). *Healthy weight.* Retrieved from CDC.gov: http://www.cdc.gov/healthyweight/assessing/index.html

CDC. (2015, January). *Maps of diagnosed diabetes and obesity in 1994, 2000, and 2013.* Retrieved from CDC.gov: http://www.cdc.gov/diabetes/statistics/slides/maps_diabetesobesity94.pdf

CDC. (2017, March 30). *Morbidity and mortality weekly report.* Retrieved from CDC.gov: https://www.cdc.gov/mmwr/volumes/66/wr/mm6612a3.htm?s_cid=mm6612a3_w

CDC. (2014, October). *Long-term trends in diabetes.* Retrieved from CDC.gov: http://www.cdc.gov/diabetes/statistics/slides/long_term_trends.pdf

CDC.gov. (2009). *Overweight.* Retrieved from CDC.gov: http://nchstats.com/category/overweight/

Center for Science in the Public Interest. (2014). *Artificial trans fat: A timeline.* Retrieved from CSPInet.org: http://cspinet.org/transfat/timeline.html

Centers for Disease Control. (1999, August 6). *Ancel keys, ph.d.* Retrieved from MMWR 48(30), 651: http://www.cdc.gov/mmwr/preview/mmwrhtml/mm4830a1box.htm

Centers for Disease Control. (2004, February 6). *Trends in intake of energy and macronutrients—united states, 1971-2000.* Retrieved from CDC.gov: http://www.cdc.gov/mmwr/preview/mmwrhtml/mm5304a3.htm

Centers for Disease Control. (2012, May 1). *Inflammatory bowel disease (ibd).* Retrieved fromCDC.gov: http://www.cdc.gov/ibd/

Centers for Disease Control and Prevention. (2011, May 23). *2011 national diabetes fact sheet.* Retrieved from Centers for Disease Control and Prevention: http://www.cdc.gov/diabetes/pubs/estimates11.htm#1

Centers for Disease Control and Prevention. (2011, February 24). *Americans consume too much sodium.* Retrieved fromCDC.gov: http://www.cdc.gov/features/dssodium/

Centers for Disease Control and Prevention. (2011, July 11). *High sodium, low potassium diet linked to increased risk of death.* Retrieved fromCDC.gov: http://www.cdc.gov/media/releases/2011/p0711_sodiumpotassiumdiet.html

Centers for Disease Control and Prevention. (2013, March 20). *High blood pressure.* Retrieved fromCDC.gov: http://www.cdc.gov/bloodpressure/facts.htm

Centers for Disease Control and Prevention. (2013, June 5). *Sodium and food sources.* Retrieved July 15, 2013, from Centers for Disease Control and Prevention: http://www.cdc.gov/salt/food.htm

Centers for Disease Control and Prevention. (2014). *National diabetes statistics report: Estimates of diabetes and its burden in the united states.* Atlanta, GA: U.S. Department of Health and Human Services

Chambers, E. S., Viardot, A., Psichas, A., Morrison, D. J., Zac-Varghese, S. E., & Thomas, E. L. (2014). Effects of targeted delivery of propionate to the human colon on appetite regulation, body weight maintenance and adiposity inoverweight adults. *Gut*, doi: 10.1136/gutjnl-

Champeau, R. (2009, January 12). *Most heart attack patients' cholesterol levels did not indicate cardiac risk*. Retrieved from UCLA.edu http://newsroom.ucla.edu/releases/majority-of-hospitalized-heart-75668

Charles, D. (2012, January 9). *The forgotten, fascinating saga of crisco*. Retrieved from NPR. org: http://www.npr.org/sections/thesalt/2012/01/09/144918710/the-forgotten-fascinating-saga-of-crisco

Charles, D. (2013, July 17). *In oregon, the gmo wheat mystery deepens*. Retrievedfrom NPR. org: http://www.npr.org/blogs/thesalt/2013/07/17/202684064/in-oregon-the-gmo-wheat-mystery-deepens

Chassaing, B., K. O., Goodrich, J. K., Poole, A. C., Srinivasan, S., L. R., & Gewirtz, A. T. (2015). Dietary emulsifiers impact the mouse gut microbiota promoting colitis and metabolic syndrome. *Nature*, doi: 10.1038/nature14232

Checkoff, P. (2013). *Quick facts: The pork industry at a glance*. Iowa: National Pork Board.

Chen, G., Lv, D., Pang, Z., & Liu, Q. (2013). Red and processed meat consumption and risk of stroke: A meta-analysis of prospective cohort studies. *Eur J Clin Nutr.*, *67*, 91-95. doi: 10.1038/ejcn.2012.180

Chen, L., Caballero, B., Mitchell, D., Loria, C., Lin, P., Champagne, C.,...Appel, L. (2010). Reducing consumption of sugar-sweetened beverages is associated with reduced blood pressure: A prospective study among united states adults. *Circulation*, *121*, 2398-2406

Chen, M., Sun, Q., Giovannucci, E., Mozaffarian, D., Manson, J., Willett, W., & Hu, F. (2014). Dairy consumption and risk of type 2 diabetes: 3 cohorts of US adults and an updated meta-analysis. *BMC Med.*, *12*, 215. doi: 10.1186/s12916-014-0215-1.

Chiu, S., Bergeron, N., Williams, P., Bray, G., Sutherland, B., & Krauss, R. (2016). Comparison of the dash (dietary approaches to stop hypertension) diet and a higher-fat dash diet on blood pressure and lipids and lipoproteins: a randomized controlled trial. *Am J Clin Nutr*, *103*, 341-7

Chiu, Y.-F., Hsu, C.-C., Chiu, T. H., Lee, C.-Y., Liu, T.-T., Tsao, C. K.,...Hsiung, C. A. (2015). Cross-sectional and longitudinal comparisons of metabolic profiles between vegetarian and non-vegetarian subjects: A matched cohort study. *British Journal of Nutrition*, *114*(8), 1313-1320

Choi, C. (2015, December 11). *Yum ceo says pizza hut needs to be more like uber*. Retrieved from ap.org: http://bigstory.ap.org/article/99d47250ef45434186c37a0c974c9632/yum-ceo-says-pizza-hut-needs-be-more-uber

Chopra, M. (2017). Yes, You Can Live with Intent. *Time: Mindfulness: The new science of health and happiness*, 58-61

Chowdhury, R., Warnakula, S., Kunutsor, S., Crowe, F., Ward, H., Johnson, L.,...Di Angelantonio, E. (2014). Association of dietary, circulating, and supplement fatty acids with coronary risk: A systematic review and meta-analysis. *Ann Intern Med.*, *160*, 398-406

Cohen, S., Janicki-Deverts, D., Doyle, W. J., Miller, G. E., Frank, E., Rabin, B. S., & Turner, R. B. (2012). Chronic stress, glucocorticoid receptor resistance, inflammation, and disease risk. *Proceedings of the National Academy of Science*, *109*(16), 5995-5999

Coleman, M., Ebel, E., Goldin, N., Hogue, A., Kadry, A., Kause, J.,...Schroeder, C. (2017, June 23). *Risk assessments of salmonella enteritidis in shell eggs and salmonella.* Retrieved from USDA.gov: https://www.fsis.usda.gov/shared/PDF/SE_Risk_Assess_Oct2005.pdf

Committee on Nutrition. (1964). Factors affecting food intake. *Pediatrics, 33,* 135

Congressional research service. (2015, March 25). *H.R.1599—Safe and accurate food labeling act of 2015.* Retrieved from Congress.gov: Congress.gov: https://www.congress. gov/bill/114th-congress/house-bill/1599

Connolly, S. J., Sheldon, R., Roberts, R. S., Gent, M., & Investigators, T. V. (1999). The north american vasovagal pacemaker study (vps) §2: A randomized trial of permanent cardiac pacing for the prevention of vasovagal syncope. *JACC, 33*(1), 16-20

Connolly, S., Sheldon, R., Thorpe, K. E., Roberts, R. S., Ellenbogen, K., Wilkoff, B.,... Investigators, T.V. (2003). Pacemaker therapy for prevention of syncope in patients with recurrent severe vasovagal syncope: Second vasovagal pacemaker study (vps ii): A randomized trial. *JAMA, 289* (17), 2224-2229

Corbille, A.-G., Clairembault, T., Coron, E., Leclaire-Visioneau, L., Preterre, C., Neunlist, M., & Derkinderen, D. (2016). What a gastrointestinal biopsy can tell us about Parkinson's disease *Neurogastroenterology and Motility, 28*(7), 966-974

Cordain, L. (1999). Cereal grains: Humanity's double edge sword. *World Rev Nutr Diet, 84,* 19-73

Cordain, L. (2002). The nutritional characteristics of a contemporary diet based upon paleolithic food groups. *J Am Neutraceutical Assoc., 5,* 15-24

Cordain, L. (2002). *The paleo diet.* New York: Wiley, Inc.

Cordain, L., Brand-Miller, J., Eaton, S., Mann, N., Holt, S., & Speth, J. (2000). Plant to animal subsistence ratios and macronutrient energy estimations and worldwide hunter-gatherer diets. *Am J Clin Nutr., 71,* 682-692

Cordain, L., Eades, M., & Eades, M. (2003). Hyperinsulinemic disease of civilization: More than just syndrome x. *Comp Biochem Physiol Part A, 136,* 95-112

Cordain, L., Eaton, S. B., Sebastian, A., Mann, N., Lindeberg, S., Watkins, B. A., ... Brand-Miller, J. (2005). Origins and evolution of the Western diet: health implications for the 21st century. *The American Journal of Nutrition, 81,* 341-354

Cordain, L., Eaton, S., & Brand-Miller, J. (2002). The Paradoxical Nature of Hunter-Gatherer Diets: Meat-based, yet Non-Atherogenic. *Eur J Clin Nutr, 56* (supplement 1), S42-S52

Cordain, L., Eaton, S., Brand-Miller, J., Lindeberg, S., & Jensen, C. (2002). An evolutionary analysis of the etiology and pathogenesis of juvenile onset myopia. *Acta Opthamol Scand, 80,* 125-135

Cordain, L., Lindeberg, S., Hurtado, M., Hill, K., Eaton, S., & Brand-Miller, J. (2002). Acne vulgaris: A disease of western civilization. *Arch Dermatol, 138,* 1584-1590

Cordain, L., Miller, J., Eaton, S., & Mann, N. (2000). Macronutrient estimations in hunter-gatherer diets. *Am J Clin Nutr, 72,* 1589-1590

Cordain, L., Toohey, L., Smith, M., & Hickey, M. (2000). Modulation of immune function by dietary lectins in rheumatoid arthritis. *Bt J Nutr, 83*(3), 207-217

Cordain, L., Watkins, B., & Mann, N. (2001). Fatty acid composition and energy density of foods available to african hominids. *World Rev Nutr Diet, 90,*144-161

Cordain, L., Watkins, B., Florant, G., Kehler, M., Rogers, L., & Li, Y. (2002). Fatty acid analysis of wild ruminant tissues: Evolutionary implications for reducing diet-related chronic disease. *European Journal of Clinical Nutrition, 56,* 181-191

Corella, D., & Ordovas, J. (2009). Nutrigenomics in cardiovascular medicine.*Circ Cardiovasc Genet., 2,* 637-651. doi: 10.1161

Corella, D., Carrasco, P., Sorli, J. V., Estruch, R., Rico-Sanz, J., Martinez-Gonzalez, A.,...Warnberg, J. (2013). Mediterranean diet reduces the adverse effect of the tcf712-rs7903146 polymorphism on cardiovascular risk factors and stroke incidence: A randomized controlled trial in a high-cardiovascular-risk population. *Diabetes Care*, doi: 10.2337/dc13-0955

Corrales, A., Dessein, P. H., Tsang, L., Pina, T., Blanco, R., G.-J. C., & Gonzalez-Gay, M. A. (2015). Carotid artery plaque in women with rheumatoid arthritis and low estimated cardiovascular disease risk: A cross-sectional study. *Arthritis Research & Therapy, 17*(55), doi:10.1186/s13075-015-0576-7

Corsini, R. J., & f Wedding, D. (2010). *Current psychotherapies.* Belmont, Ca: Cengage Learning.

Cotillard, A., Kennedy, S. P., Kong, K. C., Prifiti, E., Pons, N., Le Chatelier, E.,...Fouqueray, C. (2013). Dietary intervention impact on gut microbial gene richness. *Nature, 500*, 585-588

Cox, P. A., & Metcalf, J. S. (2017). Traditional Food items in ogimi, okinawa: l-serine content and the potential for neuroprotection. *Curr Nutr Rep, 6*, 24-31 doi: 10.1007/s13668-017-0191-0

Craig, S. A. (2004). Betaine in human nutrition. *Am J Clin Nutr, 80*, 539-49

Crampton, L. (2015, March 11). *Polysorbate 80 food additive, gut bacteria and inflammation.* Retrieved from Hubpages.com: http://hubpages.com/hub/Polysorbate-80-Food-Additive-Inflammation-and-Health-Problems

Crippa, G., Zabunzi, D., Bravi, E., Cicognini, F. M., Bighi, E., & Rossi, F. (2016). Randomized, double-blind, placebo-controlled, cross-over study on the antihypertensive effect of dietary integration with grana padano docg cheese. *Journal of the American Society of Hypertension, 104*S: e6 doi: 10.1016/j.jash.2016.03.014

Daley, C. A., Abbot, A., Doyle, P. S., Nader, G. A., & Larson, S. (2010). A review of fatty acid profiles and antioxidant content in grass-fed and grain-fed beef. *Nutrition Journal, 9*, 10-22

Daley, C. A., Abbott, A., Doyle, P. S., Nader, G. A., & Larson, S. (2010). A review of fatty acid profiles and antioxidant content in grass-fed and grain-fed beef. *Nutrition Journal, 9*: 10

Dalmeijer, G., Struijk, E., van der Schouw, Y., Soedamah-Muthu, S., Verschuren, W., Boer, J.,...Beulens, J. (2013). Dairy intake and coronary heart disease or stroke—A population-based cohort study. *Int J Cardiol., 167*, 925-9

Danforth, A. (2014). *Butchering poultry, rabbit, lamb, goat, pork: The comprehensive photographic guide to humane slaughtering and butchering.* North Adams, MA: Storey Publishing

Daniel, C. R., Cross, A. J., Koebnick, C., & Sinha, R. (2011). Trends in meat consumption in the United States. *Public Health Nutr., 14*(4): 575-583. doi:10.1017/S1368980010002077

Danzeisen, J. L., Kim, H. B., Isaacson, R. E., Tu, Z. J., & Johnson, T. J. (2011). Modulations of the chicken cecal microbiome and metagenome in response to anticoccidial and growth promoter treatment. *PLoS One.* doi:10.1371/journal.pone.0027949

Daskalopoulou, M., George, J., Walters, K., Osborn, D. P., Batty, G. D., Stogiannis, D.,...Hemingway, H. (2016). Depression as a risk factor for the initial presentation of twelve cardiac, cerebrovascular, and peripheral arterial diseases: Data Linkage study of 1.9 million women and men. *PLoS One*, doi:10.1371/journal.pone.0153838

Daubenmier, J., Moran, P. J., Kristeller, J., Acree, M., Bacchetti, P., Kemeny, M. E.,...Hecht, F. M. (2016). Effects of a mindfulness-based weight loss intervention in adults with obesity: A randomized clinical trial. *Obesity, 24*, 794-804. doi: 10.1002/oby.21396

Davenport, L. (2016, June 30). *Diabetes raises risk of death for years after a heart attack.* Retrieved from Medscape.com: http://www.medscape.com/viewarticle/865579

Davis, C., & Saltos, E. (1999). Dietary recommendations and how they have changed over time. *America's eating H=habits: Changes and consequences* (Agriculture Information Bulletin No. *750*). Washington, DC : US Department of Agriculture, Economic Research Service

Davis, C., Bryan, J., Hodgson, J., & Murphy, K. (2015). Definition of the mediterranean diet: a literature review. *Nutrients, 7*, :9139-9153. doi: 10.3390/nu7115459

Davis, M., Price, L., Liu, C.-H., & Silbergeld, E. (2011). An ecological perspective on US industrial poultry production: The role of anthropogenic ecosystems on the emergence of drug-resistant bacteria from agricultural environments. *Curr Opin Microbiol, 14*(3):244-250

De Filippoa, C., Cavalieri, D., Di Paola, M., Ramazzotti, M., Poullet, J. B., Massart, S., & Lionetti, P. (2010). Impact of diet in shaping gut microbiota revealed by a comparative study in children from Europe and rural Africa. *PNAS*.doi: 10.1073/pnas.1005963107

de Oliveira, O. M., Nettleton, J., Lemaitre, R., Steffen, L., Kromhout, D., Rich, S.,... Mozaffarian, D. (2013). Biomarkers of dairy fatty acids and risk of cardiovascular disease in the multi-ethnic study of atherosclerosis. *J Am Heart Assoc., 2*, e000092. doi: 10.1161/JAHA.113.000092

de Souza, R. J., Mente, A., Maroleanu, A., Cozma, A. I., Ha, V., & K. T. (2015). Intake of saturated and trans unsaturated fatty acids and risk of all cause mortality, cardiovascular disease, and type 2 diabetes: Systematic review and meta-analysis. *BMJ, 351*, h397

Dean, W. F. (2017, March 20). *Food value of duck.* Retrieved from Cornell University College of Veterinary Medicine Duck Research Laboratory: http://www.duckhealth.com/foodvalu.html

Dehghan, M., Mente, A., Teo, K. K., Gao, P., Sleight, P., Dagenais, G.,...Yusuf, S. (2012). Relationship between healthy diet and risk of cardiovascular disease among patients ondrug therapies for secondary prevention: A prospective cohort study of 31,546 high-risk individuals from 40 countries. *Circulation, 126*, 2705-2712

Dehghan, M., Mente, A., Zhang, X., Swaminathan, S., Li, W., Mohan, V.,...Yusuf, S. (2017). Associations of fats and carbohydrate intake with cardiovascular disease and mortality in 18 countires from five continents (pure): A prospective cohort study. *The Lancet, .* doi: 10.1016/S0140-6736(17)32252-3

Del Gobbo, L. C., Inamura, F., Aslibekyan, S., Marklund, M., Virtanen, J. K., Wennberg, M.,...Mozzafarian, D. (2016). Omega-3 Polyunsaturated fatty acid biomarkers and coronary heart disease pooling project of 19 cohort studies. *JAMA*, doi: 10.100/jamainternmed.2016.2925

del Rincon, I., Freeman, G., Haas, R., O'Leary, D., & E. A. (2005). Relative contribution of cardiovascular risk factors and rheumatoid arthritis clinical manifestations to atherosclerosis. *Arthritis Rheum.,* 3413-23

Delbyck, C. (2017, February 4). *The 15 most ridiculous items from gwyneth paltrow's holiday wish list.* Retrieved from Huffingtonpost.com: http://www.huffingtonpost.com/entry/gwyneth-paltrow-goop-gift_us_56561d80e4b08e945feae994

Denjean, C. (Director) (2013). *The gut our second brain* [Motion Picture]

Deschanel, Z. (2017, March 30). *Zooey deschanel*. Retrieved from Quoteaddicts.com: http://quoteaddicts.com/337431

Devillard, E., McIntosh, F., & Duncan, S. W. (2007). Metabolism of linoleic acid by human gut bacteria: Different routes for biosynthesis of conjugated linoleic acid. *J Bacteriol.*, *189*(6), 2566-70

Deyoung, R. K. (2017, March 31). *The seven deadly sins*. Retrieved from Calvin.edu: https://www.calvin.edu/academic/philosophy/virtual_library/articles/deyoung_rebecca_k/7deadlysins.pdf

Diaz-Lopez, A., Bullo, M., Martinez-Gonzalez, M., Corella, D., Estruch, R., Fito, M.,... Salas-Salvado, J. (2015). Dairy product consumption and risk of type 2 diabetes in an elderly spanish mediterranean population at high cardiovascular risk. *Eur J Nutr.*, doi:10.1007/s00394-015-0855-8

Dietary Guidelines Advisory Committee. (2015, March 25). *Scientific report of the 2015 dietary guidelines advisory committee*. Retrieved from Health.gov: http://www.health.gov/dietaryguidelines/2015-scientific-report/

Dilli, D., Aydin, B., Zenciroglu, A., Ozyazici, E., Beken, S., & Okumus, N. (2013). Treatment outcomes of infants with cyanotic congenital heart disease treated with synbiotics. *Pediatrics*, *132*(4),932-8

DiMarco, D. M., Norris, G. H., Millar, C. L., Blesso, C. N., & Fernandez, M. L. (2017). Intake of up to 3 Eggs per day is associated with changes in hdl function and increased plasma antioxidants in healthy, young adults. *The Journal of Nutrition*. doi: 10.3945/jn.116.241877

Dimond, E., Kittle, C., & Crockett, J. (1960). Comparison of internal mammary artery ligation and sham operation for angina pectoris. *Am J Cardiol*, *5*, 483-486

DiNicolantonio, J. J. (2014). The cardio metabolic consequences of replacing saturated fats with carbohydrates or Omega six polyunsaturated fats: Did the dietary guidelines have it wrong? *Open Heart BMJ*.v doi:10.1136/openhrt-2013-000032

DiNicolantonio, J. J., & Lucan, S. C. (2014). The wrong white crystals: Not salt but sugar as aetiological in hypertension and cardiometabolic disease. *Open Heart BMJ*, *1*,e000167. doi:10.1136/openhrt-2014-000167

DiNicolantonio, J., Lavie, C. J., Fares, H., Menezes, A. R., & O'Keefe, J. H. (2013). Lcarnitine in the secondary prevention of cardiovascular disease: systematic review and meta-analysis. *Mayo Clin. Proc.*, i,544-551

Djoussé, L., Akinkuolie, A., Wu, J., Ding, E., & Gaziano, J. (2012). Fish consumption, omega-3 fatty acids and risk of heart failure: A meta-analysis. *Clin Nutr. 31*, 846-853. doi: 10.1016/j.clnu.2012.05.010

Dobarganes, C., & Márquez-Ruiz, G. (2015). Possible adverse effects of frying with vegetable oils. *Br J Nutr.*, *113*(suppl 2), S49-S57. doi: 10.1017/S0007114514002347

Domingo, J., & Gine-Bordonaba, J. (2011). A Literature review on the safety assessment of genetically modified plants. *Enviromn Int*, *37*, 734-742

Dreon, D., Fernstrom, H., & Campos, H. (1998). Change in dietary saturated fat intake is correlated with change in mass of large low-density-lipoprotein particles in men. *Am J Clin Nutr*, *67*,828-36

Drouin-Chartier, J., Brassard, D., Tessier-Grenier, M., Côté, J., Labonté, M.-È., Desroches, S.,...Lamarche, B. (2016). Systematic review of the association between dairy product consumption and risk of cardiovascular related clinical outcomes. *Advan Nutr*, *7*,1026-40

Drouin-Chartier, J.-P., Côté, J. A., Labonté, M.-È., Brassard, D., Tessier-Grenier, M., Desroches, S.,... Lamarche, B. (2016). Comprehensive review of the impact of dairy foods and dairy fat on cardiometabolic risk. *Advances in Nutrition, 7*, 1041-51. doi:10.3945/an.115.011619

Droulez, V., Williams, P., Levy, G., Stobaus, T., & Sinclair, A. (2006). Composition of australian red meat 2002. 2. Fatty. *Food Australia*, i(7), 335-341

Dunn, J. (2017). Save yourself from stress. *Time: Mindfulness, The New Science of Health and Happiness*, 17-23

Dunn, J. (2017). The Art of meditation. *Time: Mindfulness: the New Science of Health and Happiness*, 44-49

Dunn, R. (2012, July 23). *Human ancestors were nearly all vegetarians*. Retrieved from Scientific American: http://blogs.scientificamerican.com/guest-blog/human-ancestors-were-nearly-all-vegetarians/

Durtschi, A. (2001). *Nutritional content of whole grains versus their refined flours*. Washington, DC: United States Department of Agriculture Economic Research Service

Eaton, S., Cordain, L., & Lindeberg, S. (2002). Evolutionary health promotion: A consideration of common counter arguments. *Prev Med, 34*(2), 119-123

Ebbeling, C., Swain, J., Feldman, H., Wong, W., Hachey, D., Garcia-Lago, E., & Ludwig, D. (2012). Effects of dietary composition on energy expenditure during weight-loss maintenance. *JAMA., 307*, 2627-2634. doi:10.1001/jama.2012.6607

Einstein, A. (2007). *The world as i see it*. San Diego, California: The Book Tree

Einstein, A. (2017, March 31). *Albert einstein*. Retrieved from Today in Science History: https://todayinsci.com/E/Einstein_Albert/EinsteinAlbert-Quotations.htm

Einstein, A. (2017, April 26). *Albert einstein quotes*. Retrieved from Goodreads.com: https://www.goodreads.com/quotes/32930-look-deep-into-nature-and-then-you-will-understand-everything

Einstein, A. (2017, June 23). *Einstein*. Retrieved from Goodreads.com: https://www.goodreads.com/quotes/7666163-spooky-action-at-a-distance

Einstein, A. (2017, March 25). *Everything should be made as simple as possible, but not simpler*. Retrieved from Quote investigator: http://quoteinvestigator.com/2011/05/13/einstein-simple/

Eisenberg, T., Abdellatif, A., Schroeder, S., Primessning, U., Stekovic, S., Pendl, T.,... Pietrocola, F. (2016). Cardioprotection and lifespan extension by the natural polyamine spermidine. *Nature, 22*:=, 1428-1438. doi:10.1038/nm.4222

Eiwegger, T., Stahl, B., Schmitt, J., Boehm, G., Gerstmayr, M., Pichler, J.,... Szepfalusi, Z. (2004). Human milk-derived oligosaccharides and plant-derived oligosaccharides stimulate cytokine production of cord blood t-cells in vitro. *Pediatr Res., 56*. 536-40

Eliade, M. (1964). *Shamanism: Archaic techniques of ecstasy (W. Trask, Trans.)*. Princeton, NJ: Princeton University Press

Elliott, S., Keim, N., Stern, J., Teff, K., & Havel, P. (2002). Fructose, weight gain, and the insulin resistance syndrome. *Am J Clin Nutr, 76*, 911-922

El-Sheikh, M., El-Senaity, M., Youssef, Y., Shahein, N., & Abd Rabou, N. (2011). Effect of ripening conditions on the proprieties of blue cheese produced from cow's and goat's milk. *J Am Sci., 7*, 485-90

Ely, A. V., Childress, A., Jagannathan, K., & Lowe, M. (2015). The way to her heart? Response to romantic cues is dependent on hunger state and dieting history: An fMRI pilot study. *Appetite, 95*, 126-31. doi: 10.1016/j.appet.2015.06.022

Emerging Technology from the ArXiv. (2012, March 8). *Einstein's "spooky action from a distance" paradox older than thought*. Retrieved from MIT Technology Review: https://www.technologyreview.com/s/427174/einsteins-spooky-action-at-a-distance-paradox-older-than-thought/

Epel, E., Daubenmier, J., Moskowitz, J. T., Folkman, S., & Blackburn, E. (2009). Can meditation slow rate of cellular aging? Cognitive stress, mindfulness, and telomeres. *Ann N Y Acad Sci.*, *1172*, 34-53

Ericson, U., Hellstrand, S., Brunkwall, L., Schulz, C., Sonestedt, E., Wallström, P.,... Orho-Melander, M. F. (2015). Food sources of fat may clarify the inconsistent role of dietary fat intake for incidence of type 2 diabetes. *Am J Clin Nutr.*, *101*, 1065-1080. doi: 10.3945/ajcn.114.103010

Estruch, R., Ros, E., Salas-Salvadó, J., Covas, M., Corella, D., Arós, F.,...Investigators, P. S. (2013). Primary prevention of cardiovascular disease with a M=mediterranean diet. *N Engl J Med.*, *368*(14), 1279-90. doi: 10.1056/NEJMoa1200303

Estruch, R., Sacanella, E., Badia, E., Antunez, E., Nicolas, J., Fernandez-Sola, J.,...Urbano-Marquez, A. (2004). Different effects of red wine and gin consumption on inflammatory biomarkers of atherosclerosis: A prospective randomized crossover trial. Effects of wine on inflammatory markers. *Atherosclerosis*, *175*, 117-123

Everard, A. B., Geurtsa, L., Ouwerkerkb, J. P., Druarta, C., Bindelsa, L. B., & Cani, P. D. (2013). Cross-talk between akkermansia muciniphila and intestinal epithelium controls diet-induced obesity. *PNAS*, *110*(22), 9066-9071

Everard, A., Lazarevic, V., Derrien, M., Girard, M., Muccioli, G. G., Neyrinck, A. M., & Cani, P. D. (2011). Responses of gut microbiota and glucose and lipid metabolism to prebiotics in genetic obese and diet-induced leptin-resistant mice. *Diabetes*, *60*: 2775-2786

Evert, A., Boucher, J., Cypress, M., Dunbar, S., Franz, M., Mayer-Davis, E.,...Yancy Jr., W. (2014). Nutrition therapy recommendations for the management of adults with diabetes. *Diabetes Care*, i(suppl 1), S120-S143. doi: 10.2337/dc14-S120

Fan, J., Song, Y., Wang, Y., Hui, R., & Zhang, W. (2012). Dietary glycemic index, glycemic load, and risk of coronary heart disease, stroke, and stroke mortality: A systematic review with meta-analysis. *PLoS One*, *7*, e52182. doi: 10.1371/journal.pone.0052182

Fardet, A. (2015). A shift toward a new holistic paradigm will help to preserve and better process grain products' food structure for improving their health effects. *Food Funct.*, *6*, 363-382. doi: 10.1039/c4fo00477a

Farvid, M., Ding, M., Pan, A., Sun, Q., Chiuve, S., Steffen, L.,...Hu, F. (2014). Dietary linoleic acid and risk of coronary heart disease: A systematic review and meta-analysis of prospective cohort studies. *Circulation*, *130*, 1568-1578. doi: 10.1161/CIRCULATIONAHA.114.010236

FDA. (2013, June 1). *Code of federal regulations title 21.* Retrieved December 16, 2013, from US FDA: http://www.accessdata.fda.gov/scripts/cdrh/cfdocs/cfcfr/CFRSearch.cfm?fr=101.12

FDA. (2014, September 1). *CFR- code of federal regulations title 21:sec. 172.840 polysorbate 80.* Retrieved from FDA.gov: http://www.accessdata.fda.gov/scripts/cdrh/cfdocs/cfCFR/CFRSearch.cfm?fr=172.840

FDA. (2015, June 6). *FDA Cuts Trans Fat in Processed Foods.* Retrieved from FDA.gov: http://www.fda.gov/downloads/ForConsumers/ConsumerUpdates/UCM451467.pdf

FDA. (2016, August 5). *Update: gel spice, inc. issues expanded recall of ground tumeric powder due to elevated lead levels.* Retrieved from FDA.gov: https://www.fda.gov/Safety/Recalls/ucm515328.htm

FDA. (2017, March 25). *How u.s. fda's gras notification program works.* Retrieved from www.fda.gov: https://www.fda.gov/food/ingredientspackaginglabeling/gras/ucm083022.htm

FDA. (2017, April 26). *Whole grains make a difference.* Retrieved from USDA.gov: https://www.fns.usda.gov/sites/default/files/how_to_tell_whole_grain.pdf

FDA.gov. (2016, May 2). *Questions and answers: Gluten-free food labeling final rule.* Retrieved from FDA.gov: http://www.fda.gov/Food/GuidanceRegulation/ GuidanceDocumentsRegulatoryInformation/Allergens/ucm362880.htm

Feder, A., Nestler, E. J., & Charney, D. S. (2009). Psychobiology and molecular genetics of resilience. *Nat Rev Neurosci., 10*(6): 446-457

Federal Register. (2014). *Food labeling: nutrition labeling of standard menu items in restaurants and similar retail food establishments.* Retrieved from Federal Register: https:// www.federalregister.gov/regulations/0910-AG57/food-labeling-nutrition-labeling-of-standard-menu-items-in-restaurants-and-similar-retail-food-estab

Feinman R, F. E. (2004). A calorie is a calorie violates the second law of thermodynamics. *Nutr J, 3,* 9

Fenster, M. (2014, May). *The mediterranean to modern western diet: What in hades happened? Lessons from the mediterranean.* (M. Fenster, Performer) Field to Plate Series, Crete, Greece.

Fenster, M. S. (2014). *The fallacy of the calorie: Why the modern western diet is killing us and how to stop it.* New York, NY: Koehler Books

Fenster,M.S.(2015,July28).*10healthyfoodsthatprotectyourbrain.* RetrievedfromMSN:http:// www.msn.com/en-us/health/wellness/10-healthy-foods-that-protect-your-brain/ ss-BBlGze3#image=6

Fenster, M. S. (2016). *Ancient eats (volume 1): The greeks and vikings.* New York: Koehler Books.

Fernández-Real, J. M., P. d., Luche, E., M.-N. J., W. A., Serino, M., & Zorzano, A. (2011). CD14 modulates inflammation-driven insulin resistance. *Diabetes, 60,* 2179-2186

Fine, L., Philogene, S., Gramling, R., Coups, E., & Sinha, S. (2004). Prevalence of multiple chronic disease risk factors: 2001 National Health Interview Survey. *Am J Prev Med., 27*(suppl 2), 18-24. doi: 10.1016/jamepre.2004.04.017

Finniss, D. G., Kaptchuk, T. J., Miller, F., & Benedetti, F. (2010). Placebo effects: Biological, clinical and ethical advances. *Lancet., 20; 375*(9715), 686-695. doi:10.1016/S0140-6736(09)61706-2

Firestein, S. (2017). *Big think interview with stuart firestein.* Retrieved from BigThink.com: http://bigthink.com/videos/big-think-interview-with-stuart-firestein

Firestein, S. (2017). *From tongue to brain the neurology of taste.* Retrieved from BigThink. com: http://bigthink.com/videos/from-tongue-to-brain-the-neurology-of-taste

Firestein, S. (2017). *The difference between taste and flavour.* Retrieved from BigThink.com: http://bigthink.com/videos/the-difference-between-taste-and-flavor

Firestein, S. (2017). *The evolutionary paradox of our sense of smell.* Retrieved from BigThink. com: http://bigthink.com/videos/the-evolutionary-paradox-of-our-sense-of-smell

Firestein, S. (2017). *The neurology of smell.* Retrieved from BigThink.com: http://bigthink. com/videos/from-nose-to-brain-the-neurology-of-smell

Fisher, A., Enser, M., & Richardson, R. (2000). Fatty acid composition and eating quality of lamb types derived from four diverse breed x production systems. *Meat Science, 55,* 141-147

Flores, G. E., Caporaso, J. G., Henley, J. B., Rideout, J. R., Domogala, D., Chase, J.,... Fierer, N. (2014). Temporal variability is a personalized feature of the human microbiome. *Genome Biology, 15,* 531 http://genomebiology.com/2014/15/12/531

Food and Agricultural Organisation of The United Nations. (2010). Sustainable diets and biodiversity: Directions and solutions for policy, research and action. *Proceedings of The International Scientific Symposium: Biodiversity and sustainable diets united against hunger*

Food and agricultural organization of the United Nations. (2014, November 25). *Agriculture and Consumer Protection Department.* Retrieved from Animal Production and Health:

Sources of Meat: http://www.fao.org/ag/againfo/themes/en/meat/backgr_sources.html

Food Standards Australia New Zealand. (2003). *Erucic acid in food: A toxicological review and risk assessment technical report series no. 21.* Wellington, NZ: Food Standards Australia New Zealand

Ford, A. (2017). The faith factor. *Time: Mindfulness: The New Science of Health and Happiness*, 62-65

Forouhi, N., Koulman, A., Sharp, S., Imamura, F., Kröger, J., Schulze, M.,...Wareham, N. (2014). Differences in the prospective association between individual plasma phospholipid saturated fatty acids and incident type 2 diabetes: The epic-interact case-cohort study. *Lancet Diabetes Endocrinol.*, 2, 810-818. doi: 10.1016/S2213-8587(14)70146-9

Forsythe, C., Phinney, S., & Fernandez, M. (2008). Comparison of low-fat and low carbohydrate diets on circulating fatty acid composition and markers of inflammation. *Lipids*, 43(1): 65-77

Foster, G., Wyatt, H., & Hill, J. (2003). A randomized trial of a low-carbohydrate diet for obesity. *N Engl J Med, 348,* 2082-90

Fox, R. (2016). *Food and eating: An athropological perspective.* Retrieved from Social Issues Research Centre: http://www.sirc.org/publik/food_and_eating_8.html

Franz, M., VanWormer, J., & Crain, A. (2007). Weight-loss outcomes: A systematic review and meta-analysis of weight-loss clinical trials with a minimum 1-year follow-up. *J Am Dietetic Assoc, 107,* 1755-1767

Frassetto, L., & Morris, R. S. (1997). Potassium bicarbonate reduces urinary nitrogen excretion in postmenopausal women. *Journal of Clinical Endocrinology and Metabolism, 82,* 254-259

Freed, C. R., Greene, P. E., Breeze, R. E., Tsai, W.-Y., DuMouchel, W., Kao, K.,...Fahn, S. (2001). Transplantation of embryonic dopamine neurons for severe parkinson's disease. *N Engl J Med 2001, 344,* 710-719. doi: 10.1056/NEJM200103083441002

Freeman, A. M., Morris, P. B., Barnard, N., Esselstyn, C. B., Ros, E., Agatston, A.,....Kris-Etherton, P. (2017). Trending cardiovascular nutrition controversies. *Journal of the American College of Cardiology, 69*(9), 1172-1187 doi: 10.1016/j.jacc.2016.10.086

Freeman, S. (2015, August 14). *The way to a woman's heart? It's through her stomach! Feed your partner well and 'she'll be more interested in romance'.* Retrieved from Daily Mail: http://www.dailymail.co.uk/health/article-3197484/The-way-woman-s-heart-s-stomach-Feed-partner-ll-interested-romance.html

Fruit, V. A; Miller, V.; Mente, A.; Dehghan, M.; Rangarajan, S.; Zhang, X.,...Yusef, S. (2017). *The Lancet.* doi: 10.1016/S0140-6736(17)32253-5

Fry, J. P., Love, D. C., MacDonald, G. K., West, P. C., Engstrom, P. M., Nachman, K. E., & Lawrence, R. S. (2016). Environmental health impacts of feeding crops to farmed fish. *Environmental International, 91,* 201-214

Fuller, N. R., Caterson, I. D., Sainsbury, A., Denyer, G., Fong, M., Gerofi, J.,...Markovic, T. P. (2015). The effect of a high-egg diet on cardiovascular risk factors in people with type 2 diabetes: The diabetes and egg (diabegg) study—A 3-mo randomized controlled trial. *The American Journal of Clinical Nutrition, 101,* 705-13

Gadgil, M., Appel, L., Yeung, E., Anderson, C., Sacks, F., & Miller, E. 3. (2013). The effects of carbohydrate, unsaturated fat, and protein intake on measures of insulin sensitivity: Results from the omniheart trial. *Diabetes Care, 36,* 1132-1137. doi: 10.2337/dc12-0869

Gadsby, P., & Steele, L. (2004, October 1). *The inuit paradox*. Retrieved from Discover: http://discovermagazine.com/2004/oct/inuit-paradox

Gaede, P., Vedel, P., Larsen, N., Jensen, G., Parving, H., & Pedersen, O. (2003). Multifactorial intervention and cardiovascular disease in patients with type 2 diabetes. *N Engl J Med.*, *348*(5), 383-393. doi: 10.1056/NEJMoa021778

Gan, Y., Tong, X., Li, L., Cao, S., Yin, X., Gao, C.,...Lu, Z. (2015). Consumption of fruit and vegetables and risk of coronary artery disease: a meta analysis of prospective cohort studies. *Int J Cardiol, 183*, 129-137

Gao, D., Ning, N., Wang, C., Wang, Y., Li, Q., Meng, Z.,...Li, Q. (2013). Dairy products consumption and risk of type 2 diabetes: Systematic review and dose-response meta-analysis. *PLoS One, 8*, e73965. doi: 10.1371/

Gardner, C., Kiazand, A., & Alhassan, S. (2007). Comparison of the atkins, zone, ornish, and learn diets for change in weight and related risk factors among overweight premenopausal women. *JAMA, 297*, 969-77

Garfinkel, P. (2011, November 17). *Four noble buddha quotes*. Retrieved from Huffington Post: http://www.huffingtonpost.com/perry-garfinkel/four-noble-buddha-quotes_b_86728.html

Gill, S. P., Deboy, R., Eckburg, P., Turnbaugh, P., Samuel, B., & Nelson, K. (2006). Metagenomic analysis of the human distal gut microbiome. *Science, 312*(5778), 1355-9

Gillam, C. (2015, July 234). *UPDATE 2-u.s. house passes anti-gmo labeling law*. Retrieved from CNBC.com: http://www.cnbc.com/2015/07/23/reuters-america-update-2-us-house-passes-anti-gmo-labeling-law.html

Giraffa, G. (2014). Lactobacillus helveticus: Importance in food and health. *Front Microbiol, 5*(388)doi: 10.3389/fmicb.2014.00338

Glassman, H. A. (2007). Depression and cardiovascular comorbidity. *Dialogues Clin Neurosci., 9*(1), 9-17

Goebel, M., Trebst, A., Steiner, J., Xie, Y., Exton, M., Frede, S., ...Schedlowski, M. (2002). Behavioral conditioning of immunosuppression is possible in humans. *FASEB J., 16*(14), 1869-73

Goldstein, J. (1983). *The experience of insight*. Boston: Shambhala

Goodspeed, D., Liu, J. D., Chehab, E. W., Sheng, Z., Francisco, M., Kliebenstein, D. J., & Braam, J. (2013). Post harvest circadian entrainment enhances crop pest resistance and phytochemical cycling. *Current Biology, 23*, 1235-1241

Google. (2017, May 30). *Gratitude*. Retrieved from Google.com: https://www.google.com/search?q=gratitude&ie=&oe=

Gould, S. (2002). *The structure of evolutionary theory*. Cambridge, MA: Harvard University Press

Gower, B., & Goss, A. (2015). A lower-carbohydrate, higher-fat diet reduces abdominal and intermuscular fat and increases insulin sensitivity in adults at risk of type 2 diabetes. *J Nutr., 145*, 177S-183S. doi:10.3945/jn.114.195065

Graudel, N., Hubeck-Graudel, T., & Jurgens, G. (2011). Effects of low-sodium diet versus high sodium diet on blood pressure, rennin, aldosteronen, catecholamines, cholesterol and triglyceride. *Cochrane Database Syst Rev*, (11), CD004022

Griffin, C. A., Kafadar, K. A., & Paylath, G. K. (2009). MOR23 promotes muscle regeneration and regulates cell adhesion and migration. *Dev Cell., 17*(5), 649-661. doi:10.1016/j.devcel.2009.09.004

Grundy, S., Benjamin, I., Burke, G., . Chai, A., Eckel, R., Howard, B.,...Sowers, J. (1999). Diabetes and cardiovascular disease: A statement for healthcare professional from the American Heart Association. *Circulation.*, *101*(13), 1134-1146. doi:https://doi.org/10.1161/01.CIR.100.10.1134

Gu, X., Karp, P. H., Brody, S. L., Pierce, R. A., Welsh, M. J., Holtzman, M. J., & Ben-Shahar, Y. (2014). Chemosensory functions for pulmonary neuroendocrine cells. *American Journal of Respiratory Cell and Molecular Biology, 50*(3), 637-646

Guallar, E., Stranges, S., Mulrow, C., Appel, L. J., & Miller III, E. R. (2013). Enough is enough: Stop Wasting money on vitamin and mineral supplements. *Annals of Internal Medicine, 159*(12), 850-851

Gunnsteinsdottir, H., & Olafsdottir, K. (Directors). (2016). *Inn saei* [Motion Picture]

Gustavson, C., Garcia, J., Hankins, W., & Rusiniak, K. (1974). Coyote predation control by aversive conditioning. *Science.*, *184*(4136), 581-3. doi: 10.1126/science.184.4136.581

Guyenet, S. (2012). *By 2606 the us diet will be 100% sugar!* Retrieved from wholehealth source.com: http://wholehealthsource.blogspot.com/2012/02/by-2606-us-diet-will-be-100-percent.html

Haffner, S., Lehto, S., Rönnemaa, T., Pyörälä, K., & Laakso, M. (1998). Mortality from coronary heart disease in subjects with type 2 diabetes and in nondiabetic subjects with and without prior myocardial infarction. *N Engl J Med.*, *339*(4), 229-234

Hamblin, J. (2015, July 24). *No one is denying a 'right to know what's in my food'.* Retrieved from www.The Atlantic.com: http://www.theatlantic.com/health/archive/2015/07/no-one-is-denying-a-right-to-know-whats-in-my-food/399536/

Hammond, B., Dudek, R., Lemen, J., & Nemeth, M. (2004). Results of a thirteen week safety assurance study with rats fed grain from glyphosate tolerant corn. *Food Chem Toxicol, 42,*1003-1014

Hancock, G. (2007). *Supernatural: Meetings with the ancient teachers of mankind.* San Franscico, CA: Red Wheel/Weiser, LLC

Harcombe, Baker, J. S., Cooper, S. M., Davies, B., Sculthorpe, N., DiNicolantonio, J. J., & Grace, F. (2015). Evidence from randomised controlled trials did not support the introduction of dietary fat guidelines in 1977 and 1983: A systematic review and meta-analysis. *Open Heart,2*, e000196. doi:10.1136/openhrt-2014-000196

Harcombe, Z., Baker, J., & Davies, B. (2017). Evidence from prospective cohort studies did not support the introduction of dietary fat guidelines in 1977 and 1983: A systematic review. *Br J Sports Med, 51*, 1737-1742

Harner, M. (1987). The ancient wisdom in shamanic cultures. In S. Nicholson (Ed.), *Shamanism*, 3-16. Wheaton, IL: Quest

Harris, J. (2014, November 25). *FDA requires calorie counts for cocktails, theater popcorn, vended food.* Retrieved from Los Angeles Times: http://www.latimes.com/food/dailydish/la-dd-fda-restaurants-bars-vending-machines-display-calorie-counts-20141125-story.html

Harris, W., Miller, M., Tighe, A., Davidson, M., & Schaefer, E. (2008). Omega-3 fatty acids and coronary heart disease risk: Clinical and mechanistic perspectives. *Atherosclerosis, 197*(1), 12-24

Haubrich MD, W. (2005). Sippy of the sippy diet regimen. *Gastroenterology, 128*(4), 832. doi: /10.1053/j.gastro.2005.02.042

Hauser, B. (2017). Get in the sleep zone. *Time: Mindfulness, The New Science of Health and Happiness*, 24-27

Hawkes, C. (2010). The influence of trade liberalisation on global dietary change: The case of vegetable oils, meat and highly processed foods [Chapter 3]. In C. Hawkes, C.

Blouin, S. Henson, N. Drager, & L. Dubé, *Trade, Food, Diet and Health: Perspectives and Policy Options*, 35-59. Oxford, UK: Wiley Blackwell

HealthDay News. (2013, October 16). *Crohn's and colitis may be tied to risk of heart attacks, stroke*. Retrieved from healthday.com: https://consumer.healthday.com/gastrointestinal-information-15/misc-bowel-problems-news-79/crohn-s-and-colitis-may-be-tied-to-risk-of-heart-attack-stroke-681075.html

Heart.org. (2017, March 9). *Low gluten diets may be associated with higher risk of type 2 diabetes*. Retrieved from Heart.org: http://newsroom.heart.org/news/low-gluten-diets-may-be-associated-with-higher-risk-of-type-2-diabetes?preview=f1be

Heid, M. (2016, January 8). *Experts say lobbying skewed the u.s. dietary guidelines*. Retrieved from Time.com: http://time.com/4130043/lobbying-politics-dietary-guidelines/

Helmenstine Ph.D., A. M. (2017, March 24). *How much are the elements in your body worth?* Retrieved from ThoughtCo.com: https://www.thoughtco.com/worth-of-your-elements-3976054

Heritage Foods, USA. (2017). *Heritage pork breed*. Retrieved from Heritage Foods, USA: http://www.heritagefoodsusa.com/porkbreeds.php

Herodotus. (2011, June 3). *Histories II, 2.92*. Retrieved July 30, 2012, from Project Gutenberg: http://www.gutenberg.org/wiki/Egypt_%28Bookshelf%29

Hite, A., Feinman, R., & Guzman, G. (2010). In the face of contradictory evidence: Report of the Dietary guidelines for americans committee. *Nutrition, 26*, 915-24

Hoffman, R., & Gerber, M. (2015). Food processing and the Mediterranean diet. *Nutrients, 7*, 7925-7964. doi: 10.3390/nu7095371

Holroyd, E. W., Sirker, A., Kwok, C. S., Kontopantelis, E., Ludman, P. F., De Belder, M. A.,...Mamas, M. A. (2017). The relationship of body mass index to percutaneous coronary intervention outcomes: Does the obesity paradox exist in contemporary percutaneous coronary intervention cohorts? insights from the british cardiovascular intervention society registry. *JACC: Cardiovascular Interventions*. doi: 10.1016/j.jcin.2017.03.013 .

Homer. (1998). *The Iliad*. (Edited by B. Kniox and R Fagles). New York: Penguin Classics

Høstmark, A., Haug, A., Tomten, S., Thelle, D., & Mosdøl, A. (2009). Serum hdl cholesterol was positively associated with cheese intake in the oslo health study. *J Food Lipids, 16*, 89-102

House Report. (2015, July 16). *House report 114-208—safe and accurate food labeling act of 2015 (parts 1 – 2)*. Retrieved from Congress.gov: https://www.congress.gov/congressional-report/114th-congress/house-report/208/1

Howard, B., Van Horn, L., Hsia, J., Manson, J., Stefanick, M., Wassertheil-Smoller, S.,...Kotchen, J. (2006). Low-fat dietary pattern and risk of cardiovascular disease: The women's health initiative randomized controlled dietary modification trial. *JAMA, 295*, 655-666. doi: 10.1001/jama.295.6.655

Hoyle, F., & Wickramasinehe, N. (1981). *Evolution from space*. New York: Simon & Schuster

Hu, D., Huang, J., Wang, Y., Zhang, D., & Qu, Y. (2014). Fruits and vegetables consumption and risk of stroke: A meta-analysis of prospective cohort studies. *Stroke., 45*, 1613-1619. doi: 10.1161/STROKEAHA.114.004836

Hu, EA, Toledo, E., Diez-Espino, J., Estruch, R., Corella, D.,...Martinez-Gonzalez, M. (2013). Lifestyles and risk factors associated with adherence to the mediterranean diet: A baseline assessment of the predimed trial. *PLoS One, 8*(4), e60166. doi: 10.1371/journal.pone.0060166

Hu, F. (2013). Resolved: There is sufficient scientific evidence that decreasing sugar-sweetened beverage consumption will reduce the prevalence of obesity and obesity-related diseases. *Obes Rev.*, *14*, 606-619. doi:10.1111/obr.12040

Huang, M., Quddus, A., Stinson, L., Shikany, J. M., Howard, B. V., Kutob, R. M.,...Eaton, C. B. (2017). Artificially sweetened beverages, sugar-sweetened beverages, plain water, and incident diabetes mellitus in postmenopausal women. *The Prospective Women's Health Initiative Observational Study*, *106*(2), 614. doi: 10.3945/ajcn.116.145391

Huffington Post. (2011, May 25). *FDA approved: The maximum amount of defects allowed in your food.* Retrieved January 2, 2014, from Huffington Post: http://www.huffingtonpost.com/2010/10/26/fda-approved-rat-hairs-an_n_773608.html#s165326&title=Pizza_Sauce_30

Human Genome Project. (2015, October 1). *All about the human genome project (hgp).* Retrieved from www.genome.gov: https://www.genome.gov/10001772/all-about-the--human-genome-project-hgp/#al-2

Human Microbiome Project. (2017, March 13). *Human microbiome project—Overview.* Retrieved from Human Microbiome Project: http://hmpdacc.org/overview/about.php

Human Microbiome Project Consortium. (2012). Structure, function and diversity of the healthy human microbiome. *Nature*, *486*(7402), 207-14. doi: 10.1038/nature11234

Hurley, T. (1985). Placebo: The hidden asset in healing. *Investigations*, *2*(1)

Huth, C., Thorand, B., Baumert, J., Kruse, J., Emeny, R., Schneider, A.,...Ladwig, K. (2014). Job strain as a risk factor for the onset of type 2 diabetes mellitus: Findings from the MONICA/KORA Augsburg cohort study. *Psychosom Med.*, *76*(7), 562-8. doi: 10.1097/PSY.0000000000000084

Huth, P., Fulgoni, V., Keast, D., Park, K., & Auestad, N. (2013). Major food sources of calories, added sugars, and saturated fat and their contribution to essential nutrient intakes in the U.S. diet: Data from the National Health and Nutrition Examination Survey (2003-2006). *Nutr J*, *12*, 116

IARC. (2015). Carcinogenicity of tetrachlorvinphos, parathion, malathion, diazinon, and glyphosate. *The Lancet Oncology.* doi:10.1016/S1470-2045(15)70134-8

Imamura, F., O'Connor, L., Ye, Z., Mursu, J., Hayashino, Y., Bhupathiraju, S., & Forouhi, N. (2015). Consumption of sugar sweetened beverages, artificially sweetened beverages, and fruit juice and incidence of type 2 diabetes: Systematic review, meta-analysis, and estimation of population attributable fraction. *BMJ*, *351*, h3576

IMDb. (2012). *House md quotes.* Retrieved from IMDb: http://www.imdb.com/title/tt0412142/quotes

IMDb. (2017, March 25). *Quotes for boromir.* Retrieved from IMDb.com: http://www.imdb.com/character/ch0000140/quotes

IMDb. (2017, March 2 29). *Tess trivia.* Retrieved from IMDb.com: http://www.imdb.com/title/tt0080009/trivia

Ingerman, S. (2013). Shamanic intervention in a cardiac rehabilitation program. In C. Carson MD, T. Cowan, B. Horrigan, & J. Stevens, *Spirited medicine: Shamanism in contemporary healthcare*, 159-168). Otter Bay Books

Ingerman, S. (2014). *Walking in light.* Boulder, Colorado: Sounds True, Inc

Ingerman, S., & Wesselman, H. (2010). *Awakening to the spirit world: The shamanic path of direct revelation.* Boulder, Co: Sounds True, Inc

Institute of Medicine. (2001). Dietary reference intakes: Proposed definition of dietary fiber. Washington, DC: Institute of Medicine

Institute of Medicine. (2010). *Evaluation of biomarkers and surrogate endpoints in chronic disease.* Washington, DC: The National Academies Press

Institute of Medicine. (2004). *Safety of genetically modified foods: Approaches to assessing unintended health effects.* Washington, DC: The National Academies Press

Institute of Medicine. (2010). *Promoting cardiovascular health in the developing world: A critical challenge to achieve global health.* Washington, DC: The National Academies Press

Jacobs, D. J., & Tapsell, L. (2007). Food, not nutrients, is the fundamental unit in nutrition. *Nutr Rev.*, *65*, 439-450

Jacobs, D., & Tapsell, L. (2013). Food synergy: the key to a healthy diet. *Proc Nutr Soc.*, *72*, 200-206 doi: 10.1017/S0029665112003011

Jaffiol, C. (2008). Milk and dairy products in the prevention and therapy of obesity, type 2 diabetes and metabolic syndrome. *Bull Acad Natl Med.*, *192*, 749-58

Jakobsen, M., O'Reilly, E., Heitmann, B., Pereira, M., Bälter, K., Fraser, G.,...Ascherio, A. (2009). Major types of dietary fat and risk of coronary heart disease: A pooled analysis of 11 cohort studies. *Am J Clin Nutr.*, *89*:1425-1432. doi: 10.3945/ajcn.2008.27124

Jala, D., Smits, G., Johnson, R., & Conchol, M. (2010). Increased fructose associates with elevated blood pressure. *Journal of the American Society of Nephrology, 21*, 1416-1418

James, D. (2004). Factors influencing food choices, dietary intake, and nutrition-related attitudes among african americans: Application of a culturally sensitive model. *Ethnicity & Health, 9*(4), 349-367

Japanese Food Safety Commission. (2007, June). *Evaluation report of food additives: Polysorbates.* Retrieved from Japanese Food Safety Commission: https://www.fsc.go.jp/english/evaluationreports/foodadditive/polysorbate_report.pdf

Javier, A. C.-N., Vega, F. E., Karaoz, U., Hao, Z., Jenkins, S., Lim, H. C., & Brodie, E. L. (2014). The core gut microbiome of h. hampei specimens collected from multiple coffee-producing countries. *Nature*, doi:10.1038/ncomms8618

Jeffery, I. B., Claesson, M. J., & Shanahan, F. (2012). Categorization of the gut microbiota: Enterotypes or gradients? *Nat. Rev. Microbiol.*, *10*, 591-592

Johnson, S. R., Strom, S., & Grillo, K. (2007). *Quantification of the impacts on us agriculture of biotechnology-derived crops planted in 2006: Executive summary.* Washington, DC: National Center for Food and Agricultural Policy

Jones, A. Z. (2016, August 22). *Question: what is quantum entanglement?* Retrieved from Thoughtco.com: https://www.thoughtco.com/what-is-quantum-entanglement-2699355

Jones, K., Eller, L., Parnell, J., Doyle-Baker, P., Edwards, A., & Reimer, R. (2013). Effect of a dairy- and calcium-rich diet on weight loss and appetite during energy restriction in overweight and obese adults: A randomized trial. *Eur J Clin Nutr, 67*, 371-6

Jones, M., Martoni, C., & Prakash, S. (2012). Cholesterol lowering and inhibition ofsterol absorption by lactobacillus reuteri ncimb 30242: A randomized controlled trial. . *Eur J Clin Nutr.*, *66*(11), 1234-41

Jones, M., Martoni, C., Parent, M., & Prakash, S. (2012). Cholesterol-lowering efficacy of a microencapsulated bile salt hydrolase-active Lactobacillus reuteri ncimb 30242 yoghurt formulation in hypercholesterolaemic adults. *Br J Nutr.*, *107*(10), 1505-13

Jones, P., Senanayake, V., Pu, S., Jenkins, D., Connelly, P., Lamarche, B.,...Kris-Etherton, P. (2014). DHA-enriched high-oleic acid canola oil improves lipid profile and lowers predicted cardiovascular disease risk in the canola oil multicenter randomized controlled trial. *Am J Clin Nutr.*, *100*, 88-97. doi: 10.3945/ajcn.113.081133

Jung, S., Lee, K., Kang, J., Yun, S., Park, H., Moon, Y., & Kim, J. (2013). Effect of lactobacillus gasseri bnr17 on overweight and obese adults: A randomized double-blind clinical trial. *Korean J Fam Med.*, *34*, 80-89. doi:10.4082/kjfm.2013.34.2.80

Kaddurah-Daouk, R., Baillie, R., Zhu, H., Zeng, Z.-B., Wiest, M., Nguyen, U.,...Krauss, R. (2011). Enteric microbiome metabolites correlate with response to simvastatin treatment. *PLoS One.*, *6*(10), e25482

Kadooka, Y., Sato, M., Imaizumi, K., Ogawa, A., Ikuyama, K., Akai, Y.,...Tsuchida, T. (2010). Regulation of abdominal adiposity by probiotics (lactobacillus gasseri SBT2055) in adults with obese tendencies in a randomized controlled trial. *Eur J Clin Nutr.*, *64*:636-643

Kadooka, Y., Sato, M., Ogawa, A., Miyoshi, M., Uenishi, H., Ogawa, H.,...Tsuchida, T. (2013). Effect of lactobacillus gasseri SBT2055 in fermented milk on abdominal adiposity in adults in a randomised controlled trial. *Br J Nutr.*, *110*, 1696-1703. doi: 10.1017/S0007114513001037

Kalantarian, S., Rimm, E., Herrington, D., & Mozaffarian, D. (2014). Dietary macronutrients genetic variation, and progression of coronary atherosclerosis among women. *Am Heart J.*, *167*, 627-635.e1. doi: 10.1016/j.ahj.2014.01.001

Kamps, L. (2017). What gratitude can do for you. *Time: Mindfulness: The New Science of Health and Happiness*, 54-57

Kaplan, H., Thompson, R. C., Trumble, B. C., Wann, L. S., Allam, A. H., Beheim, B.,...Thomas, G. S. (2017). Coronary atherosclerosis in indigenous South American Tsimane: A cross-sectional cohort study. *The Lancet.* doi: 10.1016/S0140-6736(17)30752-3

Kaptoge, S., Seshasai, S., Gao, P., Freitag, D., Butterworth, A., Borglykke, A.,...Lowe, G. (2014). Inflammatory cytokines and risk of coronary heart disease: new prospective study and updated meta-analysis. *Eur Heart J*, *35*, 578-89

Karaki, S., Tazoe, H., Hayashi, H., Kashiwabara, H., Tooyama, K., Suzuki, Y., & Kuwahara, A. (2008). Expression of the short-chain fatty acid receptor, gpr43, in the human colon. *J. Mol Histol*, *39*, 135-142

Karlsson, F. H., Fåk, F., Nookaew, I., Tremaroli, V., Fagerberg, B., Petranovic, D.,...Nielsen, J. (2012). Symptomatic atherosclerosis is associated with an altered gut metagenome. *Nature*, *2265*. doi: 10.1038/ncomms2266

Karlsson, F., Tremaroli, V., Nookaew, I., Bergstrom, G., Behre, C., Fagerberg, B.,...Backhed, F. (2013). Gut metagenome in european women with normal, impaired and diabetic glucose control. *Nature*, *498*, 99-103

Kassinen, A., Krogiuss-Kurikka, L., Makivuokko, H., Rinttila, T., Paulin, L., Corander, J.,...Pavla, A. (2007). The fecal microbiota of irritable bowel syndrome patients differs significantly from that of healthy subjects. *GASTROENTEROLOGY, 133*, 24-33

Kelly, L., & Kelly, H. B. (2016). *The healthy bones nutrition plan and cookbook.* White River Junction, Vermont: Chelsea Green Publishing

Kempner, W. (1949). Treatment of heart and kidney disease and of hypertensive and arteriosclerotic vascular disease with the rice diet. *Ann Intern Med.*, *31*(5), 821-856

Kennedy, P. J., Cryan, J. F., Dinan, T. G., & Clarke, G. (2014). Irritable bowel syndrome: A microbiome-gut-brain axis disorder? *World J Gastroenterol*, *20*(39): 14105-14125. doi: 10.3748/wjg.v20.i39.14105

Keys, A. (1970). Coronary heart disease in seven countries. I. The study program and objectives. *Circulation*, *41*(4 Suppl), I1-8

Keys, A. (1970). Coronary heart disease in seven countries. Summary. *Circulation*, *41*(4 Suppl), I186-95

Keys, A. (1971). Sucrose in the diet and coronary heart disease. *Atherosclerosis*, *14*(2), 193-202

Keys, A. (1975). Coronary heart disease—The global picture. *Atherosclerosis*, *22*(2), 149-192

Keys, A. (1980). *Seven countries: A multivariate analysis of death and coronary heart disease.* London: Harvard University Press.

Keys, A., Aravanis, C., Blackburn, H., Van Buchem, F., Buzina, R., Djordjević, B.,...Taylor, H. (1966). Epidemiological studies related to coronary heart disease: Characteristics of men aged 40-59 in seven countries. *Acta Med Scand Suppl., 460,* 1-392

Keys, A., Taylor, H., Blackburn, H., Brozek, J., Anderson, J., & Simonson, E. (1963). Coronary heart disease among Minnesota business and professional men followed 15 years. *Circulation, 28,* 381-95

Khaneja, R., Perez-Fons, L., Fakhry, S., Baccigalupi, L., Steiger, S., & To, E. (2010). Carotenoids found in bacillus. *Journal of Applied Microbiology, 108*(6), 1889-902

Khaw, K., Friesen, M., Riboli, E., Luben, R., & Wareham, N. (2012). Plasma phospholipid fatty acid concentration and incident coronary heart disease in men and women: The epic-norfolk prospective study. *PLoS Med, 9,* e1001255. doi: 10.1371/journal.pmed.1001255

Khera, A., Emdin, C., & Drake, I. (2016). Genetic risk, adherence to a healthy lifestyle, and coronary disease. *New Engl J Med, 375,* 2349-58

Kim, Y., Keogh, J., & Clifton, P. (2015). A review of potential metabolic etiologies of the observed association between red meat consumption and development of type 2 diabetes mellitus. *Metabolism., 64,* 768-779. doi:10.1016/j.metabol.2015.03.008

Kiran Krishnan, P. o. (2017, March 15). Gut check! Health, wellness and your gut microbiome. (M. Michael S. Fenster, Interviewer)

Klopfer, B. (1957). Psychological variables in human cancer. *Journal of Projective Techniques, 21,* 337-339.

Knight, J. (1998, January 14). *Deer need a little "tough love" in winter.* Retrieved from Montana State University Communication Services: http://www.montana.edu/cpa/news/wwwpb-archives/reso/toughlov.html

Knowler, W., Barrett-Connor, E., Fowler, S., & Group, t. D. (2002). Reduction in the incidence of type 2 diabetes with lifestyle intervention or metformin. *N Engl J Med., 346*(6), 393-403. doi: 10.1056/NEJMoa012512

Koestler, A. (1964). *The act of creation.* London: Hutchinson and company

Koeth, R. A., Wang, Z., Levison, B. S., Buffa, J. A., Org, E., Sheehy, B. T., & Warrier, M. (2013). Intestinal microbiota metabolism of lcarnitine, a nutrient in red meat, promotes atherosclerosis. *Nat. Med., 19,* 576-585

Koeth, R., Wang, Z., Levison, B., Buffa, J., Org, E., Sheehy, B.,...Li, L. (2013). Intestinal microbiota metabolism of l-carnitine, a nutrient in red meat, promotes atherosclerosis. *Nat Med., 19*(5), 576-85

Koletzko, B., Mrotzek, M., & Bremer, H. (1988). Fatty acid composition of mature human milk in Germany. *Am J Clin Nutr., 47*(6), 954-9

Konety, S., Horwitz, P., Lindower, P., & Olshansky, B. (2007). Arrhythmias in tako-tsubo syndrome—benign or malignant? *Int J Cardiol, 114,* 141-144

Kong, L., Holmes, B., Cotillard, A., Habi-Rachedi, F., Brazeilles, R., Gougis, S., & Clement, K. (2014). Dietary patterns differently associate with inflammation and gut microbiota in overweight and obese subjects. *PLoS ONE, 9,* e109434

Korem, T., Zeevi, D., Zmora, N., Weissbrod, O., Bar, N., Lotan-Pompan, M.,...Segal, E. (2017). Bread affects clinical parameters and induces gut microbiome-associated personal glycemic responses. *Cell Metabolism, 25,* 1243-1253. doi:10.1016/j.cmet.2017.05.002

Koren, O., Spora, A., Felin, J., Fåkb, Frida, S. J., Tremaroli, V.,...Bäckhed, F. (2011). Human oral, gut, and plaque microbiota in patients with atherosclerosis. *Proc. Natl Acad. Sci. USA, 108*, S4592-S4598

Koulivand, P. H., Ghadiri, M. K., & Gorji, A. (2013). Lavender and the nervous system. *Evidence-Based Complementary and Alternative Medicine*. doi: 10.1155/2013/681304

Kovacs, J. S. (2007, February 13). *Diets of the world: The japanese die*. Retrieved from Web MD: http://www.webmd.com/diet/diets-of-world-japanese-diet

Kratz, M., Baars, T., & Guyenet, S. (2013). The relationship between high-fat dairy consumption and obesity, cardiovascular, and metabolic disease. *Eur J Nutr., 52*, 1-24. doi: 10.1007/s00394-012-0418-1

Kratz, M., Marcovina, S., Nelson, J., Yeh, M., Kowdley, K., Callahan, H.,...Utzschneider, K. (2014). Dairy fat intake is associated with glucose tolerance, hepatic and systemic insulin sensitivity, and liver fat but not β-cell function in humans. *Am J Clin Nutr., 99*, 1385-1396. doi:10.3945/ajcn.113.075457

Kris-Etherton, P., Harris, W., & Appel, L. (2002). Fish Consumption, Fish Oil, Omega-3 Fatty Acids, and Cardiovascular Disease. *Circulation, 106*, 2747-2757.

Krishnan, K. (2017, March 15). Microbiome breakthroughs. (M. Fenster, Interviewer.) Retrieved from: http://radiomd.com/show/code-delicious/item/34950-microbiome-breakthroughs

Krishnan, K. (2017, October 11). Code delicious with dr. mike. (D. Mike, Interviewer)

Krishnan, K. (2017, March 15). The gut microbiome on code delicious with dr. mike. (M. Michael S. Fenster, Interviewer)

Kurtus, R. (2017, June 10). *Four noble truths of buddhism*. Retrieved from School for Champions:http://www.school-for-champions.com/religion/buddhism_four_noble_truths.htm#.WYXTFYWcF9A

Kuznar, W. (2015, March 30). *Chronic inflammation may stiffen arteries in psa*. Retrieved from Med Page Today: http://www.medpagetoday.com/Rheumatology/Arthritis/50712

Laaksonen, D., Lindström, J., Lakka, T., Eriksson, J., Niskanen, L., Wikström, K.,... Härkönen, P. (2005). Finnish diabetes prevention study. Physical activity in the prevention of type 2 diabetes: The Finnish diabetes prevention study. *Diabetes., 54*(1), 158-165. doi: 10.2337/diabetes.54.1.158

Labonté, M., Couture, P., Richard, C., Desroches, S., & Lamarche, B. (2013). Impact of dairy products on biomarkers of inflammation: a systematic review of randomized controlled nutritional intervention studies in overweight and obese adults. *Am J Clin Nutr, 97*, 706-17

Labonté, M., Cyr, A., Abdullah, M., Lepine, M., Vohl, M., Jones, P.,...Lamarche, B. (2014). Dairy product consumption has no impact on biomarkers of inflammation among men and women with lowgrade systemic inflammation. *J Nutr, 144*(11), 1760-7

Ladwig, K.-H., Baumert, J., Marten-Mittag, B., Lukaschek, K., Johar, H., Fang, X.,... Investigators, T.K. (2017). Room for depressed and exhausted mood as a risk predictor for all-cause and cardiovascular mortality beyond the contribution of the classical somatic risk factors in men. *Atherosclerosis, 257*, 224-231 doi: 10.1016/j.atherosclerosis.2016.12.003

Lamarche B, C. P. (2014). It is time to revisit current dietary recommendations for saturated fat. *Appl Physiol Nutr Metab, 39*(12), 1409-11

Lamarche, B., & Lewis, G. (1998). Atherosclerosis prevention for the next decade: Risk assessment beyond low density lipoprotein cholesterol. *Can J Cardiol, 14*, 841-51

Lambelet, P., Grandgirard, A., Gregoire, S., Juaneda, P., Sebedio, J., & Bertoli, C. (2003). Formation of modified fatty acids and oxyphytosterols during refining of low erucic acid rapeseed oil. *J Agric Food Chem.*, *51*, 4284-4290. doi: 10.1021/jf030091u

Landers, T. F., Cohen, B., Wittum, T. E., & Larson, E. L. (2012). A review of antibiotic use in food animals: Perspective, policy, and potential. *Public Health Rep.*, *127*(1), 4-22

Laparra, J., & Sanz, Y. (2010). Interactions of gut microbiota with functional food components and nutraceuticals. *Pharmacol Res.*, *61*(3), 219-25

Larsson, S. C., Orsini, N., & Wolk, A. (2011). Dietary potassium intake and risk of stroke: A dose-response meta-analysis of prospective studies. *Stroke.* doi: 10.1161/STROKEAHA.111.622142

Larsson, S. C., Virtamo, J., & Wolk, A. (2011). Red meat consumption and risk of stroke in Swedish men. *Am J Clin Nutr, 94*, 417-421

Larsson, S., Bergkvist, L., & Wolk, A. (2005). High-fat dairy food and conjugated linoleic acid intakes in relation to colorectal cancer incidence in the Swedish Mammography Cohort. *Am J Clin Nutr, 82*, 894-900

Larsson, S., Orsini, N., & Wolk, A. (2012). Long-chain omega-3 polyunsaturated fatty acids and risk of stroke: A meta-analysis. *Eur J Epidemiol., 27*, 895-901. doi: 10.1007/s10654-012-9748-9

Lathers, C. (2002). Clinical pharmacology of antimicrobial use in humans and animals. *J Clin Pharmacol., 42*(6), 587-600

Lê, K., & Bortolotti, M. (2008). Role of dietary carbohydrates and macronutrients in the pathogenesis of nonalcoholic fatty liver disease. *Curr Opin Clin Nutr Metab Care., 11*, 477-482. doi: 10.1097/MCO.0b013e328302f3ec

Leamy, E. (2012, February 7). *Companies not telling the whole truth about whole grains.* Retrieved from ABC News.com: http://abcnews.go.com/blogs/health/2012/02/07/companies-not-telling-the-whole-truth-about-whole-grains/

Lebwohl, B., Ludvigsson, J. F., & Green, P. H. (2015). Celiac disease and non-celiac gluten sensitivity. *BMJ, 351*, h4347. doi: 10.1136/bmj.h4347

Lecerf, J., & de Lorgeril, M. (2011). Dietary cholesterol from physiology to cardiovascular risk. *Br J Nutr, 106*(1), 6-14

LeChatelier, E., Nielsen, T., Qin, J., Prifti, E., Hildebrand, F., Falony, G., & . Pons, H. (2013). Richness of human gut microbiome correlates with metabolic markers. *Nature, 500*, 541-546

Legrand, P., & Rioux, V. (2010). The complex and important cellular and metabolic functions of saturated fatty acids. *Lipids, 45*, 941-6

Leiber, F., Kreuzer, M., Nigg, D., Wettstein, H., & Scheeder, M. (2005). A study on the causes for the elevated n-3 fatty acids in cows' milk of alpine origin. *Lipids, 40*, 191-202

Leiter, L., Fitchett, D., Gilbert, R., Gupta, M., Mancini, G., McFarlane, P.,...Anand, S. (2011). Cardiometabolic risk in Canada: A detailed analysis and position paper by the cardiometabolic risk working group. *Can J Cardiol, 27*, e1-33

Lennerz, B., Alsop, D., Holsen, L., Stern, E., Rojas, R., Ebbeling, C.,...Ludwig, D. (2013). Effects of dietary glycemic index on brain regions related to reward and craving in men. *Am J Clin Nutr, 98*, 641-647. doi: 10.3945/ajcn.113.064113

Leon, M. B., Kornowski, R., Downey, W. E., Weisz, G., Baim, D. S., Bonow, R. O.,... Kuntz, R. E. (2005). A blinded, randomized, placebo-controlled trial of percutaneous laser myocardial revascularization to improve angina symptoms in patients with severe coronary disease. *JACC, 46*(10), 1812-1819. doi:10.1016/j.jacc.2005.06.079

Leung Yinko, S., Stark, K., Thanassoulis, G., & Pilote, L. (2014). Fish consumption and acute coronary syndrome: A meta-analysis. *Am J Med.*, *127*, 848-57.e2. doi: 10.1016/j.amjmed.2014.04.016

Levy, N. (2014, October 1). *The young doctor.* Retrieved from Capitalnewyork.com: http:// www.capitalnewyork.com/article/media/2014/10/8553422/young-doctor

Lewsi, C. E., McTigue, K., Burke, L. E., Poirier, P., Eckel, R. H., Howard, B. V.,...Pi-Sunyer, F. X. (2011, June 8). *Mortality, health outcomes, and body mass index in the overweight range: A science advisory from the american heart association.* Retrieved October 7, 2011, from *Circulation*: American Heart Association: http://circ.ahajournals.org/ content/early/2009/06/08/CIRCULATIONAHA.109.192574.full.pdf+html

Ley, R., Turnbaugh, P., Klein, S., & Gordon, J. (2006). Microbial ecology: Human gut microbes associated with obesity. *Nature*, *444*, 1022-1023

Li, K., Kaaks, R., Linseisen, J., & Rohrmann, S. (2012). Associations of dietary calcium intake and calcium supplementation with myocardial infarction and stroke risk and overall cardiovascular mortality in the Heidelberg cohort of the european prospective investigation into cancer and nutrition study (EPIC-Hei). *Heart.*, *98*, 920-925

Li, L., Li, X., Zhou, W., & Messina, J. (2013). Acute psychological stress results in the rapid development of insulin resistance. *J Endocrinol*, *217*, 175-184

Li, M., Fan, Y., Zhang, X., Hou, W., & Tang, Z. (2014). Fruit and vegetable intake and risk of type 2 diabetes mellitus: Meta-analysis of prospective cohort studies. *BMJ Open*, *4*, e005497. doi: 10.1136/bmjopen-2014-005497

Li, Q., Kobayashi, M., Wakayama, Y., Inagaki, H., Katsumata, M., Hirata, Y.,...Miyazaki, Y. (2009). Effect of phytoncide from trees on human natural killer cell function. *Int J Immunopathol Pharmacol.*, *22*(4), 951-9

Libby, P., Ridker, P., & Hansson, G. (2009). Inflammation in atherosclerosis: From patho-physiology to practice. *J Am Coll Cardiol*, *54*, 2129-38

Lim, S., Vos, T., Flaxman, A., Danaci, G., Shibuya, K., Adair-Rohani, H.,...Memish, Z. (2012). A comparative risk assessment of burden of disease and injury attributable to 67 risk factors and risk factor clusters in 21 regions, 1990-2010: A systematic analysis for the Global Burden of Disease Study 2010. *Lancet*, *380*, 2224-2260. doi: 10.1016/ S0140-6736(12)61766-8

Lin, H., Frassetto, A., Kowalik, J. E., Nawrocki, A., Lu, M., Kosinski, J.,...Forrest, G. (2012). Butyrate and propionate protect against diet-induced obesity and regulate gut hormones via free fatty acid receptor 3-independent mechanisms. *PLoS One.*, *7*(4), e35240

Lindström, J., Peltonen, M., & Tuomilehto, J. (2005). Lifestyle strategies for weight con-trol: experience from the Finnish diabetes prevention study. *Proc Nutr Soc.*, *64*(1), 81-88. doi: doi: 10.1079/PNS2004394412

Lippi, G., Danese, E., Mattiuzzi, C., & F. J. (2017). The intriguing link between the intestinal microbiota and cardiovascular disease. *Semin Thromb Hemost*, doi: 10.1055/s-0036-1597903

Livni, E. (2016, October 12). *The japanese practice of 'forest bathing' is scientifically proven to improve your health.*

Lombardi, L. (2017). Being here. *Time: Mindfulness, The New Science of Health and Happiness*, 4-5

Lonn, E., Bosch, J., Lopez-Jaramillo, P., & Investigators, T. H.-3. (2016). Blood pressure lowering in intermediate-risk persons without cardiovascular disease. *New England Journal of Medicine.* doi: 10.1056/NEJMoa1600177

Loscalzo, J. (2013). Gut microbiota, the genome, and diet in atherogenesis. *New England Journal of Medicine, 368*(17): 1647-1649

Lou-Bonafonte, J., Gabás-Rivera, C., Navarro, M., & Osada, J. (2015). Pon1 and mediterranean diet. *Nutrients, 7*, 4068-4092. doi: 10.3390/nu7064068

Louve, R. (2005). *Last child in the woods: saving our children from nature-deficit disorder.* Chapel Hill, NC: Algonquin Books of Chapel Hill

Louzada, M., Baraldi, L., Steele, E., Martins, A., Canella, D., Moubarac, J.,...Monteiro, C. (2015). Consumption of ultra-processed foods and obesity in Brazilian adolescents and adults. *Prev Med., 81*, 9-15. doi:10.1016/j.ypmed.2015.07.018

Lucan, S. C. (2012). That it's red? Or what it was fed/How it was bred? The risk of meat. *The American Journal of Clinical Nutrition, 96*, 446

Ludwig, D., & Friedman, M. (2014). Increasing adiposity: Consequence or cause of overeating? *JAMA., 311*, 2167-2168. doi: 10.1001/jama.2014.4133

Luft, F. C., Fineberg, N. S., & Sloan, R. S. (1982). Estimating dietary sodium intake in individuals recieving a randomly fluctuating intake. *HTN, 4*, 805-808

Maimonides. (2017). *Maimonides quotes.* Retrieved from Brainyquote.com: https://www.brainyquote.com/quotes/quotes/m/maimonides326756.html

Main, D. (2017, June 26). *Monsanto weed-killer roundup causes cancer, says california.* Retrieved from Newsweek.com: http://www.newsweek.com/monsanto-week-killerroundup-causes-cancer-california-629227

Maine.gov. (2013). *Supplemental feeding of white-tailed deer during winter.* Retrieved from Maine. Gov Departmant of Inland Fisheries and Wildlife: http://www.maine.gov/ifw/wildlife/species/mammals/feeding_deer.html

Malhotra, A. (2013). Saturated fat is not the major issue. *BMJ, 347*

Malik, V., & Hu, F. (2015). Fructose and cardiometabolic health: What the evidence from sugar-sweetened beverages tells us. *J Am Coll Cardiol., 66*, 1615-1624. doi: 10.1016/j.jacc.2015.08.025

Mandrola MD, J. (2016, June 23). *Could ablation for af be an elaborate placebo?* Retrieved from Medscape.com: http://www.medscape.com/viewarticle/865209?pa=v6hk%2BztCXCHslB1Ya2ZubOLJeBbko42Njr8F2oQRji9lWI%2FrL29%2Fjfew04VX8B-macFrqow%2Bf2%2F37XuRaZT6JAA%3D%3D

Mao, P., Zhang, C., Tang, L., Xian, Y., Li, Y., Wang, W.,...Zhou, Y. (2013). Effect of calcium or vitamin D supplementation on vascular outcomes: A meta-analysis of randomized controlled trials. *Int J Cardiol., 169*, 106-111. doi: 10.1016/j.ijcard.2013.08.055

Maron, D. F. (2015, February 25). *Emulsifiers in food linked to obesity in mice.* Retrieved from Scientific American.com: http://www.scientificamerican.com/podcast/episode/emulsifiers-in-food-linked-to-obesity-in-mice/

Martínez Steele, E., Baraldi, L. G., da Costa Louzada, M. L., Moubarac, J.-C., Mozaffarian, D., & Monteiro, C.A. (2016). Ultra-processed foods and added sugars in the US diet: Evidence from a nationally representative cross-sectional study. *BMJ Open, 6*, 3-e009892. doi: 10.1136/bmjopen-2015-009892

Martínez-González, M. A., Salas-Salvadó, J., Estruch, R., Corella, D., Fitó, M., & Ros, E. (2015). Benefits of the mediterranean diet: Insights from the predimed study. *Progress in Cardiovascular Disease, 58*(1), 50-60 doi: 10.1016/j.pcad.2015.04.003

Maslow, A. (1971). *The farther reaches of human nature.* New York: Viking

Mason, S. (2013, July 20). *UCLA researchers find link between intestinal bacteria and white blood cell cancer.* Retrieved from newsroom, UCLA EDU: http://newsroom.ucla.edu/releases/ucla-researchers-find-link-between-245945

Maurer, D. (2017, April 18). *Waters and bourdain: The great hot dog debate.* Retrieved from Grubstreet.com: http://www.grubstreet.com/2009/05/waters_and_bourdain_the_great.html

McAuliff, M. (2015, July 23). *House votes to ban states from labeling gmo foods.* Retrieved from HuffingtonPost.com: http://www.huffingtonpost.com/entry/gmo-labels-food_55b12fabe4b08f57d5d3f393

McClelland, R. L., Chung, H., Detrano, R., Post, W., & Kronmal, R. A. (2006). Distribution of coronary artery calcium by race, gender, and age: Results from the multi-ethnic study of atherosclerosis (MESA). *Circulation, 113*, 30-3

McFarlin, B. K., Henning, A. L., Bowman, E. M., Gary, M. A., & Carbajal, K. M. (2017). Oral spore-based probiotic supplementation was associated with reduced incidence of post-prandial dietary endotoxin, triglycerides, and disease risk biomarkers. *World Journal of Gastrointestinal Pathophysiology, 8*(3), 117-126

Medicinenet.com. (2017, May 30). *http://www.medicinenet.com/script/main/art.asp?articlekey=31481.* Retrieved from medicinenet.com: http://www.medicinenet.com/script/main/art.asp?articlekey=31481

Mellen, P., Walsh, T., & Herrington, D. (2008). Whole grain intake and cardiovascular disease: A meta-analysis. *Nutr Metab Cardiovasc Dis., 18*, 283-290. doi: 10.1016/j.numecd.2006.12.008

Mennella, J. A. (2006). Development of food preferences: Lessons learned from longitudinal and experimental studies. *Food Qual Prefer., 17*(7-8), 635-637 doi:10.1016/j.foodqual.2006.01.008

Mensink, R., Zock, P., Kestor, A., & Katan, M. (2003). Effects of dietary fatty acids and carbohydrates on the ratio of serum total to hdl cholesterol and on serum lipids and apolipoproteins: A meta-analysis of 60 controlled trials. *Am J Clin Nutr, 77*, 1146-1155

Mente, A., de Koning, L., Shannon, H., & Anand, S. (2009). A systematic review of the evidence supporting a causal link between dietary factors and coronary heart disease. *Arch Intern Med., 169*, 659-669. doi: 10.1001/archinternmed.2009.38

Mente, A., Dehghan, M., Rangarajan, S., McQueen, M., Dagenais, G., Wielgosz, A.,... Yusuf, S. (2017). Association of dietary nutrients with blood lipids and blood pressure in 18 countries: A cross-sectional analysis from the pure study. *The Lancet*, doi: 10.1016/S2213-8587(17)30283-8

Mente, A., O'Donnell, M., Rangarajan, S., Dagenais, G., Lear, S., McQueen, M.,...Yusuf, S. (2016). Associations of urinary sodium excretion with cardiovascular events in individuals with and without hypertension: A polled ananlysis of data from four studies. *The Lancet*, doi: 10.1016/50140-6736(16)30467-6

Merriam-Webster. (2017, July 21). *Nocebo.* Retrieved from Merriam-Webster Dictionary: https://www.merriam-webster.com/dictionary/nocebo

Mesnager, R., Defarge, N., Spiroux De Vendomois, J., & Seralini, G. (2014). Major pesticides are more toxic to human cells and their declared active principles. *Biomed Res Int*, article ID 179691

Micha, R., & Mozaffarian, D. (2010). Saturated fat and cardiometabolic risk factors coronary heart disease, stroke, and diabetes: A fresh look at the evidence. *Lipids, 45*, 893-905. doi: 10.1007/s11745-010-3393-4

Micha, R., Afshin, A., Khatibzadeh, S., & Mozaffarian, D. (2014). Consumption of nuts and legumes and risk of incident ischemic heart disease, stroke and diabetes: A systematic review and meta-analysis. *Am J Clin Nutr., 100*, 278-288. doi: 10.3945/ajcn.113.076901

Micha, R., Michas, G., Lajous, M., & Mozaffarian, D. (2013). Processing of meats and cardiovascular risk: Time to focus on preservatives. *BMC Med, 11*, 136. doi: 10.1186/1741-7015-11-136

Micha, R., Peñalvo, J. L., Cudhea, F., Imamura, F., Rehm, C. D., & Mozaffarian, D. (2017). association between dietary factors and mortality from heart disease, stroke, and type 2 diabetes in the united states. *JAMA, 317*(9), 913-924

Micha, R., Wallace, S. K., & Mozaffarian, D. (2010). Red and processed meat consumption and risk of incident coronary heart disease, stroke, and diabetes: A systematic review and meta-analysis. *Circulation, 121*(21), 2271-2283. doi: 10.1161/CIRCULATIONAHA.109.924977

Michigan.gov. (2017). *Corn toxicity in ruminants (deer & elk)*. Retrieved from Michigan Department of Natural Resources: http://www.michigan.gov/dnr/0,4570,7-153-10370_12150_12220-26508--,00.html

Mickelborough, T., Gotshall, R., Kluka, E., Miller, C., & Cordain, L. (2001). Dietary chloride as a possible determinant of the severity of exercise induced asthma. *European Journal of Applied Physiology, 85*, 450-456

Miller, V., Mente, A., Dehghan, M., Rangarajan, S., Zhang, X., Swaminathan, S.,... Yusuf, S. (2017). Fruit, vegetable, and legume intake, and cardiovascular disease and deaths in 18 countries (pure): A prospective cohort study. *The Lancet*, doi: 10.1016/S0140-6736(17)32253-5

Missimer, A., DiMarco, D. M., Andersen, C. J., Murillo, A. G., V.-J. M., & Fernandez, M. L. (2017). Consuming two eggs per day, as compared to an oatmeal breakfast, decreases plasma ghrelin while maintaining the ldl/hdl ratio. *Nutrients, 9*(2), 89. doi: 10.3390/nu9020089

Mithril, C., Dragsted, L., & Meyer, C. (2012). Dietary composition and nutrient content of the new nordic diet. *Public Health Nutrition, 16*, 777-785

Mitrou, P., Kipnis, V., & Thiébaut, A. (2007). Mediterranean dietary pattern and prediction of all-cause mortality in a u.s. population. *Archives of Internal Medicine, 167*, 2461

Monteiro, C. A., Moubarac, J.-C., Cannon, G., Ng, S. W., & Popkin, B. (2013). Ultraprocessed products are becoming dominant in the global food system. *Obesity review, 14*(Suppl. 2), 21-28. doi: 10.1111/obr.12107

Monteiro, C., & Cannon, G. (2012). The impact of transnational 'Big Food' companies on the South: A view from Brazil. *PLoS Med, 9*, e1001252

Monteiro, C., Gomes, F., & Cannon, G. (2010). Can the food industry help tackle the growing burden of under-nutrition? The snack attack. *Am J Public Health, 100*, 975-981

Montmayeur, J.-P., & le Coutre, J. (2009). *Fat detection: Taste, texture, and post ingestive effects*. Boca Raton, FL: CRC Press

Montonen, J., Jarvinen, R., Knekt, P., Heliovaara, M., & Reunanen, A. (2007). Consumption of sweetened beverages and intakes of fructose and glucose predict type ii diabetes occurrence. *J Nutr, 137*, 1447-1454

Moodie, R., Stuckler, D., & Monteiro, C. (2013). Profits and pandemics: Prevention of harmful effects of tobacco, alcohol, and ultraprocessed. *Lancet, 381*, 670-679

Morris, M. C., Tangney, C. C., Wang, Y., Sacks, F. M., Bennett, D. A., & Aggarwal, N. T. (2015). MIND diet associated with reduced incidence of alzheimer's disease. *Alzheimer's and Dementia*, S1552-5260(15)00017-5. doi: 10.1016/j.jalz.2014.11.009

Morris, R., Sebastian, A., Forman, A., Tanaka, M., & Schmidlin, O. (1999). Normotensive salt sensitivity: Effects of race and dietary potassium. *Hypertension, 33*, 18-23

Mosca, L., Manson, J. E., Sutherland, S. E., Langer, R. D., Manolio, T., & Barrett-Connor, E. (1997). Cardiovascular disease in women: A statement for healthcare professionals from the american heart association. *Circulation, 96*, 2468-2482. doi: 10.1161/01. CIR.96.7.2468

Mozaffarian, D. (2008). Fish and and-3 fatty acids for the prevention of fatal coronary heart disease and sudden cardiac death. *Am J Clin Nutr, 87*, 1991S-1996S

Mozaffarian, D. (2009). Meat intake and mortality: Evidence for harm, no effect or benefit? *Arch Intern Med., 169*, 1537-1538

Mozaffarian, D. (2014). Nutrition and cardiovascular disease and metabolic diseases. In D. Mann, D. Zipes, P. Libby, & R. Bonow, *Braunwald's Heart Disease: A Textbook of Cardiovascular Medicine, 10th ed.* (1001-1014.). Philadelphia, PA: Elsevier/Saunders

Mozaffarian, D. (2015). Diverging global trends in heart disease and type 2 diabetes: The role of carbohydrates and saturated fats. *Lancet Diabetes Endocrinol., 3*, 586-588

Mozaffarian, D. (2015). Natural trans fat, dairy fat, partially hydrogenated oils, and cardiometabolic health: The ludwigshafen risk and cardiovascular health study. *Eur Heart J.*, doi: 10.1093/eurheartj/ehv595

Mozaffarian, D. (2016). Dietary and policy priorities for cardiovascular disease, diabetes, and obesity, a comprehensive review. *Circulation, 133*, 187-225 doi: 10.1161/ CIRCULATIONAHA.115.018585

Mozaffarian, D., & Ludwig, D. (2015). Dietary cholesterol and blood cholesterol concentrations-reply. *JAMA, 314*, 2084-2085

Mozaffarian, D., & Ludwig, D. (2010). Dietary guidelines in the 21st centurya time for food. *JAMA, 304*, 681-682. doi: 10.1001/jama.2010.1116

Mozaffarian, D., & Ludwig, D. (2015). The 2015 us dietary guidelines: Lifting the ban on total dietary fat. *JAMA, 313*, 2421-2

Mozaffarian, D., & Rimm, E. (2006). Fish intake, contaminants, and human health: Evaluating the risks and the benefits. *JAMA, 296*,1885-1899. doi:10.1001/ jama.296.15.1885

Mozaffarian, D., Appel, L., & Van Horn, L. (2011). Components of a cardioprotective diet: New insights. *Circulation, 123*, 2870-2891. doi: 10.1161/ CIRCULATIONAHA.110.968735

Mozaffarian, D., Aro, A., & Willett, W. (2009). Health effects of trans-fatty acids:experimental and observational evidence. *Eur J Clin Nutr., 63*(suppl 2), S5-S21. doi: 10.1038/sj.ejcn.1602973

Mozaffarian, D., Benjamin, E., Go, A., Arnett, D., Blaha, M., Cushman, M.,...Turner, M. (2015). American heart association statistics committee and stroke statistics subcommittee. Heart disease and stroke statistics–2015 update: A report from the american heart association. *Circulation, 131*, e29-e322. doi:10.1161/CIR.0000000000000152

Mozaffarian, D., Cao, H., King, I., Lemaitre, R., Song, X., & Siscovick, D. (2010). Trans-palmitoleic acid, metabolic risk factors, and new-onset diabetes in us adults: A cohort study. *Ann Intern Med, 153*, 790-9

Mozaffarian, D., Cao, H., King, I., Lemaitre, R., Song, X., Siscovick, D., & Hotamisligil, G. (2010). Trans-palmitoleic acid, metabolic risk factors, and new-onset diabetes in U.S. adults: A cohort study. *Ann Intern Med, 153*, 790-799. doi: 10.7326/0003-4819-153-12-201012210-00005

Mozaffarian, D., de Oliveira Otto, M., Lemaitre, R., Fretts, A., Hotamisligil, G., Tsai, M.,...Nettleton, J. (2013). Trans-palmitoleic acid, other dairy fat biomarkers, and incident diabetes: The multi-ethnic study of atherosclerosis (mesa). *Am J Clin Nutr., 97*, 854-861doi: 10.3945/ajcn.112.045468

Mozaffarian, D., Hao, T., Rimm, E., & Willett WC, H. F. (2011). Changes in diet and lifestyle and long-term weight gain in women and men. *N Engl J Med., 364,* 2392-2404. doi: 10.1056/NEJMoa1014296

Mozaffarian, D., Hao, T., Rimm, E., Willett, W., & Hu, F. (2011). Changes in diet and lifestyle and long-term weight gain in women and men. *N Engl J Med., 364,* 2392-2404. doi: 10.1056/NEJMoa1014296

Mozaffarian, D., Katan, M., Ascherio, A., Stampfer, M., & Willett, W. (2006). Trans fatty acids and cardiovascular disease. *N Engl J Med, 354,* 1601-1613. doi: 10.1056/NEJMra054035

Mozaffarian, D., Micha, R., & Wallace, S. (2010). Effects on coronary heart disease of increasing polyunsaturated fat in place of saturated fat: A systematic review and meta-analysis of randomized controlled trials. *PLoS Med., 7,* e1000252. doi: 10.1371/journal.pmed.1000252

Mulpeter, K. (2017). Can you shed pounds on a mindfulness diet? *Time: Mindfulness: The New Science of Health and Happiness,* 82-85

Murray, S., Tulloch, A., Gold, M., & Avena, N. (2014). Hormonal and neural mechanisms of food reward, eating behaviour and obesity. *Nat Rev Endocrinol, 10:* 540-552 doi: 10.1038/nrendo.2014.91

Myese, P. (1993). Intermediary metabolism of fructose. *Am J Clin Nutr, 58* (supplement), 754S-765S

Nagao, M., Iso, H., Y. K., Date, C., & Tamakoshi, A. ((2012)). The Japan collaborative cohort study: Meat consumption in relation to mortality from cardiovascular disease among japanese men and women. *European Journal of Clinical Nutrition, 66,* 687-693. doi:10.1038/ejcn.2012.6

Nandi, S., Maurer, J., Hofacre, C., & Summers, A. (2004). Gram-positive bacteria are a major reservoir of class 1 antibiotic resistance integrons in poultry. *Proc Natl Acad Sci USA, 101,* 7118-7122

National Nutrition Conference for Defense. (1941). National nutrition conference for defense. *JAMA, 116,* 2598-2599

Neltner, T. G., Alger, H. M., O'Reilly, J. T., Krimsky, S., Bero, L. A., & Maffini, M. V. (2013). Conflicts of interest in approvals of additives to food determined to be generally recognized as safe out of balance. *JAMA Intern Med, 173*(22), 2032-2036. doi:10.1001/jamainternmed.2013.10559

Nestel, P., Mellett, N., Pally, S., Wong, G., Barlow, C., Croft, K.,...Meikle, P. (2013). Effects of low-fat or full-fat fermented and non-fermented dairy foods on selected cardiovascular biomarkers in overweight adults. *Br J Nutr., 110,* 2242-2249. doi: 10.1017/S0007114513001621

Nettleton, J. E., Reimer, R. A., & Shearer, J. (2016). Low calorie sweeteners: Science and controversy. *Physiology & Behavior, 164,* 488-493

Neufeld, E., Stonik, J., Demosky, S., Knapper, C., Combs, C., & Cooney, A. (2004). The abc a1transporter modulates late endocytic trafficking: Insights from the correction of the genetic defect in tangier disease. *J Biol Chem, 79,* 15571-15578

Neuhaus, E. M., Zhang, W., Gelis, L., Deng, Y., Noldus, J., & Hatt, H. (2009). Activation of an olfactory receptor inhibits proliferation of prostate cancer cells. *The Journal of Biological Chemistry, 284,* 16218-16225. doi: 10.1074/jbc.M109.012096

Nevid, J. S. (2015). *Essentials of psychology: Concepts and applications.* Stamford, Conneticut: Cengage Learning

NIH. (2016, June 6). *Carbohydrates.* Retrieved from Medline Plus: https://www.nlm.nih.gov/medlineplus/ency/article/002469.htm

NIH. (2017, March 27). *Calcium.* Retrieved from NIH.gov factsheets: https://ods.od.nih. gov/factsheets/Calcium-HealthProfessional/

NIH Consensus Development Conference. (1985). Lowering blood cholesterol. *JAMA, 253,* 2080-2086

Nilzen, V., Babol, J., & Dutta, P. (2001). Free range rearing of pigs with access to pasture grazing-effect on fatty acid composition and lipid oxidation products. *Meat Science, 58:* 267-275

Niness, K. R. (1999). Inulin and oligofructose: What are they? *J. Nutr., 129*(7), 1402S-1406s

Nishimura, R. A., Trusty, J. M., Hayes, D. L., Ilstrup, D. M., Larson, D. R., Hayes, S. N.,... Tajik, J. (1997)Dual-chamber pacing for hypertrophic cardiomyopathy: A randomized, double-blind, crossover trial. *JACC, 29*(2), 435-41

Nissen, S. (2016). U.S. dietary guidelines: An evidence-free zone. *Ann Intern Med., 164,* 558-9

Norat, T., Romundstad, P., Vatten, L., & Aune, D. (2013). Dairy products and the risk of type 2 diabetes: A systematic review and dose-response meta-analysis of cohort studies. *Am J Clin Nutr., 98,* 1066-1083. doi: 10.3945/ajcn.113.059030

Nordestgaard, B., Chapman, M., Ray, K., Borén, J., Andreotti, F., Watts, G.,...Tybjærg-Hansen, A. (2010). European atherosclerosis society consensus panel. Lipoprotein(a) as a cardiovascular risk factor: Current status. *Eur Heart J., 31,* 2844-2853. doi: 10.1093/eurheartj/ehq386

Norton, J. D. (2007, November 15). *How did einstein think?* Retrieved from www.Pitt.edu: http://www.pitt.edu/~jdnorton/Goodies/Einstein_think/

Nuernberg, K., Dannenberger, D., & Nuernberg, G. (2005). Effect of a grass-based and a concentrate feeding system on meat quality characteristics and fatty acid composition of longissimus muscle in different cattle breeds. *Livest Prod Sci, 94,* 137-147

Nugent, R. (2015, October 10). *Bringing agriculture to the table: How agriculture and food can play a role in preventing chronic disease.* Retrieved from Chicago Council: http://www.thechicagocouncil.org/publication/bringing-agriculture-table-how-agriculture-and-food-policy-can-play-role-preventing

Nutopia (Dan Clifton, H.B. (Director). (2012). *Mankind: The story of us* [Motion Picture].

O'Brien, E. (1964). *The essential plotinus.* Indianapolis, IN: Hackett

O'Keefe, S., Gaskins-Wright, S., Wiley, V., & Chen, I.-C. (1994). Levels of trans geometrical isomers of essential fatty acids in some unhydrogenated u.s. vegetable oils. *Journal of Food Lipids,1*(3), 165-176

O'Rourke, K., VanderZanden, A., Shepard, D., & Leach-Kemon, K. (2015). Cardiovascular disease worldwide, 1990-2013. *JAMA, 314,* 1905

O'Sullivan, T., Hafekost, K., Mitrou, F., & Lawrence, D. (2013). Food sources of saturated fat and the association with mortality: A meta-analysis. *Am J Public Health, 103,* e31-e42. doi: 10.2105/AJPH.2013.301492

Obikoya, G. (2017, April 5). *The history of vitamins.* Retrieved from Vitamins-nutrition. org: http://www.vitamins-nutrition.org/vitamins/history-vitamins.html

Oches, S. (2010, March). *Local vs.organic.* Retrieved from QSR Magazine: https://www. qsrmagazine.com/health/local-vs-organic

O'Donnell, M. J., Yusef, S., Mente, A., Gao, P., Mann, J. F., & Teo, K. (2011). Urinary sodium and potassium excretion and risk of cardiovascular events. *Journal of The American Medical Association, 306*(20), 2262-2264

O'Donnell, M. O., Mente, A., Rangarajan, S., McQueen, M. J., Wang, X., Liu, L.,...Lanas, F. (2014). Urinary sodium and potassium excretion, mortality, and cardiovascular events. *New England Journal of Medicine, 371,* 612-623

Office of Disease Prevention and Health Promotion. (2016). *Dietary guidelines for americans, 2015-2020. 8th ed.* Washington, DC: USDA

Olmstead, L. (2016). *Real food, fake food.* Chapel Hill, NC: Algonquin Books of Chapel Hill

Olshansky MD, B. (2007). Placebo and nocebo in cardiovascular health: Implications for healthcare, research, and the doctor-patient relationship. *JACC, 49*(4): doi: 10.1016/j. jacc.2006.09.036

Ordovas, J., Corella, D., Cupples, L., Demissie, S., Kelleher, A., & Coltell, O. (2002). Polyunsaturated fatty acids modulate the effects of the apoa—1 g—a polymorphism on hdl cholesterol concentrations in a sex specific manner: The framingham study. *American Journal of Clinical Nutrition, 75*, 38-46

Oxford Dictionaries. (2017). *Conventional.* Retrieved from Oxford Dictionaries: https://www.bing.com/search?q=conventional&form=PRUSEN&pc=EUPP_&mk-t=en-us&httpsmsn=1&refig=d6c2bc3a56f74f73a9d6f088c0583fe5&sp=-1&pq=con-ventional&sc=8-12&qs=n&sk=&cvid=d6c2bc3a56f74f73a9d6f088c0583fe5

Ozeke, O., Cay, S., Ozcan, F., Baser, K., Topaloglu, S., & Aras, D. (2016). Similarities between the renal artery and pulmonary vein denervation trials: Do we have to use sham procedures for atrial fibrillation catheter ablation trials? *International Journal of Cardiology, 211*, 55-57 doi: 10.1016/j.ijcard.2016.02.158

Page, I. H., Allen, E. V., Chamberlain, F. L., Keys, A., Stamler, J., & Stare, F. J. (1961). Dietary fat and its relation to heart attacks and strokes: Report by the central committee for medical and community program of the aha. *Circulation, 23*

Pak, C., Fuller, C., Sakahee, K., Preminger, G., & Britton, F. (1985). Long-term treatment of calcium nephrolithiasis with potassium citrate. *Journal of Urology, 134*, 11-19

Pan, A., Sun, Q., Bernstein, A., Schulze, M., Manson, J., Willett, W., & Hu, F. (2011). Red meat consumption and risk of type 2 diabetes: 3 cohorts of US adults and an updated meta-analysis. *Am J Clin Nutr., 94*, 1088-1096. doi: 10.3945/ajcn.111.018978

Pan, X., Li, G., Hu, Y., Wang, J., Yang, W., An, Z.,...Howard, B. (1997). Effects of diet and exercise in preventing niddm in people with impaired glucose tolerance: The da qing igt and diabetes study. *Diabetes Care, 20*(4), 537-544

Park, D., Ahn, Y., Park, S., Huh, C., Yoo, S., Yu, R.,...Choi, M. (2013). Supplementation of Lactobacillus curvatus hy7601 and lactobacillus plantarum ky1032 in diet-induced obese mice is associated with gut microbial changes and reduction in obesity. *PLoS One, 8*, e59470. doi: 10.1371/journal.pone.0059470

Park, Y., Leitzmann, M., Subar, A., Hollenbeck, A., & Schatzkin, A. (2009). Dairy food, calcium, and risk of cancer in the NIH-AARP Diet and Health Study. *Arch Intern Med., 169*, 391-401

Pasini, E., Aquilani, R., Testa, C., Baiardi, P., Angioletti, S., Boschi, F., & Dioguardi, F. (2015). Pathogenic gut flora in patients with chronic heart failure. *JACC,* doi: 10.1016/j.jchf.2015.10.009

Patel, H. N., Freeman, A. M., & Williams, K.A. (2017, March 27). *Diabetes: An opportunity to have a lasting impact on health through lifestyle modification.* Retrieved from AJMC.com: http://www.ajmc.com/journals/evidence-based-diabetes-man-agement/2017/march-2017/diabetes-an-opportunity-to-have-a-lasting-im-pact-on-health-through-lifestyle-modification/P-1#undefined.uxfs

Patel, R. M., & Pinto, J. M. (2014). Olfaction: Anatomy, physiology, and disease. *Clinical Anatomy, 27*, 54-60

Patel, S., & Hu, F. (2008). Short sleep duration and weight gain: A systematic . *review. Obesity (Silver Spring)., 16*(3), 643-653. doi: 10.1038/oby.2007.118

Patterson, E., Larsson, S., Wolk, A., & Akesson, A. (2013). Association between dairy food consumption and risk of myocardial infarction in women differs by type of dairy food. *J Nutr., 143*, 74-9

Paul-Labrador, M., Polk, D., Dwyer, J., Velasquez, I., Nidich, S., Rainforth, M.,...Merz, C. (2006). Effects of a randomized controlled trial of transcendental meditation on components of the metabolic syndrome in subjects with coronary heart disease. *Arch Intern Med., 166*(11), 1218-1224. doi: 10.1001/archinte.166.11.1218

PBS. (2015, July 23). *Genetically modified tomatoes.* Retrieved from PBS.org: http://www.pbs.org/wnet/dna/pop_genetic_gallery/

Pepino, M. (2015). Metabolic effects of non-nutritive sweeteners. *Physiol Behav., 152*(pt B), 450-455. doi: 10.1016/j.physbeh.2015.06.024

Peppa, M., Goldberg, T., Cai, W., Rayfield, E., & Vlassara, H. (2002). Glycotoxins: A missing link in the 'relationship of dietary fat and meat intake in relation to risk of type 2 diabetes in men. *Diabetes Care, 25*, 1898-9

Perez-Fons, L., Steiger, S., Khaneja, R., Bramley, P. M., Cutting, S. M., & Sandmann, G. (2011). Identification and the developmental formation of carotenoid pigments in the yellow/orange bacillus spore former. *Biochimica et Biophysica Acta, 1811*, 177-185

Pflughoeft, K., & Versalovic, J. (2012). Human microbiome in health and disease. *Annu Rev Pathol, 7*, 99-122

Piernas, C., & Popkin, B. (2010). Snacking increased among US adults between 1977 and 2006. *J Nutr, 140*, 325-332

Pimpin, L., Wu, J. H., Haskelberg, H., Del Gobbo, L., & Mozaffarian, D. (2016). Is butter back? A systematic review and meta-analysis of butter consumption and risk of cardiovascular disease, diabetes, and total mortality. *PLoS One, 11*(6), e0158118. doi:10.1371/journal.pone.0158118

Pluznicka, J. L., Zoub, D.-J., Zhangb, X., Yana, Q., Rodriguez-Gilc, D. J., Eisnerd, C.,...Caplana, M.J. (2009). Functional expression of the olfactory signaling system in the kidney. *PNAS, 106*(6), 2059-2064. doi10.1073pnas.0812859106

Pollan, M. (2002, March 31). *Power Steer.* Retrieved July 14, 2013, from *New York Times*: http://www.nytimes.com/2002/03/31/magazine/power-steer.html?pagewanted=all&src=pm

Pollan, M. (2006). *The omnivore's dilemma: A natural history of four meals.* New York, NY: Penguin Press

Pollan, M. (2008). *In defense of food: An eater's manifesto.* New York, NY: Penguin Press

Poutahidis, T., Kleinewietfeld, M., Smillie, C., Levkovich, T., Perrotta, A., Bhela, S.,...Erdman, S. (2013). Microbial reprogramming inhibits Western diet-associated obesity. *PLoS One, 8*, e68596. doi: 10.1371/

Powell, A. (2012, February 2). *Decoding keys to a healthy life.* Retrieved from HravardGazette: http://news.harvard.edu/gazette/story/2012/02/decoding-keys-to-a-healthy-life/

Power, S., O'Toole, P., Stanton, C., Ross, R., & Fitzgerald, G. (2014). Intestinal microbiota, diet and health. *Br J Nutr., 111*, 387-402. doi: 10.1017/S0007114513002560

Prandovszky, E., Gaskell, E., Martin, H., Dubey, J., Webster, J. P., & McConkey, G.A. (2011). The neurotropic parasite toxoplasma gondii increases dopamine metabolism. *PLoS One, 6*(9): e23866 https://doi.org/10.1371/journal.pone.0023866

Pray, L., Pillsbury, L., & Tomayko, E. (2013). *The human microbiome, diet, and health: Workshop summary.* Washington, DC: THE NATIONAL ACADEMIES PRESS

Preminger, G., Sakhaee, K., Skurla, C., & Pak, C. (1985). Prevention of recurrent calcium stone formation with potassium citrate therapy in patients with distal renal tubular acidosis. *Journal of Urology, 134*, 20-23

Price, S. A., Hopkins, S. S., Smith, K. K., & Roth, V. L. (2012). Tempo of trophic evolution and its impact on. *Proceedings of the National Academy of Sciences, 109*(18),
7008-7012

Psouni, E., Janke, A., & Garwicz, M. (2012). Impact of carnivory on human development
and evolution revealed by a new unifying model of in mammals. *PLoS One, 7*(4):
e32452doi: 10.1371/journal.pone.0032452

Psychology Today. (2017, May 30). *Gratitude.* Retrieved from PsychologyToday.com:
https://www.psychologytoday.com/basics/gratitude

Qin, L., Xu, J., Han, S., Zhang, Z., Zhao, Y., & Szeto, I. (2015). Dairy consumption and
risk of cardiovascular disease: An updated meta-analysis of prospective cohort studies.
Asia Pac J Clin Nutr., 24, 90-100

Quinn, E., & Young, C. (2014, April 14). *Why the fda has never looked at some of the
additives in our food.* Retrieved from NPR.org: http://www.npr.org/sections/the-
salt/2015/04/14/399591292/why-the-fda-is-clueless-about-some-of-the-additives-
in-our-food

Ramsden, C. E., Zamaora, D., Boonseng, L., Majchrzak-Hong, S., Faurot, K. R., Suchindran,
C. M.,...Hibbeln, J. R. (2013). Use of dietary linoleic acid for secondary prevention of
coronary heart disease and death: Evaluation of recovered data from the Sydney diet
heart study and updated meta-analysis. *BMJ, 346,* e8707. doi: 10.1136/bmj.e8707

Ramsden, C. E., Zamora, D., Leelarthaepin, B., Majchrzak-Hong, S. F., Faurot, K. R.,
Suchindran, C. M.,... Hibbel, J.R. (2013). Use of dietary linoleic acid for secondary
prevention of coronary heart disease and death: Evaluation of recovered data from
the sydney diet heart study and updated meta-analysis. *British Medical Journal, 346,*
e8707. doi: 10.1136/bmj.e8707

Ramsden, C. E., Zamora, D., Majchrzak-Hong, S., Faurot, K. R., Broste, S. K., Frantz,
R. P.,... Hibbeln, J. R. (2016). Re-evaluation of the traditional diet-heart hypothesis:
Analysis of recovered data from minnesota coronary experiment (1968-73). *BMJ,
353,* i1246 doi: 10.1136/bmj.i1246

Ramsden, C., Faurot, K., & Carrera-Bastos, P. (2001). Dietary fat quality and coronary
heart disease prevention: A unified theory based on evolutionary, historical, global,
and modern perspectives. *Curr Treat Options Cardiovasc Med, 11*(4), 289-301

Ramsden, C., Hibbeln, J., & Majchrzak, S. (2010). N-6 fatty acid-specific and mixed poly-
unsaturate dietary interventions have different effects on CHD risk: A meta-analysis
of randomised controlled trials. *Br J Nutr, 104,* 1586-600

Ramsey, D., & Graham, T. (2012, April 26). *How vegetable oils replaced animal fats in the american
diet.* Retrieved from *The Atlantic:* http://www.theatlantic.com/health/archive/2012/04/
how-vegetable-oils-replaced-animal-fats-in-the-american-diet/256155/

Randerson, J. (2008, May 13). *Childish superstition: Einstein's letter makes view of religion
relatively clear.* Retrieved from *The Guardian:* https://www.theguardian.com/sci-
ence/2008/may/12/peopleinscience.religion

Ranken, M., Krill, R., & Baker, C. G. (1997). *Food industries manual.* New York, NY:
Blackie Academic and Professional Press

Rankin MD, L. (2013). *Mind over medicine: Scientific proof that you can heal yourself.*
Carlsbad, California: Hay House

Rapp, J. R. (1982). Dahl salt-susceptible and salt-resistant rats: A review. *Hypertension, 4,*
753-763

Ras, R., Streppel, M., Draijer, R., & Zock, P. (2013). Flow-mediated dilation and cardiovascular risk prediction: A systematic review with meta-analysis. *Int J Cardiol, 168,*
344-51

Ravnskov, U. (1998). The questionable role of saturated and polyunsaturated fatty acids and cardiovascular disease. *J Clin Epidemiol, 51*, 443-460

Ravnskov, U. (2002). Hypothesis out-of-date. the diet-heart idea. *J Clin Epidemiol, 55*, 1057-1063

Ravnskov, U., Allen, C., Atrens, D., Enig, M., Groves, B., Kauffman, M.,...Worm, N. (2002). Studies of dietary fat and heart disease. *Science, 295*, 1464-1465

Rayner, G., Hawkes, C., Lang, T., & Bello, W. (2006). Trade liberalization and the diet transition: A public health response. *Health Promot Int, 21*, 67-74

Remy, M. (2017). Finding your flow. *Time: Mindfulness: The New Science of Health and Happiness*, 92-94.

Renaud, S., & de Lorgeril, M. (1992). Wine, alcohol, platelets, and the French paradox for coronary heart disease. *Lancet, 339*(8808), 1523-1526

Representatives, U. H. (2018). *Minority staff report: Spinning science & silencing scientists: A case study in how the chemical industry attempts to influence science.* Washington, DC: U.S. House of Representatives Committee on Science, Space & Technology

Reuell, P. (2011, November 7). *Why cooking counts.* Retrieved from Harvard Gazette: http://news.harvard.edu/gazette/story/2011/11/why-cooking-counts/

Richard, C., Cristall, L., Fleming, E., Lewis, E., Ricupero, M., Jacobs, R., & Field, C. (2017). Impact of egg consumption on cardiovascular risk factors in individuals with type 2 diabetes and at risk for developing diabetes: A systematic review of randomized nutritional intervention studies. *Can J Diabetes, 2671*(16), 30562-30567. doi: 10.1016/j.jcjd.2016.12.002

Ridaura, V. F., Rey, F., Cheng, J., Duncan, A., K. A., & . Walters, W. (2013). Gut microbiota from twins discordant for obesity modulate metabolism in mice. *Science, 341*, 1241214

Rister, R. (2011, May 5). *Eating less salt does not necessarily cut high blood pressure and heart disease risks.* Retrieved December 17, 2011, from SteadyHealth.com: http://www.steadyhealth.com/articles/Eating_Less_Salt_Does_Not_Necessarily_Cut_High_Blood_Pressure_and_Heart_Disease_Risks_a1787.html

Ritz, E. (2005). Salt—Friend or foe? *Nephrol Dial Transplant*, doi: 10.1093/ndt/gfi256

Rizos, E., Ntzani, E., Bika, E., Kostapanos, M., & Elisaf, M. (2012). Association between omega-3 fatty acid supplementation and risk of major cardiovascular disease events: A systematic review and meta-analysis. *JAMA, 308*, 1024-1033. doi: 10.1001/2012.jama.11374

Robertson, J. (2003). Dietary salt and hypertension: Ascientific issue or a matter of faith? *J Eval Clin Pract, 9*(1), 1-22

Rohrmann, S., Overvad,K, Bueno-de-Mesquita, H., Jakobsen, M., Egeberg, R., Tjønneland, A.,...Crowe, F. (2013). Meat consumption and mortality—results from the european prospective investigation into cancer and nutrition. *BMC Med, 11*, 63. doi: 10.1186/1741-7015-11-63

Romero-Corral, A. S., Sierra-Johnson, J., Korenfeld, Y., Boarin, S., Korinek, J., Jensen, M. D.,...Lopez-Jimenez, F. (2009). Normal weight obesity: A risk factor for cardiometabolic dysregulation and cardiovascular mortality. *European Heart Journal.* doi:10.1093/eurheartj/ehp487

Rong, Y., Chen, L., Zhu, T., Song, Y., Yu, M., Shan, Z.,...Liu, L. (2013). Egg consumption and risk of coronary heart disease and stroke dose-response meta-analysis of prospective cohort studies. *BMJ, 346*, e8539

Rosell, M., Hakansson, N., & Wolk, A. (2006). Association between dairy food consumption and weight change over 9 y in 19,352 perimenopausal women. *Am J Clin Nutr*, *84*: 1481-1488

Rosmond, R. (2005). Role of stress in the pathogenesis of the metabolic syndrome. *Psychoneuroendocrinology*, *30*, 1-10

Roth, G. A., Forouzanfar, M. H., Moran, A. E., Barber, R., Nguyen, G., Feigin, V. L.,... Murray, C. J. (2015). Demographic and epidemiologic drivers of global cardiovascular mortality. *N Engl J Med.*, *372*, 1333-41

Round, J. L., & Mazmanian, S. K. (2009). The gut microbiome shapes intestinal immune responses during health and disease. *Nat Rev Immunol.*, *9*(5): 313-323. doi:10.1038/nri2515

Rovelli, C. (2017). *Reality is not what it seems: The journey to quantum gravity.* New York: Riverhead Books

Ryan, P.M., London, L.E., Bjorndahl, T.C., Mandal, R., Murphy, K., & Fitzgerald, G.F. (2017). Microbiome and metabolome modifying effects of several cardiovascular disease interventions in apo-E-/- mice. *Microbiome*, *5*, 30. doi: 10.1186/s40168-017-0246-x

Ryan, P., London, L., Bjorndahl, T., Mandal, R., Murphy, K., Fitzgerald, G.,... Stanton, C. (2017). Microbiome and metabolome modifying effects of several cardiovascular disease interventions in apo-E-/- mice. *Microbiome*, *5*, 30. doi: 10.1186/s40168-017-0246-x

Ryan, P., Ross, R., Fitzgerald, G., Caplice, N., & Stanton, C. (2015). Functional food addressing heart health: Do we have to target the gut microbiota? *Curr Opin Clin Nutr Metab Care*, *18*(6), 566-71

Sachdeva, Cannon, C. P., D. P., LaBresh, K. A., Smith, S. C., Dai, D., & Fonarrow, G. C. (2008). Lipid levels in patients hospitalized with coronary artery disease: An analysis of 136,905 hospitalizations in get with the guidelines. *American Heart Journal, 157*(1), 111-117e2. doi: 10.1016/j.ahj.2008.08.010.

Sacks, F. M., Lichtenstein, A. H.,. Wu, J. H., Appel, L. J., Creager, M. A., Kris-Etherton, P. M.,...Van Horn, L. V. (2017). On behalf of the American Heart Association. Dietary fats and cardiovascular disease: A Presidential advisory from the american heart association. *Circulation.* doi: 10.1161/CIR.0000000000000510 Circulation. 2017;CIR.0000000000000510

Sacks, F., Svetkey, L., Vollmer, W., Appel, I., Bray, G., & Harsha, D. (2001). effects on blood pressure of reduce dietary sodium and the dietary approaches to stop hypertension (dash) diet. *New England Journal of Medicine, 344*(1), 3-10

Sadrzadeh-Yeganeh, H., Elmadfa, I., Djazayery, A., Jalali, M., Heshmat, R., & Chamary, M. (2010). The effects of probiotic and conventional yoghurt on lipid profile in women. *Br J Nutr, 103*, 1778-83

Salas-Salvadó, J., Bulló, M., Babio, N., Martínez-González, M., Ibarrola-Jurado, N., Basora, J.,...Investigators., P. S. (2011). Reduction in the incidence of type 2 diabetes with the mediterranean diet: Results of the predimed-reus nutrition intervention randomized trial. *Diabetes Care, 34*(1), 14-9. doi: 10.2337/dc10-1288.

Salas-Salvadó, J., Bulló, M., Estruch, R., Ros, E., Covas, M., Ibarrola-Jurado, N.,...Martínez-González, M. (2014). Prevention of diabetes with mediterranean diets: A subgroup analysis of a randomized trial. *Ann Intern Med.*, *160*, 1-10. doi: 10.7326/M13-1725

Salmerón, J., Manson, J., Stampfer, M., Colditz, G., Wing, A., & Willett, W. (1997). Dietary fiber, glycemic load, and risk of non-insulin dependent diabetes in women. *JAMA, 277*(6), 472-477

Samara, R. A. (2010). Fats and satiety. In J. Montmayeur, *Fat detection: Taste, texture, and post ingest of effects*. Boca Raton, Florida: CRC Press

Sanchez, M., Darimont, C., Drapeau, V., Emady-Azar, S., Lepage, M., Rezzonico, E.,... Tremblay, A. (2014). Effect of lactobacillus rhamnosus CGMCC1.3724 supplementation on weight loss and maintenance in obese men and women. *Br J Nutr.*, *111*, 1507-1519. doi: 10.1017/S0007114513003875

Sandek, A., Bauditz, J., Swidsinski, A., B. S., Weber-Eibel, J., v. H., & . Anker, S. (2007). Altered intestinal function in patients with chronic heart failure. *JACC, 50*(16), 1561-1569. doi: 10.1016/j.jacc.2007.07.016.

Sarich, C. (2015, January 23). *GMO-free russia? Government approves bill that would ban gmo cultivation, breeding and imports*. Retrieved from Global Research:http://www. globalresearch.ca/gmo-free-russia-government-approves-bill-that-would-ban-gmo-cultivation-breeding-and-imports/5426431

Satija, A., Bhupathiraju, S. N., Spiegelman, D., Chiuve, S. E., Manson, J. E., Willett, W.,... Hu, F. B. (2017). Healthful and unhealthful plant-based diets and the risk of coronary heart disease in u.s. adults. *JACC, 70*(4), 411-422. doi: 10.1016/j.jacc.2017.05.047

Satprem. (1968). *Sri Aurobindo or the adventure of consciousness (L. Venet, Trans.)*.New York: Harper & Row

Sauve, S. (2014). Time to revisit arsenic regulations: Comparing drinking water and rice. *BMC Public Health, 14*, 465

Scharf, R., Demmer, R., & DeBoer, M. (2013). Longitudinal evaluation of milk type consumed and weight status in preschoolers. *Arch Dis Child 1.*, *98*, 335-340. doi: 10.1136/archdischild-2012-302941

Schlosser, E. (2001). *Fast food nation: The dark side of the all-American meal*. Boston, MA: Houghton Mifflin

Schmidt, C. (2015, March 1). *Mental health may depend on creatures in the gut: The microbiome may yield a new class of psychobiotics for the treatment of anxiety, depression and other mood disorders*. Retrieved from Scientific American.com: https://www.scientificameri-can.com/article/mental-health-may-depend-on-creatures-in-the-gut/

Schneider, R. H., Grim, C. E., Rainforth, M. V., Kotchen, T., Nidich, S. I., Gaylord-King, C.,...Alexander, C.N. (2012). Stress reduction in the secondary prevention of cardiovascular disease: Randomized, controlled trial of transcendental meditation and health education in blacks. *Circ Cardiovasc Qual Outcomes, 5*, 750-758. doi: 10.1161/ CIRCOUTCOMES.112.967406

Schwingshackl, L., & Hoffmann, G. (2013). Long-term effects of low-fat diets either low or high in protein on cardiovascular and metabolic risk factors: A systematic review and meta-analysis. *Nutr J.*, *12*, 48. doi: 10.1186/1475-2891-12-48

Schwingshackl, L., & Hoffmann, G. (2014). Monounsaturated fatty acids, olive oil and health status: Asystematic review and meta-analysis of cohort studies. *Lipids Health Dis.*, *13*, 154. doi: 10.1186/1476-511X-13-154

Schwingshackl, L., Missbach, B., König, J., & Hoffmann, G. (2015). Adherence to a mediterranean diet and risk of diabetes: A systematic review and meta-analysis. *Public Health Nutr.*, *18*(7), 1292-9. doi: 10.1017/S1368980014001542

Science Daily. (2015, February 25). *Widely used food additives promotes colitis, obesity and metabolic syndrome, shows study of emulsifiers*. Retrieved from Science Daily: http:// www.sciencedaily.com/releases/2015/02/150225132105.htm

Scotece, M., Conde, J., Abella, V., Lopez, V., Pino, J., Lago, F.,...Gualillo, O. (2015). New drugs from ancient natural foods. Oleocanthal the natural occurring spicy compound of olive oil: A brief history. Drug. *Drug Discov Today, 20,* 406–410. doi: 10.1016/j.drudis.2014.10.017

Sebastian, A., Frassetto, L., Sellmeyer, D., Merriam, R., & Morris, R. (2002). Estimation of the net acid load of the diet of ancestral preagricultural homo sapiens and their hominid ancestors. *American Journal of Clinical Nutrition, 76,* 1308-1316

Sebastian, A., Harris, S., Ottaway, J., Todd, K., & Morris, R. (1994). Improvement in mineral balance and skeletal metabolism in postmenopausal women treated with potassium bicarbonate. *New England Journal of Medicine, 330,* 1776-1781

Seekatz, A. M., Rao, K., Santhosh, K., & Young, V. B. (2016). Dynamics of the fecal microbiome in patients with recurrent and nonrecurrent Clostridium difficile infection. *Genome Medicine, 8,* 47 doi: 10.1186/s13073-016-0298-8

Seidman, E. (2017). Fourteen ways to eat in the moment (and love it). *Time: Mindfulness: The New Science of Health and Happiness,* 86-91

Selhub, E., & Logan, A. (2012). *Your brain on nature: The science of nature's influence on your health, happiness and vitality.* New York, NY: Wiley

Senate, Select committee on nutrition and human needs of the united states. (1977). *Dietary goals for the United States. 2nd ed.* Washington, DC: US Government Printing Office

Seralini, G.-E., Clair, E. M., R., G., S., D., N., & Malatesta, M. (2014). Long term toxicity of a roundup herbicide and a roundup-toerant genetically modified maize. *Environmental Sciences Europe, 26,* 14

Seven Countries Study. (2015). *Ancel keys.* Retrieved from Seven Countries Study: http://sevencountriesstudy.com/about-the-study/investigators/ancel-keys

Shadan, S. (2009). Molecular biology: Taste of umami. *Nature, 457*(160): doi:10.1038/457160a. Retrieved from Cambridge Dictionary. Cambridge University Press.

Shakepeare, W. (2003). *Hamlet.* London: Wordsworth Editions

Shakespeare, W. (2014, May 18). *Shakespeare quotes on greed.* Retrieved from Shakespeare Quotes Online: http://www.shakespeare-online.com/quotes/shakespeareongreed.html

Shankar, P., Ahuja, S., & Sriram, K. (2013). Non-nutritive sweeteners: Review and update. *Nutrition., 29,* 1293-1299. doi: 10.1016/j.nut.2013.03.024

Shantha, N., Moody, W., & Tabeidi, Z. (1997). Conjugated linoleic acid concentration in semimembranosus muscle of grass- and grain-fed and zeranol zeranolimplanted beef cattle. *J Muscle Foods, 8,* 105-10

Sharafedtinov, K., Plotnikova, O., Alexeeva, R., Sentsova, T., Songisepp, E., Stsepetova, J.,…Mikelsaar, M. (2013). Hypocaloric diet supplemented with probiotic cheese improves body mass index and blood pressure indices of obese hypertensive patients—A randomized double-blind placebo-controlled pilot study. *Nutr J, 12,* 138. doi:10.1186/1475-2891-12-138

Sharma, A., Kribben, A., Schattenfroh, S., Cetto, C., & Distler, A. (1990). Salt sensitivity in humans is associated with abnormal acid base regulation. *Hypertension, 16,* 407-413

Shen, J., Shang, Q., Li, E. K., Leung, Y.-Y., Kun, E. W., Kwok, L.-W., & . Tam, L.-S. (2015). Cumulative inflammatory burden is independently associated with increased arterial stiffness in patients with psoriatic arthritis: A prospective study. *Arthritis Res Ther,* doi: 10.1186/s13075-015-0570-0

Shepherd, G. M. (2004). The human sense of smell: Are we better than we think? *PLoS Biology, 2*(5), 572-575 DOI: 10.1371/journal.pbio.0020146

Shin, J., Xun, P., Nakamura, Y., & He, K. (2013). Egg consumption in relation to risk of cardiovascular disease and diabetes: A systematic review and meta-analysis. *Am J Clin Nutr., 98,* 146-159. doi: 10.3945/ajcn.112.051318

Shin, N., Lee, C., Lee, H., Kim, M., W. T., Lee, M., & Bae, J. (2014). An increase in the akkermansia spp. population induced by metformin treatment improves glucose homeostasis in diet-induced obese mice. *Gut, 63,* 727-735

Sider, T. (2001). *Four-dimensionalism: An ontology of persistence and time.* New York: Oxford University Press

Siegel, T., & Betz, J. (Directors). (2017). *Seed: The untold story* [Motion Picture]

Simopoulos, A. (2001). The mediterranean diets: What is so special about the diet of greece? The scientific evidence. *J Nutr, 131,* 3065S-3073S

Simopoulos, A. (2002). The importance of the ratio of omega-6/omega-3 essential fatty acids. *Biomed Pharmacother, 56(8),* 365-79

Simopoulos, A. (2006). Evolutionary aspects of diet, the omega-6/omega-3 ratio and genetic variation: Nutritional implications for chronic diseases. *Biomedicine & Pharmacotherapy, 60,* 502-507

Simopoulos, A. P. (1999). Essential fatty acids in health and chronic disease. *The American Journal of Nutrition, 70(3),* 560S-569S

Simopoulos, A. P. (2004). Omega-6/omega-3 essential fatty acid ratio and chronic diseases. *FOOD REVIEWS INTERNATIONAL, 20(1),* 77-90

Singh, G., Micha, R., Khatibzadeh, S., Lim, S., Ezzati, M., & Mozaffarian, D. (2015). Estimated global, regional, and national disease burdens related to sugar-sweetened beverage consumption in 2010. *Circulation, 132,* 639-666. doi: 10.1161/CIRCULATIONAHA.114.010636

Siri-Tarino, P. W., Sun, Q., . Hu, F. B., & Krauss, R. M. (2010). Meta-analysis of prospective cohort studies evaluating the association of saturated fat with cardiovascular disease. *The American Journal of Clinical Nutrition, 91(3),* 535-546

Siri-Tarino, P., & Krauss, R. (2005). Influence of dietary carbohydrate and fat on ldl and hdl particle distributions. *Curr Atheroscler Rep, 7(6),* 455-459.

Siri-Tarino, P., Sun, Q., Hu, F., & Krauss, R. (2010). Meta-analysis of prospective cohort studies evaluating the association of saturated fat with cardiovascular disease. *Am J Clin Nutr, 91(3),* 535-546

Skeaff, C., & Miller, J. (2009). Dietary fat and coronary heart disease: Summary of evidence from prospective cohort and randomised controlled trials. *Anal Nutr & Metab, 55,* 173-201 doi: 10.1159/000229002

Skelly, A., Hashimoto, R., Al-Khatib, S., Sanders-Schmidler, G., F. R., Brodt, E., & McDonagh, M. (2015). *AHRQ technology assessments. Catheter ablation for treatment of atrial fibrillation.* Rockville, MD: Agency for Healthcare Research and Quality.

Sluijs, I., Forouhi, N., Beulens, J., van der Schouw, Y., Agnoli, C., Arriola, L.,...Wareham, N. (2012). InterAct consortium. The amount and type of dairy product intake and incident type 2 diabetes: results from the EPIC-InterAct Study. *Am J Clin Nutr., 96,* 382-390. doi: 10.3945/ajcn.111.021907

Smith, J., Hou, T., Ludwig, D., Rimm, E., Willett, W., Hu, F., & Mozaffarian, D. (2015). Changes in intake of protein foods, carbohydrate amount and quality, and long-term weight change: Results from 3 prospective cohorts. *Am J Clin Nutr., 101,* 1216-1224. doi: 10.3945/ajcn.114.100867

Smith, P. A. (2015). The tantalizing links between gut microbes and the brain. *Nature, 526,* 312-314

Smith-Spangler, C., Brandeau, M., & Hunter, G. (2012). Are organic foods safer or healthier than conventional alternatives?: A systematic review. *Ann Intern Med, 157,* 348-366

Snell, C., Bernheim, A., Berge, J., Kuntz, M., Pascal, G., & Paris, A. (2012). Assessment of the health impact of gm plant diets in long-term in multi generational animal feeding trials: A literature review. *Food Chem Toxicol, 50,* 1134-1148

Snowdon, R., Luhs, W., & Friedt, W. (2007). Oilseeds oilseed rape. In C. Kole (ed.), *Genome Mapping and Molecular Breeding in Plants,* 55-114. New York: Springer-Verlag

Soedamah-Muthu, S., Verberne, L., Ding, E., Engberink, M., & Geleijnse, J. (2012). Dairy consumption and incidence of hypertension: A dose response meta-analysis of prospective cohort studies. *Hypertension, 60,* 1131-1137. doi: 10.1161/ HYPERTENSIONAHA.112.195206

Sofi, F., Cesari, F., Abbate, R., Gensini, G., & Casini, A. (2008). Adherence to mediterranean diet and health status: Meta-analysis. *BMJ, 337,* a1344. doi: 10.1136/bmj. a1344

Sofi, F., Dinu, M., Pagliai, G., Cesari, F., Gori, A. M., Sereni, A.,...Casini, A. (2018). Low-calorie vegetarian versus mediterranean diets for reducing body weight and improving cardiovascular risk profile: CARDIVEG study (cardiovascular prevention with vegetarian diet). *Circulation,* doi: /10.1161/CIRCULATIONAHA.117.030088

Sofi, F., Whittaker, A., Cesari, F., Gori, A., Fiorillo, C., Becatti, M.,...Benedettelli, S. (2013). Characterization of khorasan wheat (kamut) and impact of a replacement diet on cardiovascular risk factors: cross-over dietary intervention study. *Eur J Clin Nutr,* 67(2), 190-195

Song, C., Ikei, H., & Miyazaki, Y. (2016). Physiological effects of nature therapy: A review of the research in japan. *Int J Environ Res Public Health, 13*(8), pii, E781. doi: 10.3390/ijerph13080781

Sousa, T., Paterson, R., Moore, V., Carlsson, A., Abrahamsson, B., & Basit, A. (2008). The gastrointestinal microbiota as a site for the biotransformation of drugs. *Int J Pharm., 363*(1-2), 1-25

Spehr, M., Gisselmann, G., Poplawski, A., & Hatt, H. (2003). Identification of a testicular odorant receptor mediating human sperm chemotaxis. *Science, 299*(5615), 2054-8

Spiegel, A. (2014, January 23). *Chicken more popular than beef in u.s. for first time in 100 years.* Retrieved from Huffingtonpost.com: http://www.huffingtonpost.com/2014/01/02/ chicken-vs-beef_n_4525366.html

Spiroux de Vendomois, J., Rouiller, F., Cellier, D., & Seralini, G. (2009). A comparison of the effects of three gm corn varieties of mammalian health. *Int J Biol Sci, 5,* 706-726

Srednicka-Tober, D., Baranski, M., Seal, C. J., Sanderson, R., Benbrook, C., Steinshamn, H.,...Jordan, T. (2016). Composition difference between organic and convential meat: A systematic literature review and meta-analysis. *British Journal of Nutrition, 115,* 994-1011

Srednicka-Tober, D., Baranski, M., Seal, C. J., Sanderson, R., Benbrook, C., Steinshamn, H.,...Nigg. (2016). Higher pufa and n-3 pufa, conjugated linoleic acid, alpha tocopherol and iron, but lower iodine and selenium concentrations in organic milk: A sytematic literature review and meta analysis. *British Journal of Nutrition, 115,* 1043-1060

Srednicka-Tober, D., Barański, M., Seal, C., Sanderson, R., Benbrook, C., Steinshamn, H.,...Leifert, C. (2016). Composition differences between organic and conventional meat: A systematic literature review and meta-analysis. *British Journal of Nutrition, 115,* 994-1011. doi: 10.1017/S0007114515005073

Stancliffe, R., Thorpe, T., & Zemel, M. (2011). Dairy attenuates oxidative and inflammatory stress in metabolic syndrome. *Am J Clin Nutr, 94,* 422-430

Stanhope, K. (2015). Sugar consumption, metabolic disease and obesity: The state of the controversy. *Crit Rev Clin Lab Sci.,* doi: 10.3109/10408363.2015.1084990

Stanhope, K., & Havel, P. (2010). Fructose composition: recent results and their potential implications. *Annals of the New York Academy of Science, March 1190*(1), 15-24

Stanhope, K., Bremer, A., Medici, V., Nakajima, K., Ito, Y., Nakano, T.,... Havel, P. (2011). Consumption of fructose and high fructose corn syrup increase postprandial triglycerides, ldl-cholesterol, and apolipoprotein-B in young men and women. *J Clin Endocrinol Metab, 96*(10),e1596-1605

Steed, A. (2010). *Living at the edge of the world: In the center of our own story.* United Kingdom: Sacredoutcast.com Publishing

Steed, A. (2016, June 15). Code delicious with dr. mike: What is a shaman? (http://radiomd.com/show/code-delicious/item/32168-what-is-a-shaman). (D. Mike, Interviewer)

Steed, A. (2016). *Powering Up Our Life Stories.* United Kingdom: Sacredoutcast.com Publishing

Steed, A. (2017). Personal communication. (M. Fenster, Interviewer)

Stettler, D.D., & Axel, R. (2009). Representations of odor in the piriform cortex. *Neuron, 63,* 854-864 doi: 10.1016/j.neuron.2009.09.005

Stewart, R. A., Wallentin, L., Benatar, J., Danchin, N., Hagstrom, E., Held, C.,...White, H.D. (2016). Dietary patterns and the risk of major adverse cardiovascular events in a global study of high-risk patients with stable coronary heart disease. *European Heart Journal,* doi: 10.1093/eurheartj/ehw125

Stewart, R., Wallentin, L., Benatar, J., Danchin, N., Hagström, E., Held, C.,...White, H. (2016). Dietary patterns and the risk of major adverse cardiovascular events in a global study of high-risk patients with stable coronary heart disease. *Eur Heart Journal, 37*(25), 1993-2001. doi: 10.1093/eurheartj/ehw125

Stoneoct, A. (2014, October 14). *Smell turns up in unexpected places.* Retrieved from ny times.com: http://www.nytimes.com/2014/10/14/science/smell-turns-up-in-unexpected-places.html?ref=health&_r=0

Stuart, C. (2013, February 6). *Generics to push statin revenues down by $7B.* Retrieved from Cardiovascular Business: http://www.cardiovascularbusiness.com/topics/health care-economics/slides-generics-push-statin-revenues-down-7b

Stuckrad, K. (2002). Reenchanting nature: Modern western shamanism and nineteenth-century thought. *Journal of the American Academy of Religion, 70*(4), 771-799

Subhan, F. B., & Chan, C. B. (2016). Review of dietary practices of the 21st century: Facts and fallacies. *Canadian Journal of Diabetes, 40,* 348-354

Suez, J., Korem, T., Zeevi, D., Zilberman-Schapira, G., Thaiss, C. A., Maza, O.,...Elinav, E. (2014). Artificial sweeteners induce glucose intolerance by altering the gut microbiota. *Nature, 514,* 181-186. doi: 10.1038/nature13793

Sullivan, W. (1972, March 29). *The einstein papers: A man of many parts.* Retrieved from *The New York Times:* http://www.nytimes.com/1972/03/29/archives/the-einstein-papers-a-man-of-many-parts-the-einstein-papers-man-of.html

Swaminathan, S., Fonseca, V., Alam, M., & Shah, S. (2007). The role of iron in diabetes and its complications.. *Diabetes Care, 30,* 1926-1933. doi: 10.2337/dc06-2625

Swithers, S., Martin, A., & Davidson, T. (2010). High-intensity sweeteners and energy balance. *Physiol Behav. 100,* 55-62. doi: 10.1016/j

Taillie, L. S., Ng, S. W., Xue, Y., Busey, E., & Harding, M. (2017). No fat, no sugar, no salt...No problem? prevalence of "low-content" nutrient claims and their associations with the nutritional profile of food and beverage purchases in the united states. *Journal of Academy of Nutrition and Dietetics,* doi: 10.1016/j.jand.2017.01.011

Tang, G., Wang, D., Long, J., Yang, F., & Si, L. (2015). Meta-analysis of the association between whole grain intake and coronary heart disease risk. *Am J Cardiol.*, *115*, 625-629. doi: 10.1016/j.amjcard.2014.12.015

Tang, W., Wang, Z., Kennedy, D., Yuping, W., Buffa, J., Agatisa-Boyle,...Hazen, S. (2015). Gut microbiota-dependent trimethylamine Noxide (TMAO) pathway contributes to both development of renal insufficiency and mortality risk in chronic kidney disease. *Circ. Res.*, *116*, 448-455

Tang, W., Wang, Z., Levison, B., Koeth, R., Britt, E., & Fu, X. (2013). Intestinal microbial metabolism of phosphatidylcholine in cardiovascular risk. *New England Journal of Medicine*, *368*(17), 1575-1584

Taren, A. A., Gianaros, P. J., Greco, C. M., Lindsay, E. K., Fairgrieve, A., Brown, K. W.,... Creswel, J. D. (2015). Mindfulness meditation training alters stress-related amygdala resting state functional connectivity: A randomized controlled trial. *Social Cognitive and Affective Neuroscience*, 1758-1768 doi: 10.1093/scan/nsv066.

Taubes, G. (2001). The soft science of dietary fat. *Science*, *291*,2535-2541

Taubes, G. (2007). *Good calories, bad calories .* New York: Alfred Knopf Publishers

Taubes, G. (2012, June 2). Salt, we misjudged you. *The New York Times*, SR8

Taubes, G. (2017, June 16). *Vegetable oils, (francis) bacon, bing crosby, and the american heart association.* Retrieved from Cardiobrief.org: http://www.cardiobrief.org/2017/06/16/guest-post-vegetable-oils-francis-bacon-bing-crosby-and-the-american-heart-association/

Tavares, L., Fonseca, S., Rosa, M., & Yokoo, E. (2012). Relationship between ultra-processed foods and metabolic syndrome in adolescents from a brazilian family doctor program. *Public Health Nutr*, *15*, 82-87

Taylor, K. (2016, April 21). *Why 'easy beats better' is the new motto at taco bell and pizza hut.* Retrieved April 25, 2016, from Yahoo Finance: http://finance.yahoo.com/news/taco-bell-pizza-hut-focusing-160957778.html

Taylor, S. (2017, February 27). *Harvard happiness study reveals 7 factors to a happy, long & healthy life.* Retrieved from ezinearticles.com: http://ezinearticles.com/?Harvard-Happiness-Study-Reveals-7-Factors-to-a-Happy,-Long-and-Healthy-Life&id=9653778

Teff, K. L., Grudziak, J., Townsend, R. R., Dunn, T. N., Grant, R. W., Adams, S. H.,... Havel, P. J. (2009). Endocrine and metabolic effects of consuming fructose-and glucose-sweetened beverages with meals in obese men and women: Influence of insulin resistance on plasma triglyceride responses. *J Clin Endocrinol Metab*, *94*(5), 1562-1569

Teff, K., Elliott, S., Tschop, M., Kieffer, T., Rader, D., Heiman, M.,...Havel, P. (2004). Dietary fructose reduces circulating insulin and leptin, attenuates postprandial suppression of ghrelin, and increases triglycerides in women. *J Clin Endocrinol Metab*, *89*, 2963-2972

Teicholz, N. (2014, May 6). *The questionable link between saturated fat and heart disease.* Retrieved from The Wall Street Journal.com: http://www.wsj.com/articles/SB10001424052702303676404579533760760481486

Tennyson, A. L. (2003). *Idylls of the king and a selection of poems.* New York: Penguin Putnam

The Asiatic Society. (2017). *Full text of "transactions of the asiatic society of japan* Retrieved from Archive.org: https://archive.org/stream/transactionsasi18japagoog/transactionsasi18japagoog_djvu.txt

The Commonwealth Fund. (2015, March 29). *U.S. health care from a global perspective: Spending, use of services, prices, and health in 13 countries.* Retrieved from CommonwealthFund.org: http://www.commonwealthfund.org/publications/issue-briefs/2015/oct/us-health-care-from-a-global-perspective

The CP Journal. (2012, October 12). *Breaking down the limbic system*. Retrieved from The CP Journal: http://www.cp-journal.com/breaking-down-the-limbic-system-2/

The European Food Information Council. (2017, March 27). *The determinants of food choice*. Retrieved from EUFIC review 2005: http://www.eufic.org/article/en/expid/review-food-choice/

The European Food Safety Authority. (2003). Opinion of the scientific panel on genetically modified organisms on request from the commission related to the safety of food and food ingredients derived from herbicide-tolerant genetically modified maize in nk 603 for which a request for placing on the. *EFSA J, 9*, 1-14

The Holy Bible: King James Version. (2004). *The holy bible: king james version*. Dallas, TX: Brown Books Publishing

The J. M. Smucker Company. (2001). *Pursuant to rule 425 under the securities act of 1933*. Retrieved from SEC.gov: http://www.sec.gov/Archives/edgar/data/91419/000095015201505889/l91378ae425.txt

The Mellman Group. (2015). *Support for requiring labels on gmo foods*. Retrieved from Agri-pulse.com: http://www.agri-pulse.com/Uploaded/Mellman-GMO-poll.pdf

The National Law Review. (2015, July 25). *The safe and accurate food labeling act restricts state and local government from regulating gmo in food*. Retrieved from The National Law Review: http://www.natlawreview.com/article/safe-and-accurate-food-labeling-act-restricts-state-and-local-government-regulating

Thomas, L. (1980). *The medusa and the snail*. New York: Bantam Books

Thompson, M. (2015, March 29). *WHO: long-cleared round-up ingredient 'probably' causes cancer*. Retrieved from PBS.org: http://www.pbs.org/newshour/rundown/roundup-ingredient-probably-carcinogenic-humans/

Thompson, M. (2015, March 29). *WHO: Long-cleared Roundup ingredient 'probably' causes cancer*. Retrieved from Pbs.org: http://www.pbs.org/newshour/rundown/roundup-ingredient-probably-carcinogenic-humans/

Thorning, T., Raziani, F., Bendsen, N., Astrup, A., Tholstrup, T., & A.,R. (2015). Diets with high-fat cheese, high-fat meat, or carbohydrate on cardiovascular risk markers in overweight postmenopausal women: A randomized crossover trial. *Am J Clin Nutr, 102*(3), 573-81

Tillisch, K., Labus, J., Kilpatrick, L., Jiang, Z., Stains, J., Ebrat, B.,...Mayer, E. A. (2013). Consumption of fermented milk product with probiotic modulates brain activity. *Gastroenterology, 144*(7), 1394-1401

Tinker, L., Bonds, D., Margolis, K., Manson, J., Howard, B., Larson, J.,...Parker, L. (2008). Women's health initiative. Low-fat dietary pattern and risk of treated diabetes mellitus in postmenopausal women: The women's health initiative randomized controlled dietary modification trial. *Arch Intern Med., 168*, 1500-1511. doi: 10.1001/archinte.168.14.1500

Tolle, E. (1999). *The power of now: A guide to spiritual enlightenment*. Novato, CA: New World Library.

Tollefson, L., & Miller, M. (2000). Antibiotic use in food animals: Controlling the human health impact. *J AOAC Int., 83*(2), 245-54

Tollefson, L., Altekruse, S., & Potter, M. (1997). Therapeutic antibiotics in animal feeds and antibiotic resistance. *Rev Sci Tech., 16*(2), 709-15

Tremaroli, V., & Backhed, F. (2012). Functional interactions between the gut microbiota and host metabolism. *Nature, 489*, 242-249

Trichopoulou, A., Bamia, C., & Trichopoulos, D. (2009). Anatomy of health effects of mediterranean diet: Greek epic prospective cohort study. *BMJ, 338*, b2337 doi: 10.1136/bmj.b2337

Tscholl, V., Lsharaf, A. K.-A., Lin, T., Bellman, B., Biewener, S., Nagel, P.,...Rillig, A. (2016). Two years outcome in patients with persistent atrial fibrillation after pulmonary vein isolation using the second-generation 28-mm cryoballoon. *Heart Rhythm*, *13*, 1817-1822 doi: doi: 10.1016/j.hrthm.2016.05.022

Tuomilehto, J., Lindström, J., Eriksson, J., Valle, T., Hämäläinen, H., Ilanne-Parikka, P.,... Uusitupa (2001). Finnish diabetes prevention study group. Prevention of type 2 diabetes mellitus by changes in lifestyle among subjects with impaired glucose tolerance. *N Engl J Med.*, *344*(18), 1343-1350. doi: 10.1056/NEJM2

Tuomilehto, J., Schwarz, P., & Lindström, J. (2011). Long-term benefits from lifestyle interventions for type 2 diabetes. *Diabetes Care*, *34*(suppl 2), S210-S214. doi: 10.2337/dc11-s222

Turnbaugh, P. J., & Gordon, N. J. (2009). The core gut microbiome, energy balance and obesity. *J Physiol.*, *587*(Pt 17), 4153-4158. doi: 10.1113/jphysiol.2009.174136

Turnbaugh, P. J., Ley, R.E., Hamady, M., Fraser-Liggett, C., Knight, R., & Gordon, J.I. (2007). The human microbiome project: Exploring the microbial part of ourselves in a changing world. *Nature*, *449*(7164), 804-810. doi: 10.1038/nature06244

Turnbaugh, P. J., Ley, R. E., Mahowald, M. A., Magrini, V., Mardis, E. R., & Gordon, J.I. (2006). An obesity-associated gut microbiome with increased capacity for energy harvest. *Nature*, *444*, 1027-1031. doi:10.1038/nature05414

Turnbaugh, P. J., Ridaura, V. K., Faith, J. J., Rey, F. E., Knight, R., & Gordon, J.I. (2009). The effect of diet on the human gut microbiome: A metagenomic analysis in humanized gnotobiotic mice. *Sci Transl Med.*, *1*(6), 6ra14. doi:10.1126/scitranslmed.3000322

Turnbaugh, P., Backhed, F., Fulton, L., & Gordon, J. (2008). Diet-induced obesity is linked to marked but reversible alterations in the mouse distal gut microbiome. *Cell Host Microbe*, *3*, 213-223

Turner, K., Keogh, J., & Clifton, P. (2015). Dairy consumption and insulin sensitivity: A systematic review of short- and long-term intervention studies. *Nutr Metab Cardiovasc Dis*, *25*(1), 3-8

U.S. Food and Drug Administration. (2014, November 26). *Overview of fda labeling requirements for restaurants, similar retail food establishments and vending machines.* Retrieved from FDA.gov: http://www.fda.gov/Food/IngredientsPackagingLabeling/LabelingNutrition/ucm248732.htm

Ueyama, T. (2004). Emotional stress-induced tako-tsubo cardiomyopathy: Animal model and molecular mechanism. *Ann N Y Acad Sci*, *1018*, 437-44

United Nations Educational Social and Cultural Organisation. (2017, March 27). *Intangible cultural heritage. Mediterranean diet-inscribed in 2013 (eight.com) on the representative list of in the intangible cultural heritage of humanity.* Retrieved from UNESCO.org: http://www.unesco.org/culture/ich/en/RL/mediterranean-diet-00884

United States Department of Agriculture. (2000). *USDA fact book.* Retrieved from United States Department of agriculture: http://www.usda.gov/factbook/chapter2.pdf

United States Department of Agriculture. (2005, August). *Sweetener consumption in the United States.* Retrieved from United States Department of Agriculture Economic Research Service: http://www.ers.usda.gov/publications/sssm-sugar-and-sweeteners-outlook/sss243-01.aspx

United States Department of Agriculture, Economic Research Service. (2005, August). *Food consumption (per capita).* Retrieved from US Department of Agriculture: http://www.ers.usda.gov/media/326278/sss24301_002.pdf

US Burden of Disease Collaborators. (2013). The state of us health, 1990-2010: Burden of diseases, injuries, and risk factors. *JAMA., 310,* 591-608

US Department of Agriculture. (2012). *Nutrition standards in the national school lunch and school breakfast programs.* Retrieved from Food and Nutrition Service:https://www.federalregister.gov/articles/2012/01/26/2012-1010/nutrition-standards-in-the-national-school-lunch-and-school-breakfastprograms

US Department of Health and Human Services. (2016). *Million hearts initiative.* Retrieved from Health and Human Services: https://millionhearts.hhs.gov/index.html

USDA. (2005). *Nutrition and your health: Dietary guidelines for americans.* Retrieved from Health.gov: : http://health.gov/dietaryguidelines/dga2005/report/HTML/G5_History.htm

USDA. (2010). *Report of the dgac on the dietary guidelines for americans, 2010 part d. section 6: sodium, potassium, and water.* Retrieved August 25, 2013, from Report of the DGAC on the Dietary Guidelines for Americans, 2010, http://www.cnpp.usda.gov/Publications/DietaryGuidelines/2010/DGAC/Report/D-6-SodiumPotassiumWater.pdf

USDA. (2015). *2015 dietary guidelines advisory committee.* Retrieved from www/health.gov: http://www.health.gov/dietaryguidelines/2015-binder/2015/historyCurrentUse.aspx

USDA. (2017). *Animal feeding operations.* Retrieved from USDA Natural Resources Conservation Service: https://www.nrcs.usda.gov/wps/portal/nrcs/main/national/plantsanimals/livestock/afo/#

USDA. (2017, March 3). *Animal feeding operations.* Retrieved from Natural Resources Conservation Service: https://www.nrcs.usda.gov/wps/portal/nrcs/main/national/plantsanimals/livestock/afo/

USDA Center for Nutrition Policy and Promotion. (1997, May 17). *Dietary guidance on sodium: Should we take it with a grain of salt?* Retrieved from USDA Nutrition Insights: http://www.cnpp.usda.gov/publications/nutritioninsights/insight3.pdf

Van Cappellen, P., Way, B. M., Isgett, S. F., & Fredrickson, B.L. (2016). Effects of oxytocin administration on spirituality and emotional responses to meditation. *Social cognitive and affective neuroscience,* doi: 10.1093/scan/nsw078

Van Dam, R., Willett, W., Rimm, E., Stampfer, M., & Hu, F. (2002). Dietary fat and meat intake in relation to risk of type 2 diabetes in men. *Diabetes Care, 25*(3), 417-424

Van Elswyk, M., & McNeill, S. (2014). Impact of grass/forage feeding versus grain finishing on beef nutrients and sensory quality: The u.s. experience. *Meat Sci., 96,* 535-540. doi: 10.1016/j.meatsci.2013.08.010

Van Loan, M., Keim, N., Adams, S., Souza, E., Woodhouse, L., Thomas, A.,...Bremer, A. (2011). Dairy foods in a moderate energy restricted diet do not enhance central fat, weight, and intra-abdominal adipose tissue losses nor reduce adipocyte size or inflammatory markers in overweight and obese adults: A controlled feeding study. *J Obes,* 989657

Van't Riet, J., Sijtsema, S., Dagevos, H., & De Bruijn, G. (2011). The importance of habits in eating behaviour. An overview and recommendations for future research. *Appetite, 57,* 585-596. doi: 10.1016/j.appet.2011.07.010

Varbo, A., Benn, M., Tybjaeg-Hansen, A., & Nordestgaard, B. (2013). Elevated remnant cholesterol causes both low-grade inflammation and ischemic heart disease while low-density lippoprotein cholesterol causes ischemic heart disease without inflammation. *Circulation.* doi: 10.1161/?CIRCULATIONAHA.113003008

Vaziri, N., Wong, J., Pahl, M., Piceno, Y., Yuan, J., DeSantis, T., & Andersen, G. (2013). Chronic kidney disease alters intestinal microbial flora. *Kidney Int., 83,* 308-315. doi: 10.1038/ki.2012.345

Velasco, J., Marmesat, S., Bordeaux, O., Márquez-Ruiz, G., & Dobarganes, C. (2004). Formation and evolution of monoepoxy fatty acids in thermoxidized olive and sunflower oils and quantitation in used frying oils from restaurant and fried-food outlets. *J Agric Food Chem.*, *52*, 4438-4443. doi: 10.1021/jf030753f

Verma, A., Champagne, J., Sapp, J., Essebag, V., Novak, P., Skanes, A.,...Birnie, D. (2013). Discerning the incidence of symptomatic and asymptomatic episodes of atrial fibrillation before and after catheter ablation (discern af). *JAMA*, *173*(2), 149-156. doi:10.1001/jamainternmed.2013.1561

Vighi, G., Marcucci, F., Sensi, L., Di Cara, G., & Frati, F. (2008). Allergy and the gastrointestinal system. *Clinical and Experimental Immunology*, *153*(Suppl. 1), 3-6. doi: 10.1111/j.1365-2249.2008.03713.x

Viladomiu, M., Hontecillas, R., & Bassaganya-Riera, J. (2016). Modulation of inflammation and immunity by dietary conjugated linoleic acid. *Eur J Pharmacol.*, *785*, 87-95

Villegas, R., Goodloe, R., McClellan, B. J., Boston, J., & Crawford, D. (2014). Gene-carbohydrate and gene-fiber interactions and type 2 diabetes in diverse populations from the national health and nutrition examination surveys (nhanes) as part of the epidemiologic architecture for genes linked to environment (eagle) study. *BMC Genet*, *15*, 69. doi:10.1186/1471-2156-15-69

Virtanen, J. K., Mursu, J., Virtanen, H. E., Fogelholm, M., Salonen, J. T., Koskinen, T. T.,...Tuomainen, T.P. (2016). Associations of egg and cholesterol intakes with carotid intima-media thickness and risk of incident coronary artery disease according to apolipoprotein E phenotype in men: The kuopio ischaemic heart disease risk factor study. *AJCN*, doi: 10.3945/ajcn.115.122317

Visioli, F., & Strata, A. (2014). Milk, dairy products, and their functional effects in humans: A narrative review. *Adv Nutr*, *5*, 131-143. doi: 10.3945/an.113.005025

Voelker, R. (1996). Nocebos contribute to host of ills. *JAMA*, *275*, 345-7Volek, J., & Fernandez, M.F. (2008). Dietary carbohydrate restriction induces a unique metabolic state positively affecting atherogenic dyslipidemia, fatty acid partitioning, and metabolic syndrome. *Prog Lipid Res*, *47*, 307-18

Volk, B., Kunces, L., Freidenreich, D., Kupchak, B., Saenz, C., Artistizabal, J.,...Volek, J. (2014). Effects of step-wise increases in dietary carbohydrate on circulating saturated fatty acids and palmitoleic acid in adults with metabolic syndrome. *PLoS One*, *9*, e113605. doi: 10.1371/journal

Vormund, K., Braun, J., Rohrmann, S., Bopp, M., Ballmer, P., & Faeh, D. (2015). Mediterranean diet and mortality in Switzerland: An alpine paradox? *European Journal of Nutrition*, *54*, 139-148

Vrieze, A., Van Nood, E., Holleman, F., Salojarvi, J., Kootte, R. S., Bartselman, J. F., & Van Hylckaman Vlieg, J.E. (2012). Transfer of intestinal microbiota from lean donors increases insulin sensitivity in individuals with metabolic syndrome. *Gastroenterology*, *143*, 913-916.e7

Walsh, B. (2014, June 12). *Ending the war on fat*. Retrieved from *Time*: http://time.com/2863227/ending-the-war-on-fat/

Walsh, R. (2007). *The world of shamanism: New views of an ancient tradition*. Woodbury, MN: Llewellyn Publications

Wang, F., Jiang, H., Shi, K., Zhang, P., & Cheng, S. (2012). Gut bacterial translocation is associated with microinflammation in end-stage renal disease patients. *Nephrol. (Carlton)*, *17*, 733-738

Wang, H., Troy, L., Rogers, G., Fox, C., McKeown, N., Meigs, J., & Jacques, P. (2014). Longitudinal association between dairy consumption and changes of body weight and waist circumference: the framingham heart study. *Int J Obes, 38,* 299-305. doi: 10.1038/ijo.2013.78

Wang, Y., Ames, N. P., Tun, H. M., Tosh, S. M., Jones, P. J., & Khafipour, E. (2016). High molecular weight barley β-glucan alters gut microbiota toward reduced cardiovascular disease risk. *Front Microbiol., 7,* 129. doi: 10.3389/fmicb.2016.00129

Wang, Y., Huang, J., Zhang, D., Qu, Y., & Hu, D. (2014). Dairy foods and risk of stroke: A meta-analysis of prospective cohort studies. *Nutr Metab Cardiovasc Dis., 24,* 460-469. doi: 10.1016/j.numecd.2013.12.006

Wang, Z., Klipfell, E., Bennett, B. J., Koeth, R., . Levison, B. S., DuGar, B.,...Allayee, H. (2011). Gut flora metabolism of phosphatidylcholine promotes cardiovascular disease. *Nature, 472,* 57-63

Wang, Z., Klipfell, E., Bennett, B., Koeth, R., Levison, B., DuGar, B.,...Hazen, S. (2011). Gut flora metabolism of phosphatidylcholine promotes cardiovascular disease. *Nature, 472*(7341), 57-63

Wang, Z., Roberts, A. B., Buffa, J. A., Levison, B. S., Zhu, W., Org, E.,...Hazen, S. (2015). Non-lethal inhibition of gut microbial trimethylamine production for the treatment of atherosclerosis. *Cell, 163,* 1585-1595. doi: 10.1016/j.cell.2015.11.055

Wang, Z., Tang, W., Buffa, J., Fu, X., Britt, E., Koeth, R.,,...Hazen, S. (2010). Prognostic value of choline and betaine depends on intestinal microbiota-generated metabolite trimethylamineNoxide. *Eur. Heart J., 35,* 904-910

Wang, Z., Zhai, F., Du, F., & Popkin, B. (2008). Dynamic shifts in chinese eating behaviors. *Asia Pac J Clin Nutr, 17,* 123-130

Wansink, B. (2010). From mindless eating to mindlessly eating better. *Physiol Behav, 100,* 454-463

Warber, S., Ingerman, S., Moura, V., Wunder, J., Northrop, A., Gillespie, B.,,...Rubenfire, M. (2011). Healing the heart: A randomized pilot study of a spiritual retreat for depression in acute coronary syndrome patients. *Explore, 7*(4), 222-33. doi: 10.1016/j.explore.2011.04.002

Wardle, J., Chida, Y., Gibson, E., Whitaker, K., & Steptoe, A. (2011). Stress and adiposity: A meta-analysis of longitudinal studies. *Obesity, 19,* 771-778

Warrier, M., Shih, D., Burrows, A., Ferguson, D., Gromovsky, A., Brown, A.,,...Wang, Z. (2015). The tmao-generating enzyme flavin monooxygenase 3 is a central regulator of cholesterol balance. *Cell Rep., 10*(3), 326-338

Wartolowska, K., Judge, A., Hopewell, S.C., Dean, B. J., Rombach, I., Brindle, D.,,...Carr, A.J. (2014). Use of placebo controls in the evaluation of surgery: Systematic review. *BMJ, 348,* g3253 doi: 10.1136/bmj.g3253

Washington State Department of Health. (2017, January 23). *Farmed versus wild salmon.* Retrieved from Washington State Department of Health: http://www.doh.wa.gov/CommunityandEnvironment/Food/Fish/FarmedSalmon

Weaver, R. (2009, April 7). *Ruminations on other worlds.* Retrieved from statepress.com: https://web.archive.org/web/20110724233755/http://www.statepress.com:80/archive/node/5745

WebMD. (2017). *L - Carnitine.* Retrieved from WebMD.com: http://www.webmd.com/vitamins-supplements/ingredientmono-1026-l-carnitine.aspx?activeingredientid=1026

Westman, E. C. (2002). Is dietary carbohydrate essential for human nutrition? *The American Journal of Clinical Nutrition, 75*(5), 951-953

Westman, E.C., Feinman, R.D., Marvopoulos, J.C., Vernon, M.C., Volek, J.S., Wortman, J.A., & Phinney, S.D. (2007). Low-carbohydrate nutrition and metabolism. *The American Journal of Nutrition, 89*(2), 276-284

WHO Director-General. (2013, August 10). *WHO director-general addresses health promotion conference.* Retrieved from World Health Organization: http://www.who.int/dg/ speeches/ 2013/health_promotion_20130610/en/

Whole grains Council. (2012, January 12). *Research sheds light on gluten issues.* Retrieved September 15, 2013, from Whole Grains Council: http://wholegrainscouncil.org/ newsroom/blog/2012/01/research-sheds-light-on-gluten-issues

Whole Grains Council. (2013, March 21). *Health study: Kamut wheat versus modern wheat.* Retrieved from Whole Grains Council: http://wholegrainscouncil.org/newsroom/ blog/2013/03/health-study-kamut-wheat-vs-modern-wheat

Widmer, R., Flammer, A. J., Lerman, L. O., & Lerman, A. (2015). The mediterranean diet, its components, and cardiovascular disease. *Am J Med., 128*(3): 229-238

Wilber, K. (2011). *A brief history of everything.* Boston: Shambala

Williams, G., Kroes, R., & Munro, I. (2000). Safety evaluation and risk assessment of the herbicide roundup in its active ingredient, glyphosate, for humans. *Regul Toxicol Pharmacol, 31,* 117-165

Winkelman, M. (2002). Shamanism and cognitive evolution. *Cambridge Archaeological Journal, 12*(1),71-101

Wittenbecher, C., Mühlenbruch, K., Kröger, J., Jacobs, S., Kuxhaus, O., Floegel, A.,... Schulze, M. (2015). Amino acids, lipid metabolites, and ferritin as potential mediators linking red meat consumption to type 2 diabetes. *Am J Clin Nutr., 101,* 1241-1250. doi: 10.3945/ajcn.114.099150

Wittstein, I., Thiemann, D., & Lima, J. (2005). Neurohumoral features of myocardial stunning due to sudden emotional stress. *N Engl J Med, 352,* 539-48

Wlliams, M.E. (2017). Why every mind needs mindfulness. *Time: Mindfulness, The New Science of Health and Happiness,* 8-15

Wrangham, R. (2009). *Catching fire: How cooking made us human.* New York: Basic Books

Wrangham, R. (2009, August 28). Did cooking give humans an evolutionary edge? (P. Raeburn, Interviewer)

Wrangham, R., & Carmody, R. (2010). Human adaptation to the control of fire. *Evolutionary Anthropology, 19*(5), 187-199. doi: 10.1002/evan.20275

Wrangham. R, & Conklin-Brittain, N. (2003). Cooking as a biological trait. *Comp Biochem Physiol A Mol Integr Physiol, 136,* 35-46

Wu, J., & Mozaffarian, D. (2011). Omega-3 fatty acids and cardiovascular disease: Effects on risk factors, molecular pathways, and clinical events. *J Am Coll Cardiol., 58,* 2047-2067. doi: 10.1016/j.jacc.2011.06.063

Wu, J., & Mozaffarian, D. (2014). ω-3 fatty acids, atherosclerosis progression and cardiovascular outcomes in recent trials: New pieces in a complex puzzle. *Heart, 100,* 530-533. doi: 10.1136/heartjnl-2013-305257

Wu, L., & Sun, D. (2017). Adherence to mediterranean diet and risk of developing cognitive disorders: An updated systematic review and meta-analysis of prospective cohort studies. *Sci Rep., 7,* 41317 doi: 10.1038/srep41317

Wu, Y., Qian, Y., Pan, Y., Li, P., Yang, J., Ye, X., & Xu, G. (2015). Association between dietary fiber intake and risk of coronary heart disease: A meta-analysis. *Clin Nutr., 34,* 603-611. doi: 10.1016/j.clnu.2014.05.009

Xi, B., Huang, Y., Reilly, K., Li, S., Zheng, R., Barrio-Lopez, M.,...Zhou, D. (2015). Sugar-sweetened beverages and risk of hypertension and CVD: A dose-response meta-analysis. *Br J Nutr., 113,* 709-717. doi: 10.1017/S0007114514004383

Xun, P., Wu, Y., He, Q., & He, K. (2013). Fasting insulin concentrations and incidence of hypertension, stroke, and coronary heart disease: A meta-analysis of prospective cohort studies. *Am J Clin Nutr, 98*, 1543-54

Yahoo.com. (2017, April 18). *Hunting*. Retrieved from Yahoo.com: https://answers.yahoo.com/question/index?qid=20090331194350AA8aLwe

Yang, Q., Cogswell, M.E., Flanders, W.D., Hong, Y., Zhang, Z., Loustalot, F., & Hu, F. B. (2012). Trends in cardiovascular health metrics and associations with all-cause and cvd mortality among us adults. *JAMA, 307*(12), 1273-1283. doi: 10.1001/jama.2012.339

Yao, B., Fang, H., Xu, W., Yan, Y., Xu, H., Liu, Y.,...Zhao, Y. (2014). Dietary fiber intake and risk of type 2 diabetes: A dose-response analysis of prospective studies. *Eur J Epidemiol., 29*, 79-88. doi: 10.1007/s10654-013-9876-x

Yatsunenko, T., Rey, F., Manary, M., Trehan, I., Dominguez-Bello, M., Contreras, M., & Gordon, J. (2012). Human gut microbiome viewed across age and geography. *Nature, 486*, 222-227

Yeats, W. (1996). *The collected poems of w.b. yeats*. New York: Simon and Schuster

Yeoman, C. J., Chia, N., Jeraldo, P., Sipos, M., Goldenfeld, N. D., & White, B.A. (2012). The microbiome of the chicken gastrointestinal tract. *Animal Health Research Reviews, 13*(1), 89-99 doi: 10.1017/S1466252312000138

Yerushalmy, J. H. (1957). Fat in the diet and mortality from heart disease. A methodologic note. *NY State J Med, 57*, 2343-54

Yi, W., Fischer, J., Krewer, G., & Akoh, C. (2005). Phenolic compounds from blueberries can inhibit colon cancer cell proliferation and induce apoptosis. *J Agric Food Chem., 53*(18), 7320-9

Yuan, T. T., Toy, P., McClary, J. A., Lin, R. J., Miyamoto, N. G., & Kretschmer, P. J. (2001). *Genecloning and genetic characterization of an evolutionarily conserved human olfactory receptor that is differentially expressed across species, 278*, 41-51

Yusuf, S. (2013). *The need for balance in evaluating the evidence on na and cvd*. Retrieved from Institute of Medicine: http://www.iom.edu/~/media/Files/Activity%20Files/Nutrition/ConsequencesSodiumReduction/2012-DEC-04/Presentations/13_Salim%20Yusuf.pdf

Zhang, X., Shen, D., Fang, Z., Jie, Z., Qiu, X., Zhang, C., & Ji, L. (2013). Human gut microbiota changes reveal the progression of glucose intolerance. *PLoS ONE, 8*, e71108

Zhang, X., Zhang, G., Zhang, H., Karin, M., Bai, H., & Cai, D. (2008). Hypothalamic ikkβ/nf-b and er stress link overnutrition to energy imbalance and obesity. *Cell, 135*(1), 61-73

Zhao, Z., Li, S., Liu, G., Yan, F., Ma, X., Huang, Z., & Tian, H. (2012). Body iron stores and heme-iron intake in relation to risk of type 2 diabetes: A systematic review and meta-analysis. *PLoS One, 7*, e41641. doi: 10.1371/journalpone.0041641

Zheng, H., Yde, C. C., Clausen, M. R., Kristensen, M., Lorenzen, J., Astrup, A., & Bertram, H.C. (2015). Metabolomics investigation to shed light on cheese as a possible piece in the french paradox puzzle. *Journal of Agricultural and Food Chemistry, 63*, 2830-2839 doi: 10.1021/jf505878a

Zheng, J., Huang, T., Yu, Y., Hu, X., Yang, B., & Li, D. (2012). Fish consumption and CHD mortality: an updated meta-analysis of seventeen cohort studies. *Public Health Nutr., 15*, 725-737. doi: 10.1017/S1368980011002254

Zong, G., Gao, A., Hu, F., & Sun, Q. (2016). Whole grain intake and mortality from all causes, cardiovascular disease, and cancer: A meta-analysis of prospective cohort studies. *Circulation, 133*, 2370-2380

ACKNOWLEDGMENTS

Acknowledgments for a work such of this—drawing on so many people and diverse skills and practices from a vast gamut of experiences—is difficult. We only see further, and with a broader, wiser perspective because we stand on the shoulders of the Ancestors. This is the Way of the Shaman. It is also the Way of Science; learning, incorporating, and evolving knowledge by synthesis, transformation, and occasionally repudiation. With such a debtor's list, if I have left anyone unmentioned, it is purely oversight. Any and all omissions are squarely upon my shoulders.

I thank my parents; my mother for showing me a sanctuary and temple within the confines of an everyday kitchen. To my father, for opening the doors of science and their exacting rigor, and passing along the moral conviction to follow where the data leads; not where you want it to go. To my martial arts brethren, a word of thanks. To Soke Masaaki Hatsumi, for sharing his martial art and tradition that changes lives. To my mentors and friends; Kevin, Phil, Mark, Morton, Roger and my training *tomodachi*, Wild Bill, I would never have gotten the lessons, or the bruises, without you.

To my spiritual guides, teachers, and friends, Andrew and Joy, you have welcomed me into your world with wild, free abandon. You never mentioned we punched a one-way ticket! To Wendy and Tim, what foreign fruits have we plucked on this long, strange trip? To my culinary comrades, Luca and Aine, I thank you for your unwavering support and continued inspiration. To Glenn, we all miss your quirky wisdom dispensed over rusty nails.

A special thanks to my agent, Leticia Gomez who works ceaselessly and with an unending pool of enthusiasm to help spread the gospel. To my publishers and editors, Deb and Maddie; thank you for your patience, understanding, and genius in solving the mystery of the unending references! A special thanks to my friend and incredibly talented artist, Jayde Hilliard-Simpson, for life-saving graphics at a moment's notice.

And of course, to Jennifer, without whom there is no sunrise.

ENDNOTES

1   (Ingerman, Walking in Light, 2014)
2   (Ingerman, Walking in Light, 2014)
3   (Ingerman, Walking in Light, 2014)
4   (Freeman, 2015)
5   (Ely, Childress, Jagannathan, & Lowe, 2015)
6   For more detail on ancient cuisines and the health imbuing aspects of indigenous foods and diets please refer to *Ancient Eats (Volume 1): The Greeks and Vikings* and *The Fallacy of the Calorie: Why the Modern Western Diet Is Killing Us and How to Stop It.*
7   (Emerging Technology from the ArXiv, 2012)
8   (Ingerman & Wesselman, Awakening to the Spirit World: The Shamanic Path of Direct Revelation, 2010)
9   (Helmenstine Ph.D., 2017)
10   (Ladwig, et al., 2017)
11   (Ladwig, et al., 2017)
12   (Taylor, 2017)
13   (Wrangham, Catching Fire: How Cooking Made Us Human, 2009)
14   (Wilber, 2011)
15   (Ingerman, Walking in Light, 2014)
16   (Winkelman, 2002)
17   (Ingerman & Wesselman, Awakening to the Spirit World: The Shamanic Path of Direct Revelation, 2010)
18   (Ingerman, Walking in Light, 2014)
19   (Ingerman & Wesselman, 2010)
20   (Hancock, Supernatural: Meetings with the Ancient Teachers of Mankind, 2007)
21   (Ingerman, Walking in Light, 2014)
22   (Ingerman & Wesselman, 2010)
23   (Ingerman & Wesselman, 2010)
24   (Harner, 1987)
25   (Hancock, Supernatural: Meetings with the ancient teachers of mankind, 2007)
26   (Wilber, 2011)
27   (Steed, Code Delicious with Dr. Mike: What is a Shaman? (http://radiomd.com/show/code-delicious/item/32168-what-is-a-shaman), 2016)

28 (Wilber, 2011)
29 (Wilber, 2011)
30 (Martínez Steele, et al., 2016)
31 (Monteiro, Moubarac, Cannon, Ng, & Popkin, 2013)
32 (Wilber, 2011)
33 (Brillat-Savarin & Robinson, 2014)
34 (Wilber, 2011)
35 (Walsh R., 2007)
36 (Finniss, Kaptchuk, Miller, & Benedetti, 2010)
37 (Ingerman, Walking in Light, 2014)
38 (Ingerman, Walking in Light, 2014)
39 (Ingerman & Wesselman, 2010)
40 (Ingerman, Shamanic Intervention in a Cardiac
    Rehabilitation Program, 2013)
41 (Warber, et al., 2011)
42 (Glassman MD, 2007)
43 (Ingerman, Walking in Light, 2014)
44 (Norton, 2007)
45 (Einstein, 2017)
46 (Norton, 2007)
47 (Walsh R., 2007)
48 (Ingerman & Wesselman, 2010)
49 (Gunnsteinsdottir & Olafsdottir, 2016)
50 (Wilber, 2011)
51 (Wilber, 2011)
52 (Ingerman, Walking in Light, 2014)
53 (Montmayeur & le Coutre, 2009)
54 (Shadan, 2009)
55 (Montmayeur & le Coutre, 2009)
56 (Stettler & Axel, 2009)
57 (Patel & Pinto, 2014)
58 (Patel & Pinto, 2014)
59 (Fox, 2016)
60 (Patel & Pinto, 2014)
61 (Fox, 2016)
62 (Fox, 2016)
63 (Deyoung, 2017)
64 (Fox, 2016)
65 (Fox, 2016)
66 (Gustavson, Garcia, Hankins, & Rusiniak, 1974)
67 (Nevid, 2015)
68 (Wilber, 2011)
69 (Ader & Cohen, 1985)
70 (Ader, Cohen, & Felten, Psychoneuroimmunology: Interaction
    between the Nervous System and and Immune System, 1995)
71 (Ader, Cohen, & Felten, Psychoneuroimmunology: Interaction between the Nervous
    System and and Immune System, 1995)
72 (Goebel, et al., 2002)
73 (Shepherd, 2004)

[74] (Shepherd, 2004)
[75] (Wrangham. R & Conklin-Brittain, 2003)
[76] (Wrangham, Catching Fire: How Cooking Made Us Human, 2009)
[77] (Wrangham. R & Conklin-Brittain, 2003)
[78] (Ingerman & Wesselman, 2010)
[79] (Shepherd, 2004)
[80] (Busse, et al., 2014)
[81] (Neuhaus, et al., 2009)
[82] (Neuhaus, et al., 2009)
[83] (Pluznicka, et al., 2009)
[84] (Gu, et al., 2014)
[85] (Braun, Voland, Kunz, Prinz, & Gratzl, 2007)
[86] (Griffin, Kafadar, & Paylath, 2009)
[87] (Busse, et al., 2014)
[88] (Koulivand, Ghadiri, & Gorji, 2013)
[89] (Koulivand, Ghadiri, & Gorji, 2013)
[90] (Mennella, 2006)
[91] (Patel & Pinto, 2014)
[92] (Ely, Childress, Jagannathan, & Lowe, 2015)
[93] (Ely, Childress, Jagannathan, & Lowe, 2015)
[94] (Freeman, 2015)
[95] (Lim, et al., 2012)
[96] (US Burden of Disease Collaborators, 2013)
[97] (Bloom, et al., 2011)
[98] (Mozaffarian D., 2016)
[99] (Mozaffarian D., 2016)
[100] (Mozaffarian & Ludwig, Dietary Guidelines in the 21st Century—A Time for Food, 2010)
[101] (Obikoya, 2017)
[102] (Davis & Saltos, 1999)
[103] (National Nutrition Conference for Defense, 1941)
[104] (Mozaffarian, 2016)
[105] (Mozaffarian, 2016)
[106] (Freeman, et al., 2017)
[107] (Siri-Tarino, Sun, Hu & Krauss, 2010)
[108] (Chowdhury, et al., 2014)
[109] (Mente, et al., 2017)
[110] (Dehghan, et al., 2017)
[111] (Taubes, The Soft Science of Dietary Fat, 2001)
[112] (Jacobs & Tapsell, 2007)
[113] (US Department of Agriculture, 2012)
[114] (Mozaffarian, Hao, Rimm & Willett, 2011)
[115] (Smith, et al., 2015)
[116] (Wang, et al., 2014)
[117] (Sluijs, et al., 2012)
[118] (Drouin-Chartier, et al., 2016)
[119] (Drouin-Chartier, et al., 2016)
[120] (Mozaffarian & Ludwig, Dietary Guidelines in the 21st Century—A Time for Food, 2010)

[121] (Mozaffarian, 2016)
[122] (Brand-Miller, McMillan-Price, Steinbeck & Caterson, 2009)
[123] (Volk, et al., 2014)
[124] (Ludwig & Friedman, 2014)
[125] (Lennerz, et al., 2013)
[126] (Ebbeling, et al., 2012)
[127] For a full background on obesity, BMI, and the modern Western Diet, refer to *The Fallacy of The Calorie: Why the Modern Western Diet is Killing Us and How to Stop It*
[128] (Mozaffarian, et al., 2015)
[129] (Mozaffarian, Hao, Rimm & Willett, 2011)
[130] (Fenster, The Fallacy of The Calorie: Why the Modern Western Diet is Killing Us and How to Stop It, 2014)
[131] (Fenster, The Fallacy of The Calorie: Why the Modern Western Diet is Killing Us and How to Stop It, 2014)
[132] (Franz, VanWormer, & Crain, 2007)
[133] (APA, 2015)
[134] (Rosmond, 2005)
[135] (Li, Li, Zhou, & Messina, 2013)
[136] (Wardle, Chida, Gibson, Whitaker & Steptoe, 2011)
[137] (Wansink, 2010)
[138] (Murray, Tulloch, Gold, & Avena, 2014)
[139] (Kurtus, 2017)
[140] (Rovelli, 2017)
[141] (Dietary Guidelines Advisory Committee, 2015)
[142] (Feinman, 2004)
[143] (Afshin, Micha, Khatibzadeh, Schmidt, & Mozaffarian, 2014)
[144] (Jacobs & Tapsell, 2007)
[145] (Mozaffarian & Ludwig, Dietary Guidelines in the 21st Century—A Time for Food, 2010)
[146] (Jacobs & Tapsell, 2013)
[147] (Fardet, 2015)
[148] (USDA, 2015)
[149] (Mozaffarian, Appel, & Van Horn, Components of a Cardioprotective Diet: New Insights, 2011)
[150] (Dietary Guidelines Advisory Committee., 2015)
[151] (Mozaffarian, 2014)
[152] (Rovelli, 2017)
[153] (Sider, 2001)
[154] (Khera, Emdin, & Drake, 2016)
[155] (IMDb, 2012)
[156] (Fenster, The Fallacy of The Calorie: Why the Modern Western Diet is Killing Us and How to Stop It, 2014)
[157] (Kaplan, et al., 2017)
[158] (Kaplan, et al., 2017)
[159] (McClelland, Chung, Detrano, Post, & Kronmal, 2006)
[160] (Herodotus, 2011)
[161] (The Holy Bible: King James Version, 2004)
[162] (Fenster, Ancient Eats (Volume 1): The Greeks and Vikings, 2016)
[163] (Shakespeare, 2014)

164   (CBS News, 1977)
165   (Senate, Select Committee on Nutrition and Human Needs of the United States, 1977)
166   (Ramsden, et al., 2013)
167   (Ramsden, et al., 2016)
168   (Keys, Sucrose in the Diet and Coronary Heart Disease, 1971)
169   (Keys, Coronary Heart Disease—The Global Picture, 1975)
170   (Fenster, The Fallacy of The Calorie: Why the Modern Western Diet is Killing Us and How to Stop It, 2014)
171   (Brown, Tzoulaki, Candeias, & Elliott, 2009)
172   (O'Donnell, et al., 2011)
173   (O'Donnell, et al., 2014)
174   (Yusuf, 2013)
175   (Alderman, 2010)
176   (Graudel, Hubeck-Graudel, & Jurgens, 2011)
177   (CDC, 2017)
178   (Badkar & Lubin, 2012)
179   (Fenster, The Fallacy of The Calorie: Why the Modern Western Diet is Killing Us and How to Stop It, 2014)
180   (Guyenet, 2012)
181   (Fenster, The Fallacy of The Calorie: Why the Modern Western Diet is Killing Us and How to Stop It, 2014)
182   (Martínez Steele, et al., 2016)
183   (Hoffman & Gerber, 2015)
184   (Louzada, et al., 2015)
185   (Dobarganes & Márquez-Ruiz, 2015)
186   (Hu, 2013)
187   (Smith, et al., 2015)
188   (Imamura, et al., 2015)
189   (Xi, et al., 2015)
190   (Singh, et al., 2015)
191   (Azad, et al., 2017)
192   (Swithers, Martin, & Davidson, 2010)
193   (Shankar, Ahuja, & Sriram, 2013)
194   (Burke & Small, 2015)
195   (Pepino, 2015)
196   (Azad, et al., 2017)
197   (Huang, et al., 2017)
198   (Alhazmi, Stojanovski, McEvoy & Garg, 2012)
199   (Mente, de Koning, Shannon & Anand, 2009)
200   (Howard, et al., 2006)
201   (Tinker, et al., 2008)
202   (Micha & Mozaffarian, Saturated Fat and Cardiometabolic Risk Factors Coronary Heart Disease, Stroke, and Diabetes: A Fresh Look at the Evidence, 2010)
203   (Chowdhury, et al., 2014)
204   (Salas-Salvadó, et al., 2011)
205   (Salas-Salvadó J., et al., 2014)
206   (Estruch, et al., 2013)
207   (Appel, et al., 2005)
208   (Gadgil, et al., 2013)

209 (Suez, et al., 2014)
210 (Neltner, et al., 2013)
211 (Chassaing, et al., 2015)
212 (Moodie, Stuckler, & Monteiro, 2013)
213 (Monteiro, Moubarac, Cannon, Ng, & Popkin, 2013)
214 (Moodie, Stuckler, & Monteiro, 2013)
215 (Tavares, Fonseca, Rosa, & Yokoo, 2012)
216 (Wang, Zhai, Du, & Popkin, 2008)
217 (Piernas & Popkin, 2010)
218 (Monteiro, Gomes & Cannon, Can the Food Industry Help Tackle the Growing Burden of Under-nutrition? The Snack Attack, 2010)
219 (Rayner, Hawkes, Lang, & Bello, 2006)
220 (Hawkes, 2010)
221 (Monteiro & Cannon, 2012)
222 (WHO Director-General, 2013)
223 (The European Food Information Council, 2017)
224 (James, 2004)
225 (Committee on Nutrition, 1964)
226 (Vormund, et al., 2015)
227 (Mozaffarian, Appel & Van Horn, Components of a Cardioprotective Diet: New Insights, 2011)
228 (Dietary Guidelines Advisory Committee., 2015)
229 (Djoussé, Akinkuolie, Wu, Ding, & Gaziano, 2012)
230 (Mozaffarian, Hao, Rimm & Willett, 2011)
231 (Smith, et al., 2015)
232 (Estruch, et al., 2013)
233 (Martínez-González, et al., 2015)
234 (Fenster M. S., The Fallacy of The Calorie: Why the Modern Western Diet is Killing Us and How to Stop It, 2014)
235 (Corella, et al., 2013)
236 (Fenster, 10 Healthy Foods that Protect Your Brain, 2015)
237 (Food and Agricultural Organisation of The United Nations, 2010)
238 (Rovelli, 2017)
239 (United Nations Educational Social and Cultura lOrganisation, 2017)
240 (Howard, et al., 2006)
241 (Tinker, et al., 2008)
242 (Micha & Mozaffarian, 2010)
243 (Chowdhury, et al., 2014)
244 (Dietary Guidelines Advisory Committee, 2015)
245 (The Asiatic Society, 2017)
246 (Schwingshackl, Missbach, König & Hoffmann, 2015)
247 (Wu & Sun, 2017)
248 (Widmer, Flammer, Lerman & Lerman, 2015)
249 (Bloomfield, et al., 2016)
250 (Subhan & Chan, 2016)
251 (Vormund, et al., 2015)
252 (Chiu, et al., 2015)
253 (Satija, et al., 2017)
254 (Buettner, 2012)

[255] (Fenster, Ancient Eats (Volume 1): The Greeks and Vikings, 2016)
[256] (Subhan & Chan, 2016)
[257] (Gadsby & Steele, 2004)
[258] (Mithril, Dragsted, & Meyer, 2012)
[259] (Renaud & de Lorgeril, 1992)
[260] (Kaplan, et al., 2017)
[261] (Simopoulos, Evolutionary Aspects of Diet, the Omega-6/Omega-3 Ratio and Genetic Variation: Nutritional Implications for Chronic Diseases, 2006)
[262] (Buettner, 2012)
[263] (Fenster, The Fallacy of The Calorie: Why the Modern Western Diet is Killing Us and How to Stop It, 2014)
[264] (Micha, Wallace & Mozaffarian, Red and Processed Meat Consumption and Risk of Incident Coronary Heart Disease, Stroke, and Diabetes: A Systematic Review and Meta-Analysis, 2010)
[265] (Rohrmann, et al., 2013)
[266] (Gadsby & Steele, 2004)
[267] (Stewart, et al., 2016)
[268] (Choi, 2015)
[269] (Taylor, 2016)
[270] (Tennyson, 2003)
[271] (Einstein, Everything Should Be Made as Simple as Possible, But Not Simpler, 2017)
[272] (Haubrich, 2005)
[273] (Anderson, et al., 2016)
[274] (NIH, 2017)
[275] (Anderson, et al., 2016)
[276] (Anderson, et al., 2016)
[277] (Anderson, et al., 2016)
[278] (Li, Kaaks, Linseisen, & Rohrmann, 2012)
[279] (Bolland, et al., 2008)
[280] (Rovelli, 2017)
[281] (Carlin, 2012)
[282] (Wilber, 2011)
[283] For a more detailed description of this, refer to *The Fallacy of the Calorie: Why the Modern Western Diet Is Killing Us and How to Stop It*
[284] (Ordovas, et al., 2002)
[285] (Neufeld, et al., 2004)
[286] (Wrangham, Catching Fire: How Cooking Made Us Human, 2009)
[287] (Wrangham, Did Cooking Give Humans An Evolutionary Edge? 2009)
[288] (Adams, 2017)
[289] (Human Microbiome Project Consortium, 2012)
[290] (Human Microbiome Project Consortium, 2012)
[291] (Denjean, 2013)
[292] (Corbille, et al., 2016)
[293] (Denjean, 2013)
[294] (Vighi, Marcucci, Sensi, Di Cara & Frati, 2008)
[295] (IMDb, 2017)
[296] (Sebastian, Frassetto, Sellmeyer, Merriam & Morris, 2002)
[297] (Sebastian, Harris, Ottaway, Todd & Morris, 1994)
[298] (Bushinsky, 1996)

299   (Frassetto & Morris, 1997)
300   (Pak, Fuller, Sakahee, Preminger & Britton, 1985)
301   (Preminger, Sakhaee, Skurla & Pak, 1985)
302   (Morris, Sebastian, Forman, Tanaka & Schmidlin, 1999)
303   (Sharma, Kribben, Schattenfroh, Cetto, & Distler, 1990)
304   (Mickelborough, Gotshall, Kluka, Miller, & Cordain, 2001)
305   (Alpern & Sakhaee, 1997)
306   (Cani, et al., 2008)
307   (Cordain, Toohey, Smith, & Hickey, 2000)
308   (Human Microbiome Project, 2017)
309   (HealthDay News, 2013)
310   (Mason, 2013)
311   (Kassinen, et al., 2007)
312   (Kennedy, Cryan, Dinan & Clarke, 2014)
313   (Pflughoeft & Versalovic, 2012)
314   (Tremaroli & Backhed, 2012)
315   (Pray, Pillsbury, & Tomayko, 2013)
316   (Prandovszky, et al., 2011)
317   (Smith, 2015)
318   (Schmidt, 2015)
319   (Turnbaugh P. J., et al., 2006)
320   (Turnbaugh, Backhed, Fulton, & Gordon, 2008)
321   (Aron-Wisnewsky & Clément, 2015)
322   (Cani, et al., 2008)
323   (Ley, Turnbaugh, Klein, & Gordon, 2006)
324   (Ridaura, et al., 2013)
325   For further detail see the *Fallacy of the Calorie: Why the Modern Western Diet Is Killing Us and How to Stop It.*
326   (Vrieze, et al., 2012)
327   (Zhang, et al., 2013)
328   (Seekatz, Rao, Santhosh, & Young, 2016)
329   (Wang, et al., 2011)
330   (Koren, et al., 2011)
331   (Wang, et al., 2011)
332   (Craig, 2004)
333   (Tang, et al., 2013)
334   (Wang, et al., 2015)
335   (DiNicolantonio, Lavie, Fares, Menezes & O'Keefe, 2013)
336   (Eaton, Cordain, & Lindeberg, 2002)
337   (Krishnan, 2017)
338   (Backhed, Ley, Sonnenberg, Peterson, & Gordon, 2005)
339   (Ley, Turnbaugh, Klein, & Gordon, 2006)
340   (Ryan, et al., 2017)
341   (Catry, et al., 2015)
342   (Kaddurah-Daouk, et al., 2011)
343   (Bea, et al., 2002)
344   (Ryan, et al., 2017)

345   (Jones, Martoni, & Prakash, Cholesterol Lowering and Inhibition Of sterol Absorption
       by Lactobacillus Reuteri NCIMB 30242: A Randomized Controlled Trial, 2012)
346   (Jones, Martoni, Parent, & Prakash, 2012)
347   (Ryan, et al., 2017)
348   (Shin, et al., 2014)
349   (Cotillard A., et al., 2013)
350   (LeChatelier, et al., 2013)
351   (Wang, et al., 2016)
352   (Pasini, et al., 2015)
353   (Pasini, et al., 2015)
354   (Tang, et al., 2015)
355   (Aron-Wisnewsky & Clément, 2015)
356   (Aron-Wisnewsky & Clément, 2015)
357   (Craig, 2004)
358   (Wang, et al., 2015)
359   (Wang, et al., 2015)
360   (Wang, et al., 2015)
361   (Wang, et al., 2015)
362   (Wang, et al., 2015)
363   (Wang, et al., 2015)
364   (De Filippoa, et al., 2010)
365   (De Filippoa, et al., 2010)
366   (Yatsunenko, et al., 2012)
367   (Kong, et al., 2014)
368   (LeChatelier, et al., 2013)
369   (Alexander & Rietschel, 2001)
370   (McFarlin, Henning, Bowman, Gary & Carbajal, 2017)
371   (Aron-Wisnewsky & Clément, 2015)
372   (Aron-Wisnewsky & Clément, 2015)
373   (Rovelli, 2017)
374   (McFarlin, Henning, Bowman, Gary & Carbajal, 2017)
375   (Amar, et al., 2011)
376   (Dilli, et al., 2013)
377   (Beilharz, Kaakoush, Maniam & Morris, 2017)
378   (Tillisch, et al., 2013)
379   (Krishnan, 2017)
380   (FDA, 2017)
381   (Quinn & Young, 2014)
382   (Nettleton, Reimer & Shearer, 2016)
383   (Chassaing, et al., 2015)
384   (Chassaing, et al., 2015)
385   (Laparra & Sanz, 2010)
386   (Lippi, Danese, Mattiuzzi & Favaloro, Emmanuel, 2017)
387   (Maurer, 2017)
388   As discussed in depth in *The Fallacy of the Calorie: Why the Modern Western Diet Is
       Killing Us and How to Stop It*
389   (Yahoo.com, 2017)
390   (Kiran Krishnan, 2017)
391   (Krishnan, Code Delicious with Dr. Mike, 2017)

[392] (Wilber, 2011)
[393] (Wilber, 2011)
[394] (Rovelli, 2017)
[395] (Maine.gov, 2013)
[396] (Michigan.gov, 2017)
[397] (Knight, 1998)
[398] (Goodspeed, et al., 2013)
[399] (Braam, 2013)
[400] (Oches, 2010)
[401] (Ingerman, Walking in Light, 2014)
[402] (Micha, Wallace, & Mozaffarian, 2010)
[403] (Pan, et al., 2011)
[404] (Chen, Lv, Pang, & Liu, 2013)
[405] (Abete, Romaguera, Vieira, Lopez de Munain, & Norat, 2014)
[406] (Mozaffarian, Meat Intake and Mortality: Evidence For Harm, No Effect or Benefit, 2009)
[407] (Mozaffarian, Meat Intake and Mortality: Evidence for Harm, No Effect or Benefit? 2009)
[408] (Swaminathan, Fonseca, Alam, & Shah, 2007)
[409] (Zhao, et al., 2012)
[410] (Wittenbecher, et al., 2015)
[411] (Kim, Keogh, & Clifton, 2015)
[412] (Micha, Michas, Lajous, & Mozaffarian, 2013)
[413] (Institute of Medicine, 2010)
[414] (Daley, Abbot, Doyle, Nader, & Larson, 2010,)
[415] (Van Elswyk & McNeill, 2014)
[416] (IMDb, 2017)
[417] (Renaud & de Lorgeril, 1992)
[418] (Chowdhury, et al., 2014)
[419] (Wrangham, Catching Fire: How Cooking Made Us Human, 2009)
[420] (Carmody, Weintraub, & Wrangham, 2011)
[421] (Wrangham, Catching Fire: How Cooking Made Us Human, 2009)
[422] (Wrangham, Did Cooking Give Humans An Evolutionary Edge? 2009)
[423] (Westman, 2002)
[424] (Gadsby & Steele, 2004)
[425] (Wrangham, Catching Fire: How Cooking Made Us Human, 2009)
[426] (Carmody, Weintraub, & Wrangham, 2011)
[427] (Price, Hopkins, Smith, & Roth, 2012)
[428] (Psouni, Janke, & Garwicz, 2012)
[429] (DiNicolantonio & Lucan, The Wrong White Crystals: Not Salt But Sugar As Aetiological in Hypertension and Cardiometabolic Disease, 2014)
[430] (Harcombe, et al., 2015)
[431] (Harcombe, et al., 2015)
[432] (Heid, 2016)
[433] (Heid, 2016)
[434] (Harcombe, et al., 2015)
[435] (CDC, 2009)
[436] (Bentley, 2017)
[437] (CDC, 2014)

[438] (Malhotra, 2013)
[439] (Dreon, Fernstrom, & Campos, 1998)
[440] (Siri-Tarino, Sun, Hu, & Krauss, 2010)
[441] (Ramsden, et al., 2013)
[442] (Ramsden, Hibbeln, & Majchrzak, 2010)
[443] (DiNicolantonio, The Cardio Metabolic Consequences of Replacing Saturated Fats With Carbohydrates or Omega Six Polyunsaturated Fats: Did the Dietary Guidelines Have It Wrong? 2014)
[444] (DiNicolantonio, The Cardio Metabolic Consequences of Replacing Saturated Fats with Carbohydrates or Omega Six Polyunsaturated Fats: Did the Dietary Guidelines Have It Wrong? 2014)
[445] (The European Food Information Council, 2017)
[446] (DiNicolantonio & Lucan, The Wrong White Crystals: Not Salt But Sugar as Aetiological in Hypertension and Cardiometabolic Disease, 2014)
[447] (CDC, 2015)
[448] (Malhotra, 2013)
[449] (Mozaffarian, et al., Trans-Palmitoleic Acid, Metabolic Risk Factors, and New-Onset Diabetes in U.S. Adults: A Cohort Study, 2010)
[450] (Sachdeva, et al., 2008)
[451] (Abumrad & Davidson, 2012)
[452] (Stuart, 2013)
[453] (Teicholz, 2014)
[454] (American Heart Association, 2017)
[455] (Sacks, et al., 2017.)
[456] (Harcombe, et al., 2015)
[457] (de Souza, et al., 2015)
[458] (Siri-Tarino, Sun, Hu & Krauss, 2010)
[459] (Chowdhury, et al., 2014)
[460] (Skeaff & Miller, 2009)
[461] (Harcombe, Baker & Davies, 2017)
[462] (Forsythe, Phinney, & Fernandez, 2008)
[463] (Volek & Fernandez, 2008)
[464] (Estruch, et al., 2013)
[465] (Feinman R, 2004)
[466] (Micha & Mozaffarian, Saturated Fat And Cardiometabolic Risk Factors Coronary Heart Disease, Stroke, and Diabetes: A Fresh Look at the Evidence, 2010)
[467] (Rohrmann, et al., 2013)
[468] (Nagao, Iso, Yamagishi, Date & Tamakoshi, (2012)
[469] (IARC, 2015)
[470] (Thompson, 2015)
[471] (Aron-Wisnewsky & Clément, 2015)
[472] (Psouni, Janke, & Garwicz, 2012)
[473] (Lucan, 2012)
[474] (Danforth, 2014)
[475] (Srednicka-Tober, et al., 2016)
[476] (Oxford Dictionaries, 2017)
[477] (Checkoff, 2013)
[478] (USDA, 2017)
[479] (Snell, et al., 2012)

480 (Daley, Abbott, Doyle, Nader & Larson, 2010)
481 (Lucan, 2012)
482 (Droulez, Williams, Levy, Stobaus & Sinclair, 2006)
483 (Srednicka-Tober, et al., Composition Difference Between Organic and Convential Meat: A Systematic Literature Review and Meta-Analysis, 2016)
484 (Zheng, et al., 2012)
485 (Wu & Mozaffarian, 2011)
486 (Leung Yinko, Stark, Thanassoulis & Pilote, 2014)
487 (Larsson, Orsini & Wolk, 2012)
488 (Rizos, Ntzani, Bika, Kostapanos, & Elisaf, 2012)
489 (Mozaffarian & Rimm, Fish Intake, Contaminants, and Human Health: Evaluating the Risks and the Benefits, 2006)
490 (Wu & Mozaffarian, 2011)
491 (Wu & Mozaffarian, ω-3 fatty Acids, Atherosclerosis Progression And Cardiovascular Outcomes in Recent Trials: New Pieces in a Complex Puzzle, 2014)
492 (Wu & Mozaffarian, Omega-3 Fatty Acids and Cardiovascular Disease: Effects on Risk Factors, Molecular Pathways, and Clinical Events, 2011)
493 (Aung, et al., 2018)
494 (Anderson, et al., 2016)
495 (Fry, et al., 2016)
496 (Thompson, 2015)
497 (Tang G., Wang, Long, Yang & Si, 2015)
498 (Mellen, Walsh, & Herrington, 2008)
499 (Aune, Norat, Romundstad, & Vatten, 2013)
500 (Jakobsen, et al., 2009)
501 (Cai, et al., 2015)
502 (Alhazmi, Stojanovski, McEvoy & Garg, 2012)
503 (Bhupathiraju, et al., 2014)
504 (Wu, et al., 2015)
505 (Yao, et al., 2014)
506 (Mozaffarian, Appel & Van Horn, Components of a Cardioprotective Diet: New Insights, 2011)
507 (Ebbeling, et al., 2012)
508 (Fan, Song, Wang, Hui & Zhang, 2012)
509 (Basaranoglu, Basaranoglu, Sabuncu & Sentürk, 2013)
510 (Jala, Smits, Johnson & Conchol, 2010)
511 (Malik & Hu, 2015)
512 (Stanhope K., Sugar Consumption, Metabolic Disease and Obesity: The State of the Controversy, 2015)
513 (Stanhope, et al., 2011)
514 (Stanhope & Havel, Fructose Composition: Recent Results and Their Potential Implications, 2010)
515 (Deschanel, 2017)
516 (Delbyck, 2017)
517 (Sauve, 2014)
518 (Zong, Gao, Hu & Sun, 2016)
519 (American Heart Association, 2017)
520 The differences are discussed in detail in *The Fallacy of The Calorie Why the Modern Western Diet is Killing Us and How to Stop It*

[521] (Wang, et al., 2016)
[522] For a detailed exploration of Ancient Greek cuisine including the many different types of wheat and flours, see *Ancient Eats Volume I: The Greeks and Vikings*
[523] (Niness, 1999)
[524] (Institute of Medicine, 2001)
[525] (Whole Grains Council, 2013)
[526] (FDA, 2017)
[527] (Zong, Gao, Hu & Sun, 2016)
[528] (Zong, Gao, Hu & Sun, 2016)
[529] (Wang, et al., 2016)
[530] (Zong, Gao, Hu & Sun, 2016)
[531] (Aune, Norat, Romundstad & Vatten, 2013)
[532] (FDA.gov, 2016)
[533] (Heid, 2016)
[534] (Heid, 2016)
[535] (Dietary Guidelines Advisory Committee., 2015)
[536] (Sluijs, et al., 2012)
[537] (Soedamah-Muthu, Verberne, Ding, Engberink & Geleijnse, 2012)
[538] (Wang, Huang, Zhang, Qu & Hu, 2014)
[539] (Qin, et al., 2015)
[540] (Gao, et al., 2013)
[541] (Norat, Romundstad, Vatten & Aune, 2013)
[542] (Chen, et al., 2014)
[543] For a detailed description of the confusion surrounding milk and health effects, see *The Devil in the Milk* by Keith Woodford (2009, Chelsea Green Publishing Company, White River Junction, VT) which discusses at length the A1 versus A2 milk debate.
[544] (Sluijs, et al., 2012)
[545] (Swaminathan, Fonseca, Alam & Shah, 2007)
[546] (Zhao, et al., 2012)
[547] (Wittenbecher, et al., 2015)
[548] (Kim, Keogh & Clifton, 2015)
[549] (Micha, Michas, Lajous & Mozaffarian, 2013)
[550] (Daley, Abbot, Doyle, Nader, & Larson, 2010,)
[551] (Gao, et al., 2013)
[552] (Diaz-Lopez, et al., 2015)
[553] (Ericson, et al., 2015)
[554] (Nestel, et al., 2013)
[555] (Mozaffarian, et al., Trans-palmitoleic acid, metabolic risk factors, and new-onset diabetes in US adults: a cohort study, 2010)
[556] (Mozaffarian, et al., 2013)
[557] (Forouhi, et al., 2014)
[558] (Kratz, Baars & Guyenet, The Relationship Between High-Fat Dairy Consumption and Obesity, Cardiovascular, and Metabolic Disease, 2013)
[559] (Kratz, et al., 2014)
[560] (Khaw, Friesen, Riboli, Luben & Wareham, 2012)
[561] (de Oliveira, et al., 2013)
[562] (Sofi, et al., 2018)
[563] (Mozaffarian, 2016)
[564] (Scharf, Demmer & DeBoer, 2013)

565   (Mozaffarian, Hao, Rimm & Willett, 2011)
566   (Wang, et al., 2014)
567   (Smith, et al., 2015)
568   (Poutahidis, et al., 2013)
569   (Park, et al., 2013)
570   (Power, O'Toole, Stanton, Ross & Fitzgerald, 2014)
571   (Kadooka, et al., 2010)
572   (Kadooka, et al., 2013)
573   (Sharafedtinov, et al., 2013)
574   (Jung, et al., 2013)
575   (Sanchez, et al., 2014)
576   (Barrett, Dekker, Conwell, & Callaway, 2014)
577   (Bittman, Trust Me. Butter Is Better, 2015)
578   (The Commonwealth Fund, 2015)
579   (Pimpin, Wu, Haskelberg, Del Gobbo & Mozaffarian, 2016)
580   (Buijsse, et al., 2015)
581   (O'Sullivan, Hafekost, Mitrou & Lawrence, 2013)
582   (Wang, Huang, Zhang, Qu & Hu, 2014)
583   (Qin, et al., 2015)
584   (Pimpin, Wu, Haskelberg, Del Gobbo & Mozaffarian, 2016)
585   (Davenport, 2016)
586   (Pimpin, Wu, Haskelberg, Del Gobbo & Mozaffarian, 2016)
587   (Benbrook, Butler, Latif, Leifert, & Davis, 2013)
588   (Srednicka-Tober, et al., Higher PUFA and n-3 PUFA, Conjugated Linoleic Acid,
      Alpha Tocopherol and Iron, but Lower Iodine and Selenium Concentrations in
      Organic Milk: A Sytematic Literature Review and Meta Analysis, 2016)
589   (Renaud & de Lorgeril, 1992)
590   (Zheng, et al., 2015)
591   (Forouhi, et al., 2014)
592   (Crippa, et al., 2016)
593   (Giraffa, 2014)
594   (Høstmark, Haug, Tomten, Thelle & Mosdøl, 2009)
595   (El-Sheikh, El-Senaity, Youssef, Shahein & Abd Rabou, 2011)
596   (Wang Z, et al., 2011)
597   (Zheng, et al., 2015)
598   (Eisenberg, et al., 2016)
599   (Mozaffarian, 2016)
600   (Shin, Xun, Nakamura & He, 2013)
601   (Rong, et al., 2013)
602   (Lecerf & de Lorgeril, 2011)
603   (Fuller, et al., 2015)
604   (Richard, et al., 2017)
605   (Virtanen, et al., 2016)
606   (DiMarco, Norris, Millar, Blesso & Fernandez, 2017)
607   (America Heart Association, 2016)
608   (Freeman, et al., 2017)
609   (Missimer, et al., 2017)
610   (Ballesteros, et al., 2015)
611   (Gan, et al., 2015)

612   (Hu, Huang, Wang, Zhang & Qu, 2014)
613   (Li, Fan, Zhang, Hou & Tang, 2014)
614   (Afshin, Micha, Khatibzadeh & Mozaffarian, Consumption of Nuts and Legumes and Risk of Incident Ischemic Heart Disease, Stroke, and Diabetes: A Systematic Review and Meta-Analysis, 2014)
615   (Baranski, 2014)
616   (Yi, Fischer, Krewer & Akoh, 2005)
617   (Basu & Lyons, 2012)
618   (Micha, Afshin, Khatibzadeh & Mozaffarian, 2014)
619   (Estruch, et al., 2013)
620   (Hammond, Dudek, Lemen & Nemeth, 2004)
621   (Seralini, et al., 2014)
622   (Williams, Kroes & Munro, 2000)
623   (Mesnager, Defarge, Spiroux De Vendomois & Seralini, 2014)
624   (Domingo & Gine-Bordonaba, 2011)
625   (Snell, et al., 2012)
626   (Hammond, Dudek, Lemen & Nemeth, 2004)
627   (Spiroux de Vendomois, Rouiller, Cellier & Seralini, 2009)
628   (Hammond, Dudek, Lemen & Nemeth, 2004)
629   (The European Food Safety Authority, 2003)
630   (Seralini, et al., 2014)
631   (Representatives, 2018)
632   (Lou-Bonafonte, Gabás-Rivera, Navarro & Osada, 2015)
633   (Scotece, et al., 2015)
634   (Beauchamp, et al., 2005)
635   (Estruch, et al., 2013)
636   (Binia, Jaeger, Hu, Singh & Zimmermann, 2015)
637   (Baranski, 2014)
638   (Smith-Spangler, Brandeau & Hunter, 2012)
639   (Miller, et al., 2017)
640   (Baranski, 2014)
641   (Braun, Voland, Kunz, Prinz & Gratzl, 2007)
642   (Clifton, Nutopia, 2012)
643   (Taubes, 2017)
644   (Rovelli, 2017)
645   (Wilber, 2011)
646   (Shakepeare, 2003)
647   (Medicinenet.com, 2017)
648   (Klopfer, 1957)
649   (Hurley, 1985)
650   (Thomas, 1980)
651   (Wartolowska, et al., 2014)
652   (Google, 2017)
653   (Psychology Today, 2017)
654   (Ingerman, Walking in Light, 2014)
655   (Kamps, 2017)
656   (Algoe & Way, 2014)
657   (Van Cappellen, Way, Isgett & Fredrickson, 2016)
658   (Kamps, 2017)

MICHAEL S. FENSTER, MD

659 (Ingerman & Wesselman, Awakening to the Spirit World: The Shamanic Path of Direct Revelation, 2010)
660 (Ingerman & Wesselman, 2010)
661 (Ingerman & Wesselman, 2010)
662 (Ingerman, Walking in Light, 2014)
663 (Ingerman & Wesselman, Awakening to the Spirit World: The Shamanic Path of Direct Revelation, 2010)
664 (Ingerman, Walking in Light, 2014)
665 (Wlliams, 2017)
666 (Lombardi, 2017)
667 (Cohen, et al., 2012)
668 (Huth, et al., 2014)
669 (Epel, Daubenmier, Moskowitz, Folkman & Blackburn, 2009)
670 (Feder, Nestler & Charney, 2009)
671 (Selhub & Logan, 2012)
672 (Livni, 2016)
673 (Li, et al., 2009)
674 (Song, Ikei & Miyazaki, 2016)
675 (Atchley, Strayer & Atchley, 2012)
676 (Hauser, 2017)
677 (Dunn, 2017)
678 (Schneider, et al., 2012)
679 (Dunn, The Art of Meditation, 2017)
680 (Rankin, 2013)
681 (Rankin, 2013)
682 (Ford, 2017)
683 (Chopra, 2017)
684 (Fenster, The Fallacy of The Calorie: Why the Modern Western Diet is Killing Us and How to Stop It, 2014)
685 (Holroyd, et al., 2017)
686 (Daubenmier, et al., 2016)
687 (Mulpeter, 2017)
688 (Remy, 2017)
689 (Ingerman & Wesselman, Awakening to the Spirit World: The Shamanic Path of Direct Revelation, 2010)
690 (Walsh, 2007)
691 (Walsh, 2007)
692 (Ingerman & Wesselman, 2010)
693 (Ingerman, Walking in Light, 2014)
694 (Steed, Code Delicious with Dr. Mike: What is a Shaman? 2016)
695 (Einstein, Albert Einstein Quotes, 2017)
696 (Ingerman, Walking in Light, 2014)
697 (American Diabetes Association, 2013)
698 (Gaede, et al., 2003)
699 (Grundy, et al., 1999)
700 (Haffner, Lehto, Rönnemaa, Pyörälä & Laakso, 1998)
701 (Kempner, 1949)
702 (Patel, Freeman & Williams, 2017)
703 (Laaksonen, et al., 2005)

704   (Lindström, Peltonen & Tuomilehto, 2005)
705   (Fine, Philogene, Gramling, Coups & Sinha, 2004)
706   (Centers for Disease Control and Prevention, 2014)
707   (Tuomilehto, Schwarz & Lindström, 2011)
708   (Patel, Freeman & Williams, 2017)
709   (American Diabetes Association, 2015)
710   (Evert, et al., 2014)
711   (Food and Agricultural Organisation of The United Nations, 2010)
712   (Daniel, Cross, Koebnick, & Sinha, 2011)
713   (Barclay, 2012)
714   (Spiegel, 2014)
715   (Landers, Cohen, Wittum & Larson, 2012)
716   (Danzeisen, Kim, Isaacson, Tu & Johnson, 2011)
717   (Yeoman, et al., 2012)
718   (Lathers, 2002)
719   (Tollefson, Altekruse & Potter, 1997)
720   (Tollefson & Miller, Antibiotic Use in Food Animals: Controlling the Human Health
       Impact, 2000)
721   (Nandi, Maurer, Hofacre & Summers, 2004)
722   (Davis, Price, Liu & Silbergeld, 2011)
723   (The National Law Review., 2015)
724   (House Report, 2015)
725   (The Mellman Group, 2015)
726   (Hamblin, 2015)
727   (House Report, 2015)
728   (Representatives, 2018)
729   (Main, 2017)
730   (Domingo & Gine-Bordonaba, 2011)
731   (The National Law Review, 2015)
732   (Congressional Research Service, 2015)
733   (Congressional Research Service, 2015)
734   (House Report, 2015)
735   (Sarich, 2015)
736   (Homer, 1998)
737   (Fox, 2016)
738   (Coleman, et al., 2017)
739   (Kaplan, et al., 2017)
740   (Siegel & Betz, 2017)
741   (Siegel & Betz, 2017)
742   (Siegel & Betz, 2017)
743   (Fenster, The Fallacy of The Calorie: Why the Modern Western Diet is Killing Us and
       How to Stop It, 2014)
744   (Siegel & Betz, 2017)
745   (Walsh, 2007)
746   (Ingerman, Walking in Light, 2014)
747   (Walsh, 2007)
748   (Merriam-Webster, 2017)
749   (Ozeke, et al., 2016)
750   (Bhatt, et al., 2014)

751 (Bhatt, et al., 2014)
752 (Mandrola, 2016)
753 (Verma, et al., 2013)
754 (Tscholl, et al., 2016)
755 (Connolly, Sheldon, Roberts, Gent & Investigators, 1999)
756 (Connolly, et al., 2003)
757 (Nishimura, et al., 1997)
758 (Freed, et al., 2001)
759 (Buchbinder, et al., 2009)
760 (Leon, et al., 2005)
761 (Dimond, Kittle & Crockett, 1960)
762 (Al-Lamee, et al., 2017)
763 (Wartolowska, et al., 2014)
764 (Olshansky, 2007)
765 (Voelker, 1996)
766 (Konety, Horwitz, Lindower & Olshansky, 2007)
767 (Ueyama, 2004)
768 (Wittstein, Thiemann & Lima, 2005)
769 (Walsh, 2007)
770 (Walsh, 2007)
771 (Wilber, 2011)
772 (Walsh, 2007)
773 (Corsini & Wedding, 2010)
774 (Heart.org, 2017)
775 (Mozaffarian & Ludwig, Dietary Guidelines in the 21st Century—A Time for Food, 2010)
776 (Micha, Wallace, & Mozaffarian, Red and Processed Meat Consumption and Risk of Incident Coronary Heart Disease, Stroke, and Diabetes: A Systematic Review and Meta-Analysis, 2010)
777 (Satija, et al., 2017)
778 (Korem, et al., 2017)
779 (Harcombe, et al., 2015)
780 (Mozaffarian, Diverging Global Trends in Heart Disease and Type 2 Diabetes: The Role of Carbohydrates and Saturated Fats, 2015)
781 (Mozaffarian, Nutrition and Cardiovascular Disease and Metabolic Diseases, 2014)
782 (Appel, et al., 2005)
783 (Gadgil, et al., 2013)
784 (Estruch, et al., 2013)
785 (Salas-Salvadó, et al., 2014)
786 (Afshin, Micha, Khatibzadeh & Mozaffarian, Consumption of Nuts and Legumes and Risk of Incident Ischemic Heart Disease, Stroke, and Diabetes: A Systematic Review and Meta-Analysis, 2014)
787 (Jones, et al., 2014)
788 (Mozaffarian, Aro, & Willett, Health effects of trans-fatty acids:experimental and observational evidence, 2009)
789 (Mozaffarian, Natural Trans Fat, Dairy Fat, Partially Hydrogenated Oils, and Cardiometabolic Health: The Ludwigshafen Risk and Cardiovascular Health Study, 2015)
790 (Mente, de Koning, Shannon & Anand, 2009)

791   (Mozaffarian, Katan, Ascherio, Stampfer & Willett, 2006)
792   (US Department of Health and Human Services, 2016)
793   (Mente, et al., 2016)
794   (Schwingshackl & Hoffmann, Long-Term Effects of Low-Fat Diets Either Low or High in Protein on Cardiovascular and Metabolic Risk Factors: A Systematic Review and Meta-Analysis, 2013)
795   (Mozaffarian, Diverging Global Trends in Heart Disease and Type 2 Diabetes: The Role of Carbohydrates and Saturated Fats, 2015)
796   (Mozaffarian & Ludwig, The 2015 US Dietary Guidelines: Lifting the Ban on Total Dietary Fat, 2015)
797   (Olmstead, 2016)
798   (Walsh, 2007)
799   (Walsh, 2007)
800   (Walsh, 2007)
801   (Weaver, 2009)
802   (Hoyle & Wickramasinehe, 1981)
803   (Sullivan, 1972)
804   (Walsh, 2007)
805   (Rovelli, 2017)
806   (Randerson, 2008)
807   (Einstein, The World as I See It, 2007)
808   (Rovelli, 2017)
809   (Rovelli, 2017)
810   (Rovelli, 2017)
811   (Brillat-Savarin & Robinson, 2014)
812   (Bloom, 2015)
813   (Wilber, 2011)
814   (Wilber, 2011)
815   (Wilber, 2011)
816   (Steed, Personal Communication, 2017)
817   (Koestler, 1964)
818   (Wilber, 2011)
819   (Rovelli, 2017)
820   (Rovelli, 2017)
821   (Rovelli, 2017)
822   (Nugent, 2015)
823   (Brug, 2008)
824   (Van't Riet, Sijtsema, Dagevos & De Bruijn, 2011)
825   (Patel & Hu, 2008)
826   (Mozaffarian, Hao, Rimm, Willett, & Hu, Changes In Diet and Lifestyle and Long-Term Weight Gain in Women and Men, 2011)
827   (Nugent, 2015)
828   (Institute of Medicine, 2010)
829   (The Holy Bible: King James Version, 2004)
830   (Einstein, Einstein, 2017)
831   (Jones A. Z., 2016)
832   (Korem, et al., 2017)
833   (Krishnan, Microbiome Breakthroughs, 2017)
834   (Bae & Hong, 2014)

835   (Bai, et al., 2017)
836   (Louve, 2005)
837   (Stuckrad, 2002)
838   (Satprem, 1968)
839   (Wilber, 2011)
840   (Ingerman & Wesselman, 2010)
841   (Ingerman & Wesselman, 2010)
842   (Ingerman & Wesselman, 2010)
843   (Ingerman & Wesselman, Awakening to the Spirit World: The Shamanic Path of Direct Revelation, 2010)
844   (Ingerman & Wesselman, 2010)
845   (Garfinkel, 2011)
846   (Stettler & Axel, 2009)
847   (Patel & Pinto, 2014)
848   (Spehr, Gisselmann, Poplawski & Hatt, 2003)
849   (Spehr, Gisselmann, Poplawski & Hatt, 2003)
850   (Neuhaus, et al., 2009)
851   (Gu, et al., 2014)
852   (Griffin, Kafadar & Paylath, 2009)
853   (Busse, et al., 2014)
854   (Stoneoct, 2014)
855   (Forouhi, et al., 2014)
856   (Scharf, Demmer & DeBoer, 2013)
857   (Smith, et al., 2015)
858   (Wang, et al., 2014)
859   (Poutahidis, et al., 2013)
860   (Park, et al., 2013)
861   (Power, O'Toole, Stanton, Ross & Fitzgerald, 2014)
862   (Mozaffarian, Appel & Van Horn, Components of a Cardioprotective Diet: New Insights, 2011)
863   (Dietary Guidelines Advisory Committee, 2015)
864   (Mozaffarian, Hao, Rimm & Willett, 2011)
865   (Smith, et al., 2015)
866   (Brand-Miller, McMillan-Price, Steinbeck & Caterson, 2009)
867   (Volk, et al., 2014)
868   (Browning, et al., 2011)
869   (Lennerz, et al., 2013)
870   (Ebbeling, et al., 2012)
871   (Dietary Guidelines Advisory Committee, 2015)
872   (Fardet, 2015)
873   (Jacobs & Tapsell, 2007)
874   (Jacobs & Tapsell, 2013)
875   (Mozaffarian & Ludwig, The 2015 US Dietary Guidelines: Lifting the Ban on Total Dietary Fat, 2015)
876   (Mozaffarian, 2014)
877   (Lou-Bonafonte, Gabás-Rivera, Navarro & Osada, 2015)
878   (Taillie, Ng, Xue, Busey, & Harding, 2017)
879   (Turnbaugh, et al., 2009)
880   (Turnbaugh & Gordon, 2009)

881 (Chambers, et al., 2014)
882 (Gill, et al., 2006)
883 (Aron-Wisnewsky & Clément, 2015)
884 (Amar, et al., 2011)
885 (Vrieze, et al., 2012)
886 (Zhang, et al., 2013)
887 (Koren, et al., 2011)
888 (Karlsson, et al., 2012)
889 (Khaneja, et al., 2010)
890 (Perez-Fons, et al., 2011)
891 (Devillard, McIntosh & Duncan, 2007)
892 (Viladomiu, Hontecillas & Bassaganya-Riera, 2016)
893 (Wang, et al., 2011)
894 (Loscalzo, 2013)
895 (Tang, et al., 2013)
896 (The World Health Organisation, 2014)
897 (Aron-Wisnewsky & Clément, 2015)
898 (Koeth, et al., 2013)
899 (WebMD, 2017)
900 (Jones, Martoni, & Prakash, Cholesterol Lowering and Inhibition Ofsterol Absorption by Lactobacillus Reuteri NCIMB 30242: A Randomized Controlled Trial, 2012)
901 (Jones, Martoni, Parent & Prakash, 2012)
902 (Lin, et al., 2012)
903 (Ryan, et al., 2017)
904 (Chambers, et al., 2014)
905 (Karaki, et al., 2008)
906 (LeChatelier, et al., 2013)
907 (Cotillard, et al., 2013)
908 (Sandek, et al., 2007)
909 (Vaziri, et al., 2013)
910 (Wang, Jiang, Shi, Zhang & Cheng, 2012)
911 (Wang, Jiang, Shi, Zhang & Cheng, 2012)
912 (Wang, et al., 2015)
913 (Wang, et al., 2015)
914 (Aron-Wisnewsky & Clément, 2015)
915 (Karlsson, et al., 2013)
916 (Karlsson, et al., 2012)
917 (Jeffery, Claesson & Shanahan, 2012)
918 (Cani, et al., 2008)
919 (Cani, et al., 2008)
920 (Cani, et al., 2008)
921 (Everard, et al., 2011)
922 (Everard, et al., 2013)
923 (Mozaffarian, et al., Trans-Palmitoleic Acid, Metabolic Risk Factors, and New-Onset Diabetes in U.S. Adults: A Cohort Study, 2010)
924 (Lennerz, et al., 2013)
925 (Lê & Bortolotti, 2008)
926 (Gower & Goss, 2015)
927 (Basaranoglu, Basaranoglu, Sabuncu & Sentürk, 2013)

928 (Stanhope, 2015)
929 (Malik & Hu, 2015)
930 (Estruch, et al., 2013)
931 (Taren, et al., 2015)
932 (Estruch, et al., 2013)
933 (Bunner, et al., 2015)
934 (Van Dam, Willett, Rimm, Stampfer & Hu, 2002)
935 (Salmerón, et al., 1997)
936 (Paul-Labrador, et al., 2006)
937 (Knowler, Barrett-Connor, Fowler & Group, 2002)
938 (Pan, et al., 1997)
939 (Tuomilehto, et al., 2001)
940 (Patel, Freeman & Williams, 2017)
941 (Skelly, et al., 2015)
942 (Heart.org, 2017)
943 (Mensink, Zock, Kestor & Katan, 2003)
944 (Nordestgaard, et al., 2010)
945 (Berglund, et al., 2007)
946 (Mozaffarian, 2016)
947 (Mozaffarian, Micha, & Wallace, Effects on Coronary Heart Disease of Increasing Polyunsaturated Fat In Place Of Saturated Fat: A Systematic Review and Meta-Analysis of Randomized Controlled Trials, 2010)
948 (Schwingshackl & Hoffmann, 2014)
949 (Lambelet, et al., 2003)
950 (Velasco, Marmesat, Bordeaux, Márquez-Ruiz & Dobarganes, 2004)
951 (Trichopoulou, Bamia, & Trichopoulos, 2009)
952 (Lonn, Bosch, Lopez-Jaramillo & Investigators, 2016)
953 (Crippa, et al., 2016)
954 (Brug, Kremers, Lenthe, Ball & Crawford, 2008)
955 (Nugent, 2015)
956 (Nugent, 2015)
957 (Mozaffarian, 2016)
958 (Mozaffarian, 2016)
959 (Corella & Ordovas, 2009)
960 (Kalantarian, Rimm, Herrington & Mozaffarian, 2014)
961 (Abdullah, Jones & Eck, 2015)
962 (Villegas, Goodloe, McClellan, Boston & Crawford, 2014)
963 (Corella & Ordovas, 2009)
964 (Bae & Hong, 2014)
965 (Bai, et al., 2017)

ABOUT THE AUTHOR

Michael S. Fenster, MD, "Chef Dr. Mike," is The Food Shaman. Dr. Mike is a board-certified interventional cardiologist and professional chef. He currently holds joint faculty appointments at University of Montana College of Health Professions and Biomedical Sciences and Missoula College (part of U. of Mt.) Culinary Arts Program. He travels the world cooking and lecturing on food and health.